Lynda L. Geller, Ph.D.

ANNALS OF THE NEW YORK ACADEMY OF SCIENCES

Volume 992

The New York Academy of Sciences
2 East 63rd Street
New York, New York 10021

NEUROENDOCRINE AND NEURAL REGULATION OF AUTOIMMUNE AND INFLAMMATORY DISEASE

Molecular, Systems, and Clinical Insights

ANNALS OF THE NEW YORK ACADEMY OF SCIENCES

Volume 992

NEUROENDOCRINE AND NEURAL REGULATION OF AUTOIMMUNE AND INFLAMMATORY DISEASE

Molecular, Systems, and Clinical Insights

Edited by Esther M. Sternberg, France G. Haour, and Craig C. Smith

The New York Academy of Sciences
New York, New York
2003

∞ The paper used in this publication meets the minimum requirements of the American National Standard for Information Sciences—Permanence of Paper for Printed Library Materials, ANSI Z39.48-1984.

Library of Congress Cataloging-in-Publication Data

International Congress ISNIM (5th : 2002 : Montpellier, France)
Neuroendocrine and neural regulation of autoimmune and inflammatory disease : molecular, systems, and clinical insights / edited by Esther M. Sternberg, France G. Haour, and Craig C. Smith
p. ; cm. -- (Annals of the New York Academy of Sciences ; v. 992)
Contributions from the 5th International Congress of the International Society for NeuroImmunoModulation, held on September 9–11, 2002, in Montpellier, France.
Includes bibliographical references and index.
ISBN 1-57331-454-4-X (cloth : alk. paper) -- ISBN 1-57331-455-2 (paper : alk. paper)
1. Autoimmune diseases -- Pathophysiology -- Congresses. 2. Inflammation -- Pathophysiology -- Congresses. 3. Neuroendocrinology -- Congresses.
[DNLM: 1. Autoimmune Diseases -- immunology -- Congresses. 2. Neuroimmunomodulation -- Congresses. 3. Inflammation -- immunology -- Congresses. 4. Neurosecretory Systems -- immunology -- Congresses. WD 305 I61 2003] I. Sternberg, Esther M. II. Haour, France G. III. Smith, Craig C. IV. Title. V. Series.
Q11.N5 vol. 992
[RC600
500 s--dc21
[616.97/8 2003010296

GYAT/PCP

Printed in the United States of America

ISBN 1-57331-454-4 (cloth)
ISBN 1-57331-455-2 (paper)
ISSN 0077-8923

ANNALS OF THE NEW YORK ACADEMY OF SCIENCES

Volume 992
May 2003

NEUROENDOCRINE AND NEURAL REGULATION OF AUTOIMMUNE AND INFLAMMATORY DISEASE

Molecular, Systems, and Clinical Insights

Editors
ESTHER M. STERNBERG, FRANCE G. HAOUR, AND CRAIG C. SMITH

Conference Organizers
ESTHER M. STERNBERG, CRAIG C. SMITH, FRANCE G. HAOUR, JEAN BOUSQUET, VINCENT GEENEN, CATHERINE RIVIER, AND ANGELA VINCENT

This volume is the result of a conference entitled, **The 5th International Congress of the International Society for Neuroimmunomodulation**, held on September 9–11, 2002, in Montpellier, France.

CONTENTS

Part II. Stress Axis in Autoimmune/Inflammatory Diseases

Part III. Peripheral Neuroimmune Interactions (Basic)

Part IV. Allergy and Neuroimmunomodulation

Assistance was received from:

- **SCHERING PLOUGH CORPORATION**
- **GALAXOSMITHKLINE BIOLOGICALS**
- **PFIZER PHARMACEUTICALS-BRUSSELS**
- **SANOFI SYNTHELABO, INC.**
- **MERCK & COMPANY**
- **AMERICAN AUTOIMMUNE RELATED DISEASES ASSOCIATION, INC.**
- **REGION LANGUEDOC—ROUSSILLION**
- **VILLA DE MONTPELIER**

Preface

Neuroimmunomodulation: A Kuhnian Model of Evolution of a Scientific Field

The publication of the Proceedings of the 5th International Congress of the International Society for Neuroimmunomodulation (ISNIM) marks the continuation of an ongoing and successful relationship with the *Annals* of the New York Academy of Sciences that began in 1990 to bring cutting-edge advances in the field of neuroimmunomodulation to the global scientific community. This volume reflects not only the evolution of the field, but also the adaptation of the Society to that evolution. There have been many changes in the field since the founding of ISNIM, which traces its roots to the First International Workshop on Neuroimmunomodulation, held in Bethesda, Maryland, in 1984,[1] changes reflected in the topics, technologies, and therapeutic applications that can be found in the research papers in this volume.

The most profound change in the field since its inception has been the movement from ostracism to acceptance by its parent disciplines—immunology, neuroscience, endocrinology, and neuroendocrinology. This evolution is typical of the evolution of the development of once marginal fields, as described by the historian and philosopher of science, Thomas S. Kuhn,[2,3] and is reflected in the make-up, motivation, and membership of the scientific societies representing this field. In this sense, neuroimmunomodulation typifies a field in which individual researchers, whose integrative approaches were at odds with the reductionist doctrines of their parent disciplines, found themselves not only ignored, but also unequivocally rejected by their peers. In search of like-minded colleagues, they came together out of isolation to found a society that reflected their interests and approach to science. The make-up of the first Congress, held in Florence, Italy, in May 1990, included subcategories of research that focused on a broad range of subjects: psychoneuroimmunology, immunology, neurosciences, cell biology, genetics, physiology, chronobiology, endocrinology, pharmacology, developmental biology, and comparative biology.[1] Soon after the first International Congress of the International Society for Neuroimmunomodulation, these subgroups split apart and ISNIM in its present form evolved with a focus on neuroendocrine immunology.

Since then, acceptance into the mainstream has come relatively quickly and visibly, within the last 5 to 6 years. This was due in large part to the exponentially increasing numbers of rigorous scientific studies and publications in the field. However, the active and aggressive efforts of the ISNIM leadership in sponsoring satellite symposia at the parent disciplines' major national conferences and other international forums has greatly helped to highlight this research and has served an important role in the movement of the field to the next phase, that of acceptance.

While acceptance is a great success and gratifying, it also presents an equally great challenge for the next phase of evolution of the field, for with acceptance comes desire to participate and with that, competition. Like mushrooms after a rain, a plethora of societies, conferences, and groups have sprung up, each focusing on their particular area of neural immune interactions, with at least six simultaneous

Ann. N.Y. Acad. Sci. 992: ix–x (2003).

related conferences taking place in Europe alone at the time of this Congress. Thus, in the next phase, members must recognize that participation will not be automatic, but must be actively sought among a field of many groups competing for the attention of researchers in the field.

According to Kuhn, in the next phase, each of these many small focused groups may blend back into their parent disciplines' mainstream, resulting in dissolution of a separate identity for the field, or they may coalesce as separate and distinct entities under a federated umbrella, creating a new and stronger parent discipline of neural immune interactions. At the time of the publication of this volume, it remains to be seen in which direction the field will move. In part its direction will be determined by the degree to which scientists from different backgrounds are willing to let go of their defining territories. Certainly, coming together within a loose federation that defines a larger group, yet retains the identities of the individual components, has many merits. The most well known organization of this sort is the Federation of American Societies of Experimental Biology (FASEB). Recently, the Federation of Clinical Immune Societies (FOCIS) was formed; there is a growing list of such organizations.

Movement towards initiating such a federation for the field of Neuroimmunomodulation has already been broached, with the participation of ISNIM at the last International Congress of the International Society for Neuroimmunology (ISNI) (Edinburgh, 2001) and the active participation of the ISNI President at this Congress. The success of these initiatives will pave the way for future joint ventures, which should form the core of a larger, stronger federation of like-minded research societies, thus successfully completing the cycle suggested by Thomas Kuhn.

ESTHER M. STERNBERG, M.D.
President, ISNIM, 1999-2002

REFERENCES

1. SPECTOR, N.H. 1990. Neuroimmunomodulation Takes Off. Immunol. Today Nov: 381–383.
2. KUHN, T.S. 1962. The Structure of Scientific Revolutions. Chicago.
3. BOORBOOR, S. (BROWN, T.M., Advisor). 2002. Integrating the incompatible: the rise of the incorporated immune system. J. Undergrad. Res. (Univ. of Rochester) **1:** 19–26.

Introduction

Neuroendocrine and Neural Factors in Autoimmune, Inflammatory, Infectious, and Allergic Disease: A Summary of the Conference

ESTHER M. STERNBERG

National Institute of Mental Health, National Institutes of Health, Bethesda, Maryland 20892-1284, USA

As the field of neuroimmunomodulation has progressed from its inception, it has matured in both rigor and complexity. These changes are dramatically reflected in the papers in this volume. This conference purposefully focused on the role of neural and neuroendocrine factors in autoimmune, inflammatory, allergic, and infectious disease, in part because of the exponential growth and diversity of the field, but also in part to draw emphasis to the movement of the field towards more focused translational and clinically relevant research.

Whereas in previous volumes there was a strong focus on the hypothalamic pituitary adrenal axis and the role of its key hormones corticotrophin- releasing hormone (CRH) and glucococorticoids in inflammation, it is the intent of this volume to also emphasize the many other neural and other neuroendocrine and endocrine pathways and hormones that regulate the immune system and immune-mediated diseases. Thus, in addition to the role of the HPA axis in autoimmune, inflammatory, infectious and allergic diseases, the role of noradrenergic sympathetic factors and parasympathetic cholinergic pathways (opiates, neurotrophins), peripheral nervous system factors such as substance P, and vasoactive intestinal polypeptide (VIP) are extensively explored. The roles of sex and gender as well as sex steroids including estrogens, androgens, and testosterone are also explored.

Temporal factors and the level of inflammatory mediator exposure on HPA axis activity are explored, as in studies of the effects of acute stress on delayed-type hypersensitivity and of chronic inflammatory and autoimmune disease impact on hypothalamic CRH and AVP expression. The effects on expression of these hormones of a single exposure to interleukin-1 are also explored. Within the HPA axis, the effects of factors other than glucocorticoids from the long-ignored adrenal glands are explored; chromogranins released from the adrenal medulla exhibit important antifungal and antibacterial effects.

These interactions are explored not only at the physiological level, but also at the molecular and cellular level, including a discussion of shared transcription factors that regulate transcriptional activity of glucocorticoids, cytokines, and T cell receptors; the role of second signal factors such as nitric oxide (NO) on HPA axis activity; and the role of other mediators previously neglected, including complement.

Local neural immune interactions in immune organs such as the thymus and mucosa are explored. In this regard, studies reported here highlight the importance

Ann. N.Y. Acad. Sci. 992: xi–xii (2003). © 2003 New York Academy of Sciences.

of regional neuronal circuitry in specific organ innervation, and subsequent immune/ inflammatory or allergic disease is explored such as the role of such circuits in bronchial constriction in asthma.

The most important change in direction that has accompanied this evolution of the field has been in the area of therapeutics and diagnostics. Although many studies still focus on mechanism and much work remains to be done in this area to fully elucidate the many anatomical and molecular pathways by which the CNS and immune system communicate and regulate each other, many new studies are taking these findings to the next level of application to the treatment of disease. Thus, studies reported in this volume continue to test the usefulness of the endogenous interleukin-1 receptor antagonist (IL-1RA) in stroke. Completely novel therapeutic applications of neuroendocrine-derived molecules, the chromagranin peptides, as antibiotics and antifungals are also reported here. Careful assessment of neuroendocrine responsiveness of subgroups of patients with autoimmune diseases such as rheumatoid arthritis and multiple sclerosis suggests that such approaches may be used in the future as diagnostics and prognostics to identify subgroups of patients with these diseases and perhaps to predict their course of disease activity.

Finally, new technologies, including expression microarray gene chips and the use of complex mathematical analyses integrating multiple factors that change simultaneously, point to the direction for future research in this field. Thus, it is clear that patterns of change in the relationships of expression of many genes, hormones, and nerve products, rather than single genes, hold the key to understanding the ways in which the CNS and immune systems regulate each other at the molecular as well as the whole systems level.

The Novera Herbert Spector Lectureship Award

Since the First International Workshop on Neuroimmunomodulation, held at the National Institutes of Health, Bethesda, Maryland, in November 1984, Novera Herbert Spector has been a dynamic force in organizing the integrative field of neuroimmunomodulation and in the founding of the International Society for Neuroimmunomodulation (ISNIM).

In 1996 the Officers and Executive Committee of ISNIM voted to establish the Novera Herbert Spector Lectureship Award as a fitting tribute to the tireless efforts and accomplishments of Novera Herbert Spector. The award was first presented at the 3rd International Congress, which was held at the Natcher Conference Center, at the National Institutes of Health in November 1996, and thereafter was presented at each subsequent Congress, "To that investigator who in the estimation of the Award Committee has made significant contributions in leadership and research to the field of neuroimmunomodulation."

It is with great pleasure that the Award Committee for the 5th International Congress, comprised of individuals who in their own right have demonstrated significant leadership in international neuroimmunomodulation research, has voted to award the Lectureship for this Congress to Dr. Hugo O. Besedovsky, of the Institute of Physiology, Division of Immunophysiology, Philipps University Marburg, Marburg, Germany.

Ann. N.Y. Acad. Sci. 992: xiii (2003).

Hippocampal Interleukin-1β Gene Expression during Long-Term Potentiation Decays with Age

DETLEF BALSCHUN,[a] ANKE RANDOLF,[b] FERNANDO PITOSSI,[c]
HORST SCHNEIDER,[b] ADRIANA DEL REY,[b] AND HUGO O. BESEDOVSKY[b]

[a]*Leibniz Institute for Neurobiology, 39 118 Magdeburg, Germany*

[b]*Institute of Physiology, Division of Immunophysiology, Philipps University Marburg, 35037 Marburg, Germany*

[c]*Fundacion Instituto Leloir, University of Buenos Aires, Buenos Aires, Argentina*

KEYWORDS: **cytokines; interleukin-1 (Il-1); gene expression; long-term potentiation; hippocampus**

INTRODUCTION

Molecules originally described as intrinsic to the immune system are evidently also involved in physiological processes that are different from immunoregulation. A clear example is the proinflammatory cytokine interleukin-1 (IL-1). This cytokine is also synthesized in the brain by glial cells and certain neurons, and its receptors have been found in different regions of the CNS with the greatest abundance in the hippocampus.[1–4] These complementary findings indicate a physiological role of IL-1 in the brain. In further support of this, pharmacological and behavioral studies demonstrated the capacity of IL-1β to affect various neuroendocrine functions, to alter the release and turnover rate of certain neurotransmitters and modulators, and to induce changes in behavior.[5,6] (See Refs. 1, 7, and 8 for additional references.) However, in most cases the effects of IL-1 in the brain were tested either *in vitro* or after exogenous administration of pharmacological doses of the cytokine.

We previously described a function for physiological levels of IL-1 in long-term potentiation (LTP), the best-studied model for the cellular mechanisms underlying memory storage.[9,10] The expression of IL-1 in the hippocampus was significantly enhanced during LTP.[11] This increased production of IL-1 was not an epiphenomenon, because blockade of brain receptors for this cytokine resulted in significant inhibition of LTP maintenance.[11] Pathologically high levels of IL-1, however, achieved by external application of the cytokine were reported to impair LTP[12–16] and learning.[17–20] In continuation of our previous study,[11] we investigated the expression of IL-1 during LTP *in vivo* in older (12–16-month-old), freely moving

Address for correspondence: Hugo O. Besedovsky, Institute of Physiology, Division of Immunophysiology, Philipps University Marburg, Deutschhausstr. 3, 35037 Marburg, Germany.

Ann. N.Y. Acad. Sci. 992: 1–8 (2003).

rats. Here we report decay of IL-1 gene expression during LTP with age, which is not accompanied by impairment of LTP.

MATERIAL AND METHODS

Animals. Male Wistar rats were used for the experiments. Young rats were about 3 months old, and middle-aged rats were between 12 and 16 months old. Animals were fed ad libitum and housed in temperature- and light-controlled (12 h/day) rooms. Rats were treated in accordance with institutional guidelines.

Long-Term Potentiation in Vivo. Experiments were performed on freely moving rats. A monopolar recording electrode (coordinates AP –2.8, L 1.8) and a bipolar stimulation electrode (coordinates AP –6.9, L 4.1) were implanted stereotaxically under Nembutal anesthesia (40 mg/kg, ip) into the granule cell layer of the dentate gyrus and into the perforant path, respectively, of the right hemisphere. Animals were allowed to recover from surgery for at least 1 week. The stimulus intensity was adjusted to evoke 40% of the maximum population spike amplitude. Five test stimuli were applied every 10 minutes and the responses averaged for each set of the stimulus parameters. Once stable responses were obtained for 45 minutes, LTP was induced by strong tetanic bursts (10 bursts of 15 pulses 200 Hz, 0.2-ms duration of each stimulus, interburst interval 10 seconds), resulting in a "saturated," late LTP. Population spikes were recorded 1, 4, 7, 10, and 15 minutes after tetanization. Thereafter, recordings were taken in 15-minute intervals until the end of the experiment.

Interleukin-1β Gene Expression. To study IL-1β mRNA expression, rats were killed 8 hours after tetanic stimulation. After decapitation, ipsilateral and contralateral hippocampi were quickly dissected and processed for the evaluation of IL-1 mRNA. RNA was extracted from the hippocampi following standard protocols and reverse transcribed using a commercial kit (Superscript II RT kit, GIBCO/BRL). All conditions used in the semiquantitative reverse transcription–polymerase chain reaction (RT-PCR) using a multispecific competitive fragment (pRat6) were previously described.[21] The primer sequences were: IL-1β, sense: TCCATGAGCTTTGTACAAGG and antisense: GGTGCTGATGTACCAGTTGG. Amplicons were separated by agarose gel electrophoresis in 1.5% gels containing 5 μg/ml ethidium bromide and 10% PAGE at 80 volts for 3 hours. Bands were visualized in the agarose gels by excitation at 316 nm and documented. Signals were quantified using a Phosphorimager device (Molecular Dynamics) with an Image Quant program. Background levels were subtracted from the detected signals. Each individual sample was amplified by PCR at least three times.

RESULTS AND DISCUSSION

To test whether the expression of IL-1β during LTP is subject to age-dependent changes, we evaluated IL-1β gene expression in young and middle-aged rats. As evidenced by the values of the untetanized left hippocampi (contralateral side) (FIG. 1), basal IL-1β gene expression was slightly reduced in middle-aged rats compared to young rats (0.400 ± 0.040 vs 0.224 ± 0.040; $P < 0.05$, Student's t test). Although both groups of rats displayed significant enhancement of gene expression in

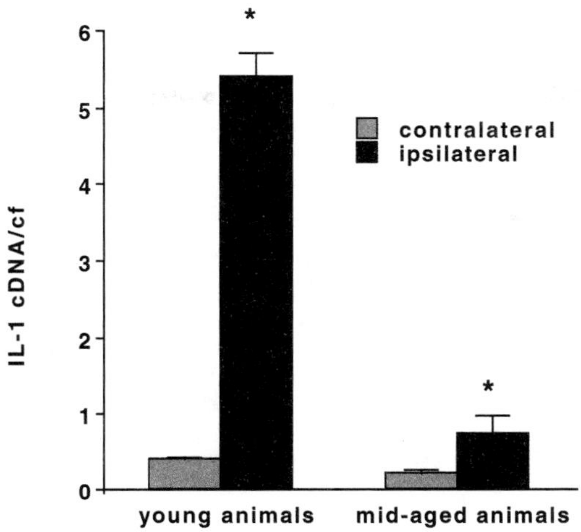

FIGURE 1. Interleukin-1β gene expression during long-term potentiation (LTP) in the dentate gyrus of freely-moving young and middle-aged rats. IL-1β gene expression during LTP *in vivo* as assessed by RT-PCR (ratio IL-1 cDNA/competitive fragment [cf], mean ± SEM). Middle-aged rats display a lower basal level (contralateral hippocampi) and a reduced upregulation of IL-1β gene expression during LTP (ipsilateral hippocampi). Young rats: $n = 4$; middle-aged rats: $n = 5$. $^{*}P < 0.05$.

the right hippocampi (ipsilateral side) during LTP, this increase was more pronounced in young than in midde-aged rats (FIG. 1). Thus, young rats showed a more than 10-fold increase (ipsilateral versus contralateral hippocampus), but the rise in middle-aged animals was only threefold. Our findings apparently contradict reports of increasing hippocampal IL-1β levels during aging.[22,23] However, because these studies were conducted with older rats (22 months old), we cannot completely rule out that the decrease in IL-1β in middle-aged rats is only temporary and is followed by upregulation in older animals.

As depicted in FIGURE 2, young and middle-aged rats attained a comparable magnitude of potentiation and did not differ significantly in the maintenance of LTP. The only discernible difference was a tendency of a faster decay of potentiation in middle-aged rats. A weakened synaptic plasticity within the hippocampus had been suggested to underlie deficits in hippocampal-dependent learning and memory in aging rodents.[24–26] However, age-dependent deterioration of potentiation does not appear to manifest before the age of about 20 months in rats. Furthermore, a decline of certain forms of LTP was mostly reported for the CA1 region,[26–31] whereas the situation in the dentate gyrus is not clear. Our results confirm a continuing capacity for the induction of dentate LTP during aging in rats, as also supported by other groups.[32–34] Impairment of dentate LTP in aged animals has been described by Lynch *et al.*[23] and O'Donnell *et al.*[35] In accordance with lacking or only mild overt deficits in dentate LTP, the capacity for morphological synaptic changes during LTP was widely preserved in the dentate gyrus of aged rats.[36] Furthermore, several signaling cascades appear to operate normally in aged rats, as indicated by an

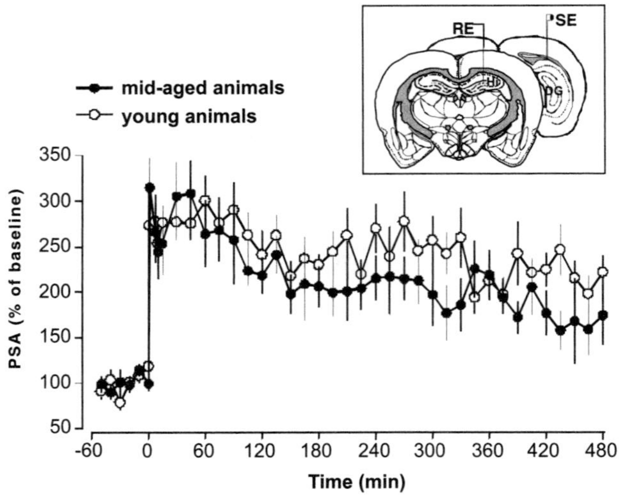

FIGURE 2. Long-term potentiation (LTP) induction in young and middle-aged rats. LTP is unchanged in middle-aged rats ($n = 5$) compared with young rats ($n = 7$). The only discernible difference was a weak tendency to faster decay of potentiation in middle-aged rats. PSA, population spike amplitude. The scheme represents placement of the stimulation electrode (SE) in the perforant path and of the recording electrode (RE) in the granule cell layer of the dentate gyrus. *DG,* dentate gyrus; *HI,* hilus of DG.

unchanged induction of an array of immediate early genes that are known to be transcriptionally activated after LTP-inducing stimuli.[37] Other pathways, however, were found to be changed in senescent animals.[25,35,37–39] Elevation of the threshold for LTP induction that has been described in aged, spatial memory-impaired rats[40] is likely to be compensated by a tetanization protocol that is sufficiently strong.

Taken together, our findings provide evidence of a reduced basal level and a decreased range of regulation of Il-1β gene expression in middle-aged animals. Since our previous investigations indicated a supportive effect of enhanced IL-1β levels on LTP maintenance, the decreased upregulation of IL-1β gene expression during LTP in middle-aged as compared to young animals would be anticipated to result in impaired maintenance of LTP in the older animals. However, this was not observed. The reasons might be the following: (1) Normal LTP only requires a "threshold" concentration of IL-1β that is also achieved in middle-aged animals. (2) The lower upregulation of IL-1β gene expression during LTP may be compensated by a greater efficacy/activity of subsequent translational cascades, resulting in about the same concentration of IL-1β protein in young and middle-aged rats. (3) The net efficacy of IL-1β in LTP does not only depend on IL-1ß concentration but is also contingent on the level of Il-1 receptors,[41] the IL-1 receptor accessory protein (IL-1RAcP),[6] and the IL-1 receptor antagonist (IL-1ra). Thus, the equilibrium of these regulatory components might be differently adjusted in older animals, while still ensuring almost normal potentiation. The preliminary findings of our laboratories support upregulation of IL-1ra during LTP. Interestingly, interleukin-6 (IL-6), which can be induced by IL-1 in the brain,[42,43] is also upregulated during hippocampal

LTP,[44,45] but it has a function opposite to that of IL-1 in LTP (Balschun *et al.*, manuscript submitted). Hence, it is tempting to speculate that in the brain a cytokine network that is activated during LTP is important for the fine-tuning of mechanisms responsible for the consolidation of potentiation. Cytokines such as IL-1 and IL-6 are known to readily diffuse from their site of release in the brain.[46,47] Therefore, their increased production triggered by potentiated neurons can be expected to result in a wave of cytokines, which spreads to surrounding neurons. Since potentiation is not confined to activated synapses but propagates to synapses on neighboring neurons,[48,49] an enhanced level of diffusing IL-1 could prevent such a propagation of potentiation as suggested by inhibition of LTP by IL-1 *in vitro*[12–16] and in freely moving rats (Ref. 16 and unpublished data). By contrast, IL-6 would tend to confine an already expressed potentiation. In this way, IL-6 and IL-1 could act as diffusible messengers that augment the input-specificity of plasticity.

In conclusion, our data exclude a simple linear relation between IL-1β gene expression and the properties of synaptic plasticity in the dentate gyrus, thereby supporting the existence of fine-tuned, cytokine-mediated regulatory mechanisms. The elucidation of age-associated changes in these processes could provide a clue to the preservation of cognitive performance in old age.

SUMMARY

Interleukin-1 is a cytokine that, apart from its contribution to immunoregulation, can affect neuroendocrine mechanisms and brain functions. We have previously shown that an increase in the endogenous production of IL-1 in the dentate gyrus during LTP is relevant for the maintenance of this process. We report here that in middle-aged rats (12 to 16 months old), enhancement of IL-1 gene expression is diminished compared to that in young animals. Furthermore, basal levels of IL-1 gene expression were slightly reduced in middle-aged rats. The reduced upregulation of IL-1 gene expression during LTP was not accompanied by overt impairment of potentiation, suggesting that either the level of the cytokine is still enough to maintain synaptic plasticity in the dentate gyrus or that compensatory, probably less efficient, mechanisms develop during aging.

ACKNOWLEDGMENT

This work was supported by the Deutsche Forschungsgemeinschaft (SFB 297) and the Nationalen Genomforschungsnetz (NGFN), NV-S14T02.

REFERENCES

1. BESEDOVSKY, H.O. & A. DEL REY. 1996. Immune-neuro-endocrine interactions: facts and hypotheses. Endocr. Rev. **17:** 64–102.
2. HAAS, H.S. & K. SCHAUENSTEIN. 1997. Neuroimmunomodulation via limbic structures: the neuroanatomy of psychoimmunology. Prog. Neurobiol. **51:** 195–222.
3. ROTHWELL, N.J. & S.J. HOPKINS. 1995. Cytokines and the nervous system. II. Actions and mechanisms of action [see comments]. Trends Neurosci. **18:** 130–136.

4. PARNET, P., K.W. KELLEY, R.M. BLUTHE & R. DANTZER. 2002. Expression and regulation of interleukin-1 receptors in the brain. Role in cytokines-induced sickness behavior. J. Neuroimmunol. **125:** 5–14.
5. MONTKOWSKI, A., R. LANDGRAF, A. YASSOURIDIS, *et al.* 1997. Central administration of IL-1 reduces anxiety and induces sickness behaviour in rats. Pharmacol. Biochem. Behav. **58:** 329–336.
6. NEVEU, P.J. & S. LIEGE. 2000. Mechanisms of behavioral and neuroendocrine effects of interleukin-1 in mice. Ann. N.Y. Acad. Sci. **917:** 175–185.
7. DUNN, A.J., J. WANG & T. ANDO. 1999. Effects of cytokines on cerebral neurotransmission. Comparison with the effects of stress. Adv. Exp. Med. Biol. **461:** 117–127.
8. ROTHWELL, N.J. & G.N. LUHESHI. 2000. Interleukin 1 in the brain: biology, pathology and therapeutic target. Trends Neurosci. **23:** 618–625.
9. BLISS, T.V. & G.L. COLLINGRIDGE. 1993. A synaptic model of memory: long-term potentiation in the hippocampus. Nature **361:** 31–39.
10. MALINOW, R., Z.F. MAINEN & Y. HAYASHI. 2000. LTP mechanisms: from silence to four-lane traffic. Curr. Opin. Neurobiol. **10:** 352–357.
11. SCHNEIDER, H., F. PITOSSI, D. BALSCHUN, *et al.* 1998. A neuromodulatory role of interleukin-1beta in the hippocampus. Proc. Natl. Acad. Sci. USA **95:** 7778–7783.
12. KATSUKI, H., S. NAKAI, Y. HIRAI, *et al.* 1990. Interleukin-1 beta inhibits long-term potentiation in the CA3 region of mouse hippocampal slices. Eur. J. Pharmacol. **181:** 323–326.
13. BELLINGER, F.P., S. MADAMBA & G.R. SIGGINS. 1993. Interleukin 1 beta inhibits synaptic strength and long-term potentiation in the rat CA1 hippocampus. Brain Res. **628:** 227–234.
14. CUNNINGHAM, A.J., C.A. MURRAY, L.A. O'NEILL, *et al.* 1996. Interleukin-1 beta (IL-1 beta) and tumour necrosis factor (TNF) inhibit long-term potentiation in the rat dentate gyrus *in vitro*. Neurosci. Lett. **203:** 17–20.
15. COOGAN, A. & J.J. O'CONNOR. 1997. Inhibition of NMDA receptor-mediated synaptic transmission in the rat dentate gyrus *in vitro* by IL-1 beta. Neuroreport **8:** 2107–2110.
16. VEREKER, E., E. O'DONNELL & M.A. LYNCH. 2000. The inhibitory effect of interleukin-1beta on long-term potentiation is coupled with increased activity of stress-activated protein kinases. J. Neurosci. **20:** 6811–6819.
17. OITZL, M.S., H. VAN OERS, B. SCHOBITZ & E.R. DE KLOET. 1993. Interleukin-1 beta, but not interleukin-6, impairs spatial navigation learning. Brain Res. **613:** 160–163.
18. GOTZ, F., G. DORNER, U. MALZ, *et al.* 1993. Short- and long-term effects of perinatal interleukin-1 beta-application in rats. Neuroendocrinology **58:** 344–351.
19. GIBERTINI, M., C. NEWTON, H. FRIEDMAN & T.W. KLEIN. 1995. Spatial learning impairment in mice infected with *Legionella pneumophila* or administered exogenous interleukin-1-beta. Brain Behav. Immun. **9:** 113–128.
20. GIBERTINI, M. 1996. IL1 beta impairs relational but not procedural rodent learning in a water maze task. Adv. Exp. Med. Biol. **402:** 207– 217.
21. PITOSSI, F., A. DEL REY, A. KABIERSCH & H. BESEDOVSKY. 1997. Induction of cytokine transcripts in the central nervous system and pituitary following peripheral administration of endotoxin to mice. J. Neurosci. Res. **48:** 287–298.
22. MURRAY, C.A. & M.A. LYNCH. 1998. Evidence that increased hippocampal expression of the cytokine interleukin-1 beta is a common trigger for age- and stress-induced impairments in long-term potentiation. J. Neurosci. **18:** 2974–2981.
23. LYNCH, M.A. 1998. Age-related impairment in long-term potentiation in hippocampus: a role for the cytokine, interleukin-1 beta? Prog. Neurobiol. **56:** 571–589.
24. DEUPREE, D.L., D.A. TURNER & C.L. WATTERS. 1991. Spatial performance correlates with in vitro potentiation in young and aged Fischer 344 rats. Brain Res. **554:** 1–9.
25. BACH, M.E., M. BARAD, H. SON, *et al.* 1999. Age-related defects in spatial memory are correlated with defects in the late phase of hippocampal long-term potentiation in vitro and are attenuated by drugs that enhance the cAMP signaling pathway. Proc. Natl. Acad. Sci. USA **96:** 5280–5285.
26. TOMBAUGH, G.C., W.B. ROWE, A.R. CHOW, *et al.* 2002. Theta-frequency synaptic potentiation in CA1 *in vitro* distinguishes cognitively impaired from unimpaired aged Fischer 344 rats. J. Neurosci. **22:** 9932–9940.

27. HORI, N., I. HIROTSU, P.J. DAVIS & D.O. CARPENTER. 1992. Long-term potentiation is lost in aged rats but preserved by calorie restriction. Neuroreport **3:** 1085–1088.
28. DEUPREE, D.L., J. BRADLEY & D.A. TURNER. 1993. Age-related alterations in potentiation in the CA1 region in F344 rats Neurobiol. Aging **14:** 249–258.
29. MOORE, C.I., M.D. BROWNING & G.M. ROSE. 1993. Hippocampal plasticity induced by primed burst, but not long-term potentiation, stimulation is impaired in area CA1 of aged Fischer 344 rats. Hippocampus **3:** 57–66.
30. SHANKAR, S., T.J. TEYLER & N. ROBBINS. 1998. Aging differentially alters forms of long-term potentiation in rat hippocampal area CA1. J. Neurophysiol. **79:** 334–341.
31. WATSON, J.B., H.K HORASANI, A. PERSSON, *et al.* 2002. Age-related deficits in long-term potentiation are insensitive to hydrogen peroxide: coincidence with enhanced autophosphorylation of Ca^{2+}/calmodulin-dependent protein kinase II. J. Neurosci. Res. **70:** 298–308.
32. CHANG, P.L., K.R. ISAACS & W.T. GREENOUGH. 1991. Synapse formation occurs in association with the induction of long-term potentiation in two-year-old rat hippocampus *in vitro*. Neurobiol. Aging **12:** 517–522.
33. DIANA, G., D.C. SCOTTI, C. FRANK, *et al.* 1994. Selective reduction of hippocampal dentate frequency potentiation in aged rats with impaired place learning. Brain Res. Bull. **35:** 107–111.
34. MAROUN, M. & G. RICHTER-LEVIN. 2002. Local circuit plasticity in the rat dentate gyrus: characterization and aging-related impairment. Neuroscience **112:** 1001–1007.
35. O'DONNELL, E., E. VEREKER & M.A. LYNCH. 2000. Age-related impairment in LTP is accompanied by enhanced activity of stress-activated protein kinases: analysis of underlying mechanisms. Eur. J. Neurosci. **12:** 345–352.
36. GEINISMAN, Y., L. TOLEDO-MORRELL, F. MORRELL, *et al.* 1992. Structural synaptic plasticity associated with the induction of long-term potentiation is preserved in the dentate gyrus of aged rats. Hippocampus **2:** 445–456.
37. LANAHAN, A., G. LYFORD, G.S. STEVENSON, *et al.* 1997. Selective alteration of long-term potentiation-induced transcriptional response in hippocampus of aged, memory-impaired rats. J. Neurosci. **17:** 2876–2885.
38. KELLY, A., C. MAGUIRE & M.A. LYNCH. 2000. Deficits in nerve growth factor release and tyrosine receptor kinase phosphorylation are associated with age-related impairment in long-term potentiation in the dentate gyrus. Neuroscience **95:** 359–365.
39. MORI, K., H. TOGASHI, M. MATSUMOTO & M. YOSHIOKA. 2000. Deficits in nitric oxide production after tetanic stimulation are related to the reduction of long-term potentiation in Schaffer-CA1 synapses in aged Fischer 344 rats. Acta Physiol. Scand. **169:** 79–85.
40. BARNES, C.A., G. RAO & F.P. HOUSTON. 2000. LTP induction threshold change in old rats at the perforant path—granule cell synapse. Neurobiol. Aging **21:** 613–620.
41. LYNCH, A.M. & M.A. LYNCH. 2002. The age-related increase in IL-1 type I receptor in rat hippocampus is coupled with an increase in caspase-3 activation. Eur. J. Neurosci. **15:** 1779–1788.
42. REYES, T.M. & C.L. CO. 1999. The proinflammatory cytokine network: interactions in the CNS and blood of rhesus monkey. Am. J. Physiol. **274:** R139–R144.
43. ZUMWALT, J.W., B.J. THUNSTROM & B.L. SPANGELO. 1999. Interleukin-1beta and catecholamines synergistically stimulate interleukin-6 release from rat C6 glioma cells in vitro: a potential role for lysophosphatidylcholine. Endocrinology **140:** 888–896.
44. BESEDOVSKY, H.O., F. PITOSSI, H. SCHNEIDER, *et al.* 1999. Cytokines in the brain as mediators of immune-endocrine interactions. J. Immunol. 31: 2.
45. JANKOWSKY, J.L., B.E. DERRICK & P.H. PATTERSON. 2000. Cytokine responses to LTP induction in the rat hippocampus: a comparison of *in vitro* and *in vivo* techniques Learn. Mem. **7:** 400–412.
46. D'ARCANGELO, G., V. TANCREDI, F. ONOFRI, *et al.* 2000. Interleukin-6 inhibits neurotransmitter release and the spread of excitation in the rat cerebral cortex Eur. J. Neurosci. **12:** 1241–1252.
47. VITKOVIC, L., J. BOCKAERT & C. JACQUE. 2000. "Inflammatory" cytokines: neuromodulators in normal brain? J. Neurochem. **74:** 457–471.

48. Schuman, E.M. & D.V. Madison. 1994. Locally distributed synaptic potentiation in the hippocampus. Science **263:** 532–536.
49. Engert, F. & T. Bonhoeffer. 1997. Synapse specificity of long-term potentiation breaks down at short distances. Nature **388:** 279–284.

Humoral Links between Sleep and the Immune System

Research Issues

JAMES M. KRUEGER AND JEANNINE A. MAJDE

Department of Veterinary and Comparative Anatomy, Pharmacology and Physiology, Washington State University, Pullman, Washington 99164, USA

ABSTRACT: In the last twenty years we have realized that the immune system synthesizes a class of peptides, termed cytokines, that play a central role in alerting the brain to ongoing inflammation in peripheral tissues. Among the brain's responses to proinflammatory cytokines, or agents that induce these cytokines, are certain alterations in sleep profiles. Characteristically there is an increase in non-rapid eye movement sleep (NREMS), and NREMS intensity is often accompanied by a decrease in rapid eye movement sleep (REMS). Cytokines appear to play a role in normal sleep regulation; during pathology, higher levels of cytokines amplify the physiological cytokine sleep mechanisms. In this review we summarize the extensive literature on the roles of interleukin-1 (IL-1) and tumor necrosis factor-α (TNF-α) in sleep regulation, and their interactions with the neuropeptides growth hormone-releasing hormone (GHRH) and corticotropin-releasing hormone (CRH). We reach the tentative conclusion that the sleep-promoting actions of IL-1 and GHRH are mediated via anterior hypothalamic neurons that are receptive to these substances. It also seems likely that TNF-α and CRH also influence these neurons. In addition, we discuss an array of research issues raised by these studies that remain to be resolved.

KEYWORDS: sleep; cytokine; interleukin-1 (IL-1); tumor necrosis factor-alpha (TNF-α); growth hormone releasing hormone (GHRH); corticotropin-releasing hormone (CRH)

INTRODUCTION

Over the last 20 years, much has been learned about molecular linkages between the immune system and the central nervous system (CNS). It is now clear that these two body systems are intricately intertwined and in close communication via humoral as well as neurological signals. One manifestation of this linkage is the well-documented relation between immune system cytokines and the fever and excess

Address for correspondence: Dr. James M. Krueger, P.O. Box 646520, Department of VCAPP, Washington State University, Pullman, WA 99164-6520. Voice: 509-335-8212; fax: 509-335-4650.

Krueger@vetmed.wsu.edu

Ann. N.Y. Acad. Sci. 992: 9–20 (2003). © 2003 New York Academy of Sciences.

sleep, or acute phase response (APR), occurring in response to infections and other inflammatory diseases. We have progressed in our thinking from the "immune system is autonomous" to the "immune system is the mobile brain"[1] and signals the brain in health and disease. Furthermore, we have detected direct neurological interactions with cells of the immune system[2] that supplement classical CNS immune regulation through endocrine and neuroendocrine hormones. However, our comprehension of these immune system-CNS interactions is still limited. In our laboratory we have focused on immune system regulation of the sleep response to infection, both to gain insights into how the immune system signals the brain and, especially, to better understand the function of sleep. In this review we summarize our current knowledge of the humoral regulators of the sleep response outside and within the brain, with an emphasis on cytokines. We also focus on defining the research remaining to be done.

CYTOKINE REGULATION OF SLEEP

Fever was the first APR to be investigated with regard to humoral mediators. Indeed, the concept of the cytokine grew out of studies directed at purifying and subsequently cloning "endogenous pyrogen," or interleukin (IL)-1,[3] induced in response to microbial cell wall components such as endotoxins.[4] The same microbial cell wall components had been shown to be somnogenic,[4] and it was quickly determined that IL-1α and IL-1β and other proinflammatory cytokines, such as tumor necrosis factor-alpha (TNF-α) were also somnogenic.[4] Microbial product-induced proinflammatory cytokines were also implicated as central mediators of the anorexic response,[5] the social withdrawal response,[6] and the hepatic acute phase proteins, hematological responses, and endocrine responses associated with infection.[7] Thus, the concept that cytokines mediated the total APR, including "sickness behavior," to inflammatory stimuli evolved.[6] The focus has currently shifted from the nature of the mediators to their mode of action on and in the brain.

Studies of direct IL-1 action on the brain led to the realization that this molecular class is remarkably potent: only 50–100 pg (3–6 fmol) of IL-1β given to rats by the intracerebroventricular (icv) route induces a systemic immune suppression within 15 minutes.[8] A dose range of 0.5–25 ng (30–1,500 fmol) of IL-1β icv induces a fever and an increase in non-rapid eye movement sleep (NREMS, also termed slow wave sleep, or SWS) in rats within 30 minutes.[9] The somnogenic dose and sleep profile depend on the time of day injected.[9] Lower doses promote sleep without corresponding fever, whereas higher doses induce fever and also suppress rapid eye movement (REM) sleep.[9] Even higher doses inhibit both NREMS and REMS in rats[9] and cats,[10] perhaps via activation of negative feedback signals such as corticotropin-releasing hormone (CRH) (see below).[11] Intracerebroventricular IL-1α is also somnogenic and pyrogenic in rabbits at a dose as low as 0.01 ng.[12] The actions of icv, intraperitoneal (ip), and intravenous (iv) IL-1 and IL-1 inhibitors on fever and sleep have been reviewed.[13] TNF-α also induces excess NREMS when introduced either intracerebroventricularly or intravenously.[13,14] It is considerably less potent on a weight basis, requiring microgram quantities[15] (although heterologous TNF was employed, which may be less potent than the homologous cytokine). As with

IL-1, TNF inhibitors also block this response.[13,14] Physiological NREMS is altered in mice with targeted deletions (knockouts) of IL-1 and TNF receptors,[13,14] indicating that these cytokines regulate sleep in the absence of inflammation.

Substantial additional evidence implicates IL-1 and TNF in physiological sleep regulation. Thus, if these cytokines are inhibited using either antibodies or their soluble receptors or, in the case of IL1, the IL1 receptor antagonist, spontaneous sleep is reduced.[13,14] Furthermore, these inhibitors also attenuate the sleep rebound that normally occurs after sleep loss.[13,14] Anti-inflammatory cytokines that inhibit production of IL-1 and/or TNF, such as IL-4, IL-10, IL-13, and transforming growth factor-beta (TGF-β), inhibit spontaneous sleep. Brain levels of IL-1β mRNA and TNF-α mRNA vary with sleep propensity in rats. For instance, levels of these RNAs are higher during the light period (sleep period) than during the dark period, and levels of both these mRNAs increase during sleep deprivation.[13,14,16] Protein levels of TNF in rat brain also vary with the light-dark cycle,[17] and IL-1 CSF levels vary with the sleep-wake cycle in cats.[18] For both proteins there is a large literature from human subjects showing their variations in disease states with sleep propensity.[13] For example, patients with pre-eclampsia[19] and sleep apnea[20] have high sleep propensity and circulating TNF levels. TNF-α, the soluble TNF receptor, and IL-1β have all been reported to increase in humans during sleep loss.[13,21] Furthermore, in normal subjects, circulating levels of TNF-α vary with EEG slow wave activity.[22]

Current evidence also suggests that IL-1β and TNF-α elicit their actions on NREMS, in part via the well-characterized NREMS-regulatory areas of the hypothalamic preoptic area and the basal forebrain area.[13] Thus, microinjection of TNF-α into this area enhances NREMS, whereas injection of a TNF inhibitor into this area reduces sleep.[23] Furthermore, IL-1β enhances the activity of sleep-active neurons in the anterior hypothalamus, while inhibiting wake-active neurons in this area.[24] Both IL-1β[25] and TNF-α[26] enhance intracellular Ca^{2+} levels in neurons. This action of TNF-α is mediated via TNF-α–enhanced AMPA receptor activity,[26] and TNF-α also potentiates AMPA-induced postsynaptic potentials.[27] The spontaneous activity of these AMPA-related TNF-α actions is inhibited by the soluble TNF-α receptor, thereby providing further evidence that TNF-α is playing a role in the physiological, spontaneous activity of neurons.[26,27] Finally, IL-1β and growth hormone-releasing hormone (GHRH), a hypothalamic hormone also implicated in sleep regulation (see below), receptors colocalize on GABAergic hypothalamic neurons.[25] Anti–IL-1β antibodies block GHRH-somnogenic activity.[28]

Several mechanisms have been implicated in the somnogenic actions of IL-1 and TNF including activation of nuclear factor kappa B (NFκB), enhanced NO production, adenosine release, and enhanced PGD_2 synthesis.[13,29,30] These and other possible mechanisms of somnogenic action are in need of clarification (see below).

NEUROHORMONAL REGULATION OF SLEEP

Plasma levels of many hormones have a relationship with the sleep-wake cycle.[31] Nevertheless, extensive evidence for the involvement of hormones in the regulation of sleep exists only for GHRH and vasoactive intestinal peptide (VIP), and for these substances, current evidence suggests that their involvement in sleep regulation is via their neurotransmitter/autocrine/paracrine roles within the brain, rather than their hormonal actions.[13] We review the evidence for GHRH's involvement in NREMS regulation here because, as just mentioned, its somnogenic actions seem to be linked to those of IL-1β. VIP is involved in REMS regulation; this has been reviewed elsewhere.[32] Evidence is beginning to accumulate that links CRH to promotion of spontaneous wakefulness, and this action has been tied to IL-1; we therefore briefly review this evidence here as well.

GHRH enhances NREMS in rats, rabbits, mice, and humans;[13] it is somnogenic via a variety of administrative routes including icv, iv, and ip injection and in humans, intranasally. In rats and rabbits, icv injection of GHRH enhances both NREMS and REMS. However, REMS-promoting action likely results from GHRH-induced pituitary release of GH, because in hypophysectomized rats, GHRH only enhances NREMS. Furthermore, intrahypothalamic microinjection of GHRH enhances NREMS, but not REMS or GH release.[33] Inhibition of GHRH using either antibodies or a GHRH peptide antagonist inhibits spontaneous NREMS. The anti-GHRH antibodies also attenuate the expected sleep rebound that occurs after sleep deprivation. Mutant rats and mice with defective GHRH signaling mechanisms have reduced spontaneous NREMS duration. In addition, a transgenic strain of mouse overexpressing GH in brain, hence producing a negative feedback signal for GHRH release, has substantially less spontaneous NREMS.[13]

The distribution of GHRH and GHRH receptors within brain is restricted to the hypothalamus and the adjacent basal forebrain.[34] As just mentioned, intra-anterior hypothalamic injection of GHRH promotes NREMS, whereas microinjection of a GHRH peptide antagonist into this site inhibits spontaneous NREMS.[33] It seems likely that these effects are mediated via GHRH-receptive IL-1–receptive GABAergic neurons by alteration in cytosolic Ca^{2+} levels.[25]

Hypothalamic GHRH mRNA levels vary with sleep propensity.[35] Thus, GHRH mRNA levels are highest at the beginning of the light period, when rats sleep the most, and are lowest during the active dark period. Hypothalamic GHRH content is also sleep related; GHRH release (lower content) is associated with higher sleep propensity.[36] Sleep loss also enhances GHRH mRNA levels and reduces hypothalamic GHRH content. Sleep loss is also associated with a reduction in hypothalamic, but not pituitary, binding of GHRH and of GHRH receptor mRNA levels.[38] GHRH downregulates expression of its receptor. These results clearly indicate that the action of sleep loss on the GHRH receptor is specific to the hypothalamus, thereby providing further evidence for the independence of GHRH somnogenic activity from GHRH-induced pituitary release of GH. Finally, IL-1β induces *in vitro* and *in vivo* enhanced production of GHRH mRNA and GHRH receptor mRNA; these effects are both dose and time dependent (Taishi *et al.,* unpublished data). Collectively, there is strong evidence for the involvement of GHRH in NREMS regulation and a close relationship with the somnogenic mechanisms of IL-1.

GHRH and IL-1 somnogenic mechanisms may include a shared feedback signal, CRH. Thus, spontaneous CRH levels apparently suppress hypothalamic GHRH mRNA levels, because a CRH antagonist enhances GHRH mRNA levels.[39] CRH also inhibits GHRH-induced GH release.[40] IL-1β enhances GHRH mRNA levels and CRH release, and CRH, in turn, inhibits IL-1β production.[41] It seems likely that the hypothalamic neurons that have both GHRH receptor and IL-1β[25] may be involved in these effects.

CRH also affects sleep; central administration of CRH to rats increases latency to sleep and decreases duration of NREMS.[42] This wakefulness effect of CRH may be mediated, in part, via IL-1, because IL-1–induced NREMS is inhibited by CRH.[11] Further, if CRH is inhibited using the CRH antagonist astressin, IL-1β mRNA increases as does NREMS, and these effects are blocked if rats are pretreated with anti–IL-1 antibodies.[43] The CRH receptor antagonists, alphahelical CRH and astressin, reduce spontaneous sleep as well.[44] Finally, Lewis rats have reduced CRH relative to Fischer 344 and Sprague-Dawley rats; Lewis rats spend more time in NREMS than do these other strains,[45] and Lewis rats are more responsive to IL-1β than are Sprague-Dawley rats in that their NREMS responses to IL-1β are greater.[46] Collectively, these data suggest that the sleep-altering actions of GHRH, IL-1β, and CRH are related. These substances seem to have a spontaneous "tone" in that inhibition of any one of them either inhibits (GHRH and IL-1β) or enhances (CRH) NREMS. They affect each other's production and release within the hypothalamus, and their direct application either enhances (GHRH and IL-1β) or inhibits (CRH) sleep.

OTHER CYTOKINE AND CYTOKINE-RELATED REGULATORS OF SLEEP WITHIN THE BRAIN

Many cytokines have the ability to either enhance or inhibit sleep (TABLE 1).[13,14,29] However, extensive evidence linking any one of them, other than IL-1β and TNF-α, to sleep regulation does not exist. Nevertheless, differences in their effects on sleep are subtle, suggesting that cytokines have partially independent mechanisms, yet share mechanisms, that lead to sleep. Furthermore, the fact that so many cytokines have receptors in brain, have well-characterized interactions outside the brain, and affect sleep suggests that the cytokine network operates in the brain to regulate sleep in health and sickness.[29]

Nerve growth factor (NGF) and brain-derived neurotrophic factor (BDNF), like IL-1β, promote NREMS and their levels in brain increase during sleep loss.[13] However, unlike IL-1, NGF[47] and BDNF[48] promote REMS at doses that promote NREMS. Furthermore, neither NGF nor BDNF is pyrogenic. Furthermore, central administration of NGF and BDNF decreases EEG slow-wave activity (a measure of the intensity of NREMS), whereas IL-1 enhances EEG delta wave activity. Such results suggest independent mechanisms for each of these parameters. Secondly, acidic fibroblast growth factor (aFGF) and basic FGF share many biological activities. However, only aFGF promotes NREMS.[49] Inhibition of IL-1β decreases spontaneous NREMS,[13] whereas inhibition of IL-18[50] does not. Administration of exogeneous IL-1 or IL-18 promotes NREMS. Furthermore, muramyl dipeptide- (a bacterial cell wall product capable of inducing proinflammatory cytokines and sleep)[29] induced sleep is attenuated if either IL-1 or IL-18 is inhibited.[13,50] These results suggest that IL-1, but not IL-18, is involved in physiological sleep regulation and that both are involved in sleep responses to infectious agents. Finally, if species-specific IL-18 is used, it is not pyrogenic, whereas IL-1β is.[13,50]

TABLE 1. Many cytokines can affect sleep[a]

Pro-somnogenic cytokines	Anti-somnogenic cytokines
IL-1β[b]	IL-4
IL-1α	IL-10
TNF-α	IL-13
TNF-β	Transforming growth factor beta
IL-2	Insulin-like growth factor[b]
IL-6[b]	Soluble TNF receptor
IL-15	Soluble IL-1 receptor
IL-18	
Epidermal growth factor	
Acidic fibroblast growth factor	
Nerve growth factor	
Brain-derived neurotrophic factor	
Neurotrophin 3	
Neurotrophin 4	
Glia-derived neurotrophic factor	
Interferon-α[b]	
Interferon-gamma	
Granulocyte-macrophage colony stimulating factor	
Granulocyte stimulating factor	

[a]See Ref. 13 for complete citations.
[b]Effect on sleep can be opposite, depending on time after injection, dose, time of day, or route of administration.

NEEDED RESEARCH

1. How do peripheral cytokines signal the brain?

Key to our understanding immune regulation of sleep or any other component of the APR is comprehending how cytokines produced in the periphery gain access to or signal the brain. This issue has been intensively investigated. Three routes have been defined to date: (1) transport from blood to brain directly via brain regions, the circumventricular organs, lacking a blood-brain barrier;[30] (2) molecular transporters through the blood-brain barrier;[51] and (3) signaling via the vagal nerve in response to localized inflammation.[52]

Whereas good evidence exists for all three mechanisms to be operating, it is not clear which mechanisms operate when. For instance, the APR begins in mouse influenza when no cytokines are detectable in the blood,[53] implying a non-blood source. Cytokines are often more concentrated in the lymph than in the blood. Although there are no lymphatics in the brain, antigen has been demonstrated to pass from the brain cerebrospinal fluid (CSF) through the cribiform plate into nasal lymphatics and thoracic root lymphatics.[54] Can this pathway reverse and take lymph components such as cytokines into the brain? There is no anatomical evidence for afferent pathways from the lymph, and they would seem unlikely based on the need to isolate the brain from environmental toxins. More likely, blood-borne cytokines at levels not readily detected by commonly employed assays or cytokines in equilibrium with serum carriers are accessing the brain through circumventricular organs or specific vascular transporters or both. In this context, it should be noted that the IL-1s are such potent activators of the APR (see above) that only femtomole amounts of these cytokines would suffice.

There is convincing evidence that localized, as opposed to systemic, inflammation can signal the brain via sensory vagal afferents.[55] The specific structure involved appears to be chemosensory paraganglia that are associated with clusters of macrophages, dendritic cells, and mast cells.[55] The initial site of neural activation appears to be the nucleus tractus solitarius, followed by the nucleus raphe magna, followed by the spinal cord dorsolateral funiculus.[55] Signaling via the vagus has been demonstrated only for the subdiaphragmatic vagus responding to intraperitoneal or subcutaneous inflammatory stimuli. Do other localized body compartments (such as the lung) signal via other branches of the vagus? Our understanding of neural pathways from the immune system to the brain is in its early stages.

2. Do single cytokines operate independently in sleep regulation?

Whereas the studies described above indicate that a single cytokine such as IL-1β can upregulate NREMS or fever, it seems unlikely that it operates independently of other proinflammatory cytokines *in vivo*. It is widely recognized that IL-1 and TNF induce each other, regulate each other's receptors, and, more importantly, synergize with each other with respect to several toxic actions.[56] Inflammatory challenges induce TNF first and IL-1β a few hours later.[56] Because an inflammatory challenge does not induce a single cytokine, it is probably more meaningful to study the sleep responses to the types of mixtures that are found in nature. Such studies have not been conducted to date.[57]

3. Where are the relevant cytokine receptors (IL-1s, TNF-α) expressed in the brain? Does their distribution correlate with what we know about sleep regulation?

As reviewed here and elsewhere,[13] there is evidence that IL-1β and TNF-α can affect sleep via anterior hypothalamic neurons that are receptive to these cytokines. This area of brain is known to be involved in sleep regulation and in the somnogenic actions of other sleep regulatory substances such as GHRH, adenosine, and prostaglandin D_2.[13] However, a theoretical view of brain organization and sleep mechanisms postulates that cytokines and other growth factors involved in sleep regulation (TABLE 1) are produced locally, throughout the brain, in response to neural use.[58] Once released from neurons or glia, they would act locally in an autocrine and paracrine fashion to alter input-output relationships of local neuronal networks and thereby cause local state shifts. In this view, the previously identified sleep regulatory circuits act to coordinate the localized state shifts of small groups of highly interconnected neurons.[58] Although there is supporting evidence for this view, further investigation is needed.

4. Do proinflammatory cytokines actually mediate the changes in sleep seen after infectious challenge?

Although the sleep profiles seen in response to IL-1s and TNF-α are similar to those seen in response to infectious challenge, direct evidence implicating these cytokines in pathological sleep is limited. We have demonstrated that NREMS responses to the bacterial peptidoglycan muramyl dipeptide (MDP) are attenuated in animals pretreated with IL-1 or TNF inhibitors.[29] However, sleep profiles have not yet been characterized for actual infections in animals deficient in one or more cytokine of interest, and this approach is complicated by the possible alterations in agent replication and/or distribution when these important immune regulators are blocked.

5. Is brain NFκB activation essential for cytokine action on the brain? If NFκB expression is a marker for cytokine activity, where does it occur in the brain?

The nuclear transcription factor NFκB is a central regulator of proinflammatory cytokine induction and is also induced by the same cytokines. The rel family of proteins, of which the p50/p65 heterodimer, commonly termed NFκB, is a member, is a highly conserved family of immune system regulatory proteins found as far back in evolution as the plants.[59] However, evidence for the direct involvement of NFκB in sleep regulation is limited. Thus, NFκB activation in the cerebral cortex increases with sleep loss,[60] its inhibition inhibits sleep,[61] and NFκB in cholinergic basal forebrain neurons may be involved in adenosine-induced sleep.[62] Because many prosomnogenic cytokines activate NFκB, further research into the role of NFκB in sleep regulation is warranted.

6. Is NO synthesis in the brain required for cytokine modulation of sleep? If so, which NOS is responsible?

Concurrent with the studies of IL-1 and TNF in sleep regulation, it was observed that nitric oxide (NO) is involved in enhancing NREMS.[14] Because proinflammatory cytokines enhance NO production through the inducible nitric oxide synthase (NOS-2), NO may in part mediate the cytokine effects. Recent studies with NOS-2 knockout mice reveal that these mice have more REMS and less NREMS than those observed in corresponding control mice.[63] Another source of NO in the brain is produced endogenously by neuronal NOS (NOS-1). These NOS-1 knockout mice have less REMS than do their controls.[63] NO is also involved in GHRH-induced pituitary release of GH,[64] which raises the possibility that NO may also be involved in GHRH-induced sleep, although no studies on this matter currently exist.

7. What is the role of "pathological" sleep? Is pathological sleep truly pathological or protective?

A primary focus of our laboratory is understanding why we sleep.[58] By characterizing the alterations in sleep that occur in pathological states, we hope to gain a better understanding of the role of sleep in physiological states. We have characterized sleep changes in response to several isolated cytokines, living and killed microbes, microbial components, virus, and a viral simulant.[4,29] Sleep changes have been examined in active and abortive infections and in acute and chronic inflammation.[4,29] A striking feature of the acute response to infectious stimuli is a consistent increase in NREMS and putative sleep intensity (as determined by EEG slow wave amplitudes) and a less consistent decrease in REMS (which may simply be a dose effect). One possible role of sleep in general is conservation of energy, and energy utilization is reduced during NREMS relative to energy utilization during wakefulness.[65] Also, more energy is consumed by the brain during REMS than during NREMS, and sometimes exceeds energy utilization during wakefulness.[65] It is well established that fever causes an increase in energy consumption, and this raises the question: does the increase in NREMS compensate for this increase? Several studies have shown that increased NREMS occurs in the absence of fever,[66] so compensating for fever is unlikely to explain the primary purpose of this sleep mode. We have proposed that sleep may have initially evolved for a primordial function involving neuronal connectivity.[58] However, it seems likely that in birds and mammals, additional functions for sleep, such as saving calories or helping host defense, have evolved. This issue of sleep function has only recently been experimentally addressed, but given its importance in neurobiology it most certainly will expand in the near future.

ACKNOWLEDGMENTS

This work was supported by the National Institutes of Health Grants NS25378, NS27250, NS31453, and HD36520.

REFERENCES

1. WEIGENT, D.A. & J.E. BLALOCK. 1995. Associations between the neuroendocrine and immune systems. J. Leuk. Biol. **57:** 137–150.
2. MADDEN, K.S., V.M. SANDERS & D.L. FELTEN. 1995. Catecholamine influences and sympathetic neural modulation of immune responsiveness. Ann. Rev. Pharmacol. Toxicol. **35:** 417–448.
3. DINARELLO, C.A., J.G. CANNON & S.M. WOLFF. 1988. New concepts on the pathogenesis of fever. Rev. Infect. Dis. **10:** 168–189.
4. KRUEGER, J.M. & J.A. MAJDE. 1994. Microbial products and cytokines in sleep and fever regulation. Crit. Rev. Immunol. **14:** 355–379.
5. TURRIN, N.P. & C.R. PLATA-SALAMAN. 2000. Cytokine–cytokine interactions and the brain. Brain Res. Bull. **51:** 3–9.
6. KENT, S., R.-M. BLUTHÉ, K.W. KELLEY & R. DANTZER. 1992. Sickness behavior as a new target for drug development. T.I.P.S. **13:** 24–28.
7. STEEL, D.M. & A.S. WHITEHEAD. 1994. The major acute phase reactants: C-reactive protein, serum amyloid P component and serum amyloid A protein. Immunol. Today **15:** 81–88.
8. WEISS, J.M., S.K. SUNDAR, K.J. BECKER & M.A. CIERPIAL. 1989. Behavioral and neural influences on cellular immune responses: effects of stress and interleukin-1. J. Clin. Psychiatry **50** (suppl): 43–53.
9. OPP, M.R., F. OBÀL, JR. & J.M. KRUEGER. 1991. Interleukin-1 alters rat sleep: temporal and dose-related effects. Am. J. Physiol. Reg., Integ. Comp. Physiol. **260:** R52–R58.
10. SUSIC, V. & S. TOTIC. 1989. 'Recovery' function of sleep: effects of purified human interleukin-1 on the sleep and febrile response of cats. Metab. Brain Dis. **4:** 73–80.
11. OPP, M., F. OBAL, JR. & J.M. KRUEGER. 1989. Corticotropin-releasing factor attenuates interleukin 1-induced sleep and fever in rabbits. Am. J. Physiol. **257:** R528–R535.

12. OBAL, F., JR., M. OPP, A.B. CADY, *et al.* 1990. Interleukin 1α and an interleukin 1β fragment are somnogenic. Am. J. Physiol. Reg., Integ. Comp. Physiol. **259:** R439–R446.
13. OBAL, F., JR. & J.M. KRUEGER. 2003. Biochemical regulation of non-rapid-eye-movement sleep. Frontiers Biosci. **8:** 520–550.
14. KRUEGER, J.M., J. FANG, P. TAISHI, *et al.* 1998. Biochemical regulation of non-rapid eye movement sleep. Ann. N.Y. Acad. Sci. **856:** 148–159.
15. KAPÁS, L., L. HONG, A.B. CADY, *et al.* 1992. Somnogenic, pyrogenic, and anorectic activities of tumor necrosis factor-α and TNFα fragments. Am. J. Physiol. **263:** R708–R715.
16. VITKOVIC, L., J. BOCKAERT & C. JACQUE. 2000. "Inflammatory" cytokines: neuromodulators in normal brain? J. Neurochem. **74:** 457–471.
17. FLOYD, R.A. & J.M. KRUEGER. 1997. Diurnal variations of TNF alpha in the rat brain. Neuroreport **8:** 915–918.
18. LUE, F.A., F.A. BAIL, J. JEPHTHAH-OCHOLO, *et al.* 1998. Sleep and cerebrospinal fluid interleukin-1 like activity in the cat. Int. J. Neurosci. **42:** 179–183.
19. EDWARDS, N., D.M. BLYTON, G.J. KESBY, *et al.* 2000. Pre-eclampsia is associated with marked alterations in sleep architecture. Sleep **23:** 619–625.
20. LIU, H., J. KIU, S. XIONG, *et al.* 2000. The change in interleukin-6 and tumor necrosis factor in patients with obstructive sleep apnea syndrome. J. Tongji Med. Univ. **20:** 200–202.
21. SHEARER, W.T., J.M. REUBEN, J.M. MULLINGTON, *et al.* 2001. Soluble TNF-alpha receptor 1 and IL-6 plasma levels in human subjected to the sleep deprivation model of spaceflight. J. Allergy Clin. Immunol. **107:** 165–170.
22. DARKO, D.F., J.C. MILLER, C. GALLEN, *et al.* 2002. Sleep electroencephalogram delta-frequency amplitude, night plasma levels of tumor necrosis factor alpha, and human immunodeficiency virus infection. Proc. Natl. Acad. Sci. USA **92:** 12080–12084.
23. KUBOTA, T., N. LI, Z. GUAN, *et al.* 2002. Intrapreoptic microinjection of TNF-alpha enhances non-REMS in rats. Brain Res. **932:** 37–44.
24. ALAM, N., D. MCGINTY, L. IMERI, *et al.* 2001. Effects of interleukin-1 beta on sleep- and wake-related preoptic anterior hypothalamic neurons in unrestrained rats. Sleep **24:** A59.
25. DE, A., L. CHURCHILL, F. OBAL, JR., *et al.* 2002. GHRH and IL1beta increase cytoplasmic Ca^{2+} levels in cultured hypothalamic GABAergic neurons. Brain Res. **949:** 209–212.
26. DE, A., S. SIMASKO & J.M. KRUEGER. 2000. TNFα increases intracellular calcium responses to KCl and AMPA in primary cultures of fetal hippocampal neurons. Soc. Neurosci. Abstr. **26:** 1363.
27. BEATTIE, E.C., D. STELLWAGEN, W. MORISHITA, *et al.* 2002. Control of synaptic strength by glial TNF alpha. Science **295:** 2282–2285.
28. OBAL, F., JR., J. FANG, L.C. PAYNE & J.M. KRUEGER. 1995. Growth hormone-releasing hormone mediates the sleep-promoting activity of interleukin-1 in rats. Neuroendocrinology **61:** 559–565.
29. KRUEGER, J.M., J. FANG & J.A. MAJDE. 2001. Sleep in health and disease. *In* Psychoneuroimmunology. R. Ader, D.L. Felten & N. Cohen, Eds. Vol. 1: 667–685. Academic Press. San Diego.
30. BLATTEIS, C.M. & E. SEHIC. 1997. Fever: how may circulating pyrogens signal the brain? News Physiol. Sci. **12:** 1–9.
31. OBÁL, F., JR. & J.M. KRUEGER. 2000. Hormones, cytokines and sleep. *In* Coping with the Environment Neural and Endocrine Mechanisms: Handbook of Physiology. B.S. McEwen, Ed. Chapt. 16. :331–349. Oxford University Press. Oxford, UK.
32. ROKY, R., F. OBÁL, JR., J.L. VALATX, *et al.* 1995. Prolactin and rapid eye movement sleep. Sleep **18:** 536–542.
33. ZHANG, J., F. OBAL, JR., T. ZHENG, *et al.* 1999. Intrapreoptic microinjection of GHRH or its antagonist alters sleep in rats. J. Neurosci. **19:** 2187–2194.
34. SAWCHENKO, P.E., L.W. SWANSON, J. RIVIER & W.W. VALE. 1985. The distribution of growth-hormone-releasing factor (GRF) immunoreactivity in the central nervous system of the rat: an immunohistochemical study using antisera directed against rat hypothalamic GRF. J. Comp. Neurol. **237:** 100–115.

35. ZHANG, J., Z. CHEN, P. TAISHI, *et al.* 1999. Sleep deprivation increases rat hypothalamic growth hormone-releasing hormone mRNA. Am. J. Physiol. **275:** R1755–R1761.
36. BREDOW, S., P. TAISHI, F. OBAL, JR., *et al.* 1996. Hypothalamic growth hormone-releasing hormone mRNA varies across the day in rats. Neuroreport **7:** 2501–2505.
37. GARDI, J., F. OBAL, JR., J. FANG, *et al.* 1999. Diurnal variations and sleep deprivation-induced changes in rat hypothalamic GHRH and somatostatin contents. Am. J. Physiol. **277:** R1339–R1344.
38. GARDI, J, P. TAISHI, R. SPETH, *et al.* 2002. Sleep loss alters hypothalamic growth hormone-releasing hormone receptors. Neurosci. Lett. **329:** 69–72.
39. MOUNIER, F., E. PELLIGRINI, C. KORDON, *et al.* 1997. Continuous intracerebroventricular administration of a corticotropin releasing hormone antagonist amplifies spontaneous growth hormone pulses in the rat. J. Endocrinol. **152:** 431–436.
40. BARBARINO, A., S.M. CORSELLO, S. DELLA CASA, *et al.* 1990. Corticotropin-releasing hormone inhibition of growth hormone-releasing hormone-induced growth hormone release in man. J. Clin. Endocrinol. Metab. **71:** 1368–1374.
41. ANGELI, A., R.G. MASERA, M.L. SARTORI, *et al.* 1999. Modulation by cytokines of glucocorticoids action. Ann. NY Acad. Sci. **876:** 210–220.
42. EHLERS, C.L., C. SOMES, E. SEIFRITZ & J.E. RIVIER. 1997. CRF-NPY interactions: a potential role in sleep dysregulation in depression and anxiety. Depress. Anxiety **6:** 1–9.
43. CHANG, F.C. & M.R. OPP. 2000. IL-1 is a mediator of increases in slow-wave sleep induced by CRH receptor blockade. Am. J. Physiol. Regul. Integr. Comp. Physiol. **279:** R793–R802.
44. CHANG, F.C. & M.R. OPP. 1998. Blockade of corticotropin-releasing hormone receptors reduces spontaneous waking in the rat. Am. J. Physiol. **275:** R793–R802.
45. OPP, M.R. 1997. Rat strain differences suggest a role for corticotropin-releasing hormone in modulating sleep. Physiol. Behav. **63:** 67–74.
46. OPP, M.R. & L. IMERI. 2001. Rat strains that differ in corticotropin-releasing hormone production exhibit different sleep-wake responses to interleukin 1. Neuroendocrinology **73:** 272–284.
47. TAKAHASHI, S. & J.M. KRUEGER. 1999. Nerve growth factor enhances sleep in rabbits. Neurosci. Lett. **264:** 149–152.
48. KUSHIKATA, T., J. FANG & J.M. KRUEGER. 1999. Brain-derived neurotrophic factor enhances spontaneous sleep in rats and rabbits. Am. J. Physiol. **276:** R1334–R1338.
49. KNEFATI, M., C. SOMOGYI, L. KAPAS, *et al.* 1995. Acidic fibroblast growth factor (FGF) but not basic FGF induces sleep and fever in rabbits. Am. J. Physiol. **269:** R87–R91.
50. KUBOTA, T., J. FANG, R.A. BROWN & J.M. KRUEGER. 2001. Interleukin-18 promotes sleep in rabbits and rats. Am. J. Physiol. **281:** R828–R838.
51. BANKS, W.A. & A.J. KASTIN. 1990. Exchange of peptides between the circulation and the nervous system: role of the blood-brain barrier. *In* Circulating Regulatory Factors and Neuroendocrine Function. J.C. Porter & D. Jezova, Eds. :59-69. Plenum Press. New York.
52. WATKINS, L.R., S.F. MAIER & L.E. GOEHLER. 1995. Cytokine-to-brain communication: a review and analysis of alternative mechanisms. Life Sci. **57:** 1011–1026.
53. CONN, C.A., J.L. MCCLELLAN, H.F. MAASSAB, *et al.* 1995. Cytokines and the acute phase response to influenza virus in mice. Am. J. Physiol. **268:** R78–R84.
54. WELLER, R.O., B. ENGELHARDT & M.J. PHILLIPS. 1996. Lymphocyte targeting of the central nervous system: a review of afferent and efferent CNS-immune pathways. Brain Pathol. **6:** 275–288.
55. WATKINS, L.R. & S.F. MAIER. 1999. Implications of immune-to-brain communication for sickness and pain. Proc. Natl. Acad. Sci. USA **96:** 7710–7713.
56. DINARELLO, C.A. 1989. Interleukin-1 and its biologically related cytokines. Adv. Immunol. **44:** 153–205.
57. KUBOTA, T., J.A. MAJDE, R.A. BROWN & J.M. KRUEGER. 2001. Tumor necrosis factor receptor fragment attenuates interferon-gamma-induced non-REMS in rabbits. J. Neuroimmunol. **119:** 192–198.
58. KRUEGER, J.M. & F. OBAL, JR. 2003. Sleep function. Frontiers Biosci. **8:** 511–519.
59. GHOSH, S., M.J. MAY & E.B. KOPP. 1998. NFκB and Ral proteins: evolutionarily conserved mediators of immune responses. Annu. Rev. Immunol. **16:** 225–260.

60. Chen, Z., J. Gardi, T. Kushikata, *et al.* 1999. Nuclear factor kappa B-like activity increases in murine cerebral cortex after sleep deprivation. Am. J. Physiol. **45:** R1812–R1818.
61. Kubota, T., T. Kushikata, J. Fang & J.M. Krueger. 2000. A nuclear factor kappa β (NFκB) inhibitor peptide inhibits spontaneous and interleukin-1β-induced sleep. Am. J. Physiol. **279:** R404–R413.
62. Basheer, R., D.G. Rainnie, T. Porkka-Heiskanen, *et al.* 2001. Adenosine, prolonged wakefulness, and A1-activated NF-κB DNA binding in the basal forebrain of the rat. Neuroscience **104:** 731–739.
63. Chen, L., J.A. Majde & J.M. Krueger. 2002. Spontaneous sleep in neuronal and inducible nitric oxide synthase knockout mice. Sleep **25:** A170–A171.
64. McCann, S.M., M. Kimura, S. Karanth, *et al.* 2000. The mechanism of action of cytokines to control the release of hypothalamic and pituitary hormones in infection. Ann. N.Y. Acad. Sci. **917:** 4–18.
65. Sawaya, R. & D.H. Ingvar. 1989. Cerebral blood flow and metabolism in sleep. Acta Neurol. Scand. **80:** 481–491.
66. Krueger, J.M. & S. Takahashi. 1997. Thermoregulation and sleep: closely linked but separable. Ann. N.Y. Acad. Sci. **813:** 281–286.

HPA Axis Activation and Neurochemical Responses to Bacterial Translocation from the Gastrointestinal Tract

ADRIAN J. DUNN,[a] TETSUYA ANDO,[a,c] RHONDA F. BROWN,[a,d] AND RODNEY D. BERG[b]

Department of Pharmacology and Therapeutics[a] and
Department of Microbiology and Immunology,[b]
Louisiana State University Health Sciences Center,
Shreveport, Louisiana 71130-3932, USA

ABSTRACT: Stress can cause migration of indigenous bacterial flora from the gut to the peritoneum, a phenomenon known as bacterial translocation. Destruction of the cell walls of gram-negative bacteria can result in the production of endotoxin (lipopolysaccharide, LPS), which is the likely cause of sepsis. Exogenously administered LPS can activate the hypothalamo-pituitary-adrenal (HPA) axis as well as brain noradrenergic and indoleaminergic systems. Thus, it is possible that activations of these systems associated with laboratory stressors in rats and mice could be attributed to bacterial translocation and LPS production. To test this hypothesis we conducted experiments on the time course of bacterial translocation in response to restraint in mice, while measuring HPA and neurochemical responses. These experiments failed to show good correlations between the occurrence of bacterial translocation and HPA and neurochemical activations, suggesting that the later responses were not linked to bacterial translocation. This conclusion was supported by the observation of normal neurochemical responses to restraint in germ-free mice. In further experiments, translocation of *Salmonella typhimurium*, a bacterium that readily translocates in unstressed animals, was associated with HPA activation and noradrenergic and indoleaminergic responses, indicating that bacterial translocation can indeed activate the HPA axis and brain amines. However, the above experiments suggest that this is not the mechanism by which restraint activates these systems.

KEYWORDS: bacterial translocation; lipopolysaccharide (LPS); corticosterone; norepinephrine; tryptophan; serotonin; stress

[c]Present address: Division of Psychosomatic Research, National Institute of Mental Health, National Center of Neurology and Psychiatry, 1-7-3 Konodai, Ichikawa, 272 Japan.

[d]Present address: Medical Psychology Unit, University of Sydney, Sydney, Australia.

Address for correspondence: Dr. Adrian J. Dunn, Department of Pharmacology and Therapeutics, Louisiana State University Health Sciences Center, P.O. Box 33932, Shreveport, LA 71130-3932. Voice: 318-675-7850; fax: 318-675-7857.

adunn@lsuhsc.edu

Ann. N.Y. Acad. Sci. 992: 21–29 (2003). © 2003 New York Academy of Sciences.

INTRODUCTION

Under stressful conditions, indigenous bacterial flora in the gut can enter the peritoneum, a phenomenon known as bacterial translocation.[1] Bacterial translocation can result in sepsis, which is a major cause of death in patients undergoing major surgery. Destruction of the cell walls of gram-negative bacteria can result in the production of endotoxin (lipopolysaccharide, LPS), which is the likely cause of sepsis, although other stimulators of the immune system may be involved. Exogenously administered LPS can activate the hypothalamo-pituitary-adrenal (HPA) axis as well as brain noradrenergic and indoleaminergic systems,[2] and there is a strong similarity between these responses to LPS and those to commonly used laboratory stressors,

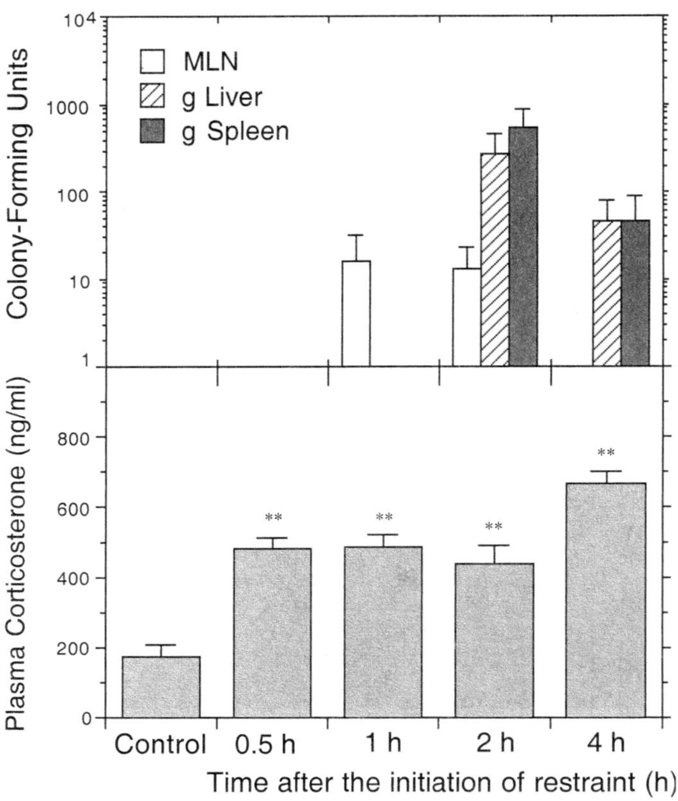

FIGURE 1. Effect of restraint for various periods of time on translocation of indigenous gastrointestinal microflora from the gastrointestinal tract. Mice (n = 9–10) were restrained for 0.5, 1, 2, or 4 hours. Immediately after their release, they were killed and homogenates of MLN, liver, and spleen were plated on blood agar and MacConkey agar for determination of bacterial colony-forming units (CFU). (*Upper panel*) Mean CFUs for the whole MLN or per gram of liver or spleen. (*Lower panel*) Plasma concentrations of corticosterone. **Significantly different from the unrestrained control (P <0.01; Fisher's LSD test). Modified from Ando *et al.*[5]

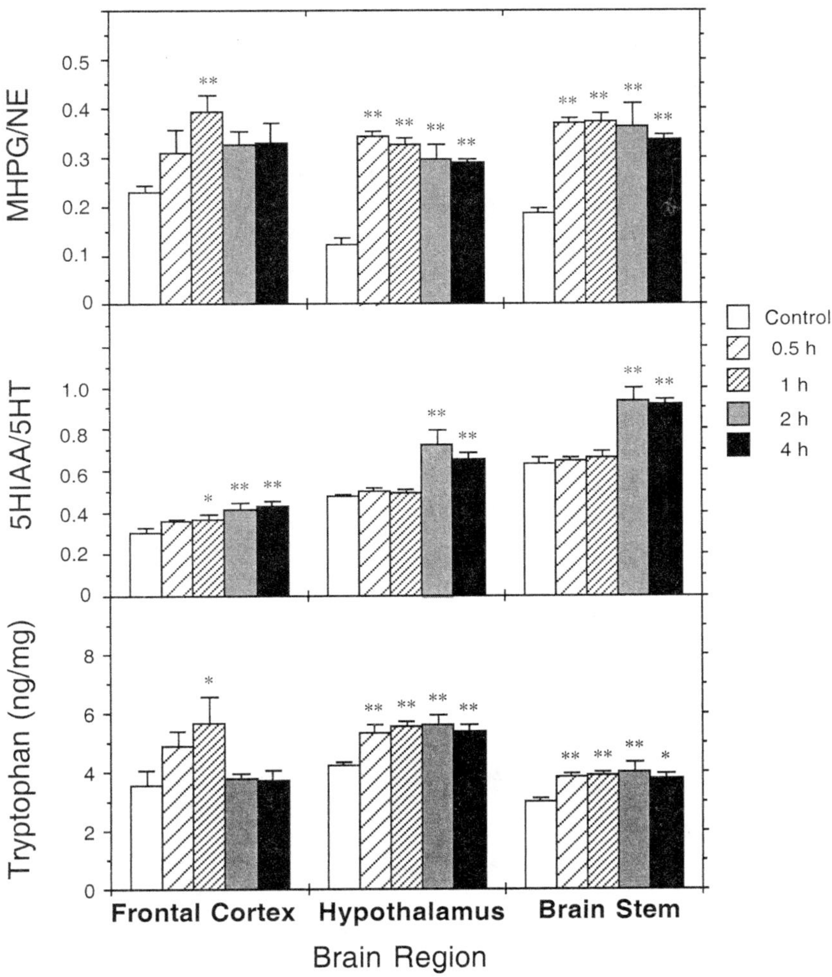

FIGURE 2. Effects of restraint for various periods of time on brain MHPG/NE, 5-HIAA/5-HT, and tryptophan in frontal cortex, hypothalamus, and brain stem. Mice (n = 9–10) were restrained for 0.5 to 4 hours in the same experiment as in FIGURE 1. *Significantly different from the unrestrained control (*P <0.05, **P <0.01; Fisher's LSD test). Modified from Ando *et al.*[5]

such as footshock and restraint.[3,4] Therefore, the HPA and neurochemical activations associated with footshock and restraint may be attributable to bacterial translocation and LPS production.

MATERIAL AND RESULTS

To test this hypothesis, we studied the effect of restraint on bacterial translocation to the mesenteric lymph node (MLN) complex, liver, and spleen in mice. Translocation was assessed by plating samples of the excised tissues on plates that would reveal the presence of live gram-negative and gram-positive bacteria. Plasma corticosterone and brain catecholamines and indoleamines were measured in the same animals immediately after various periods of restraint.[5] (For all experimental details,

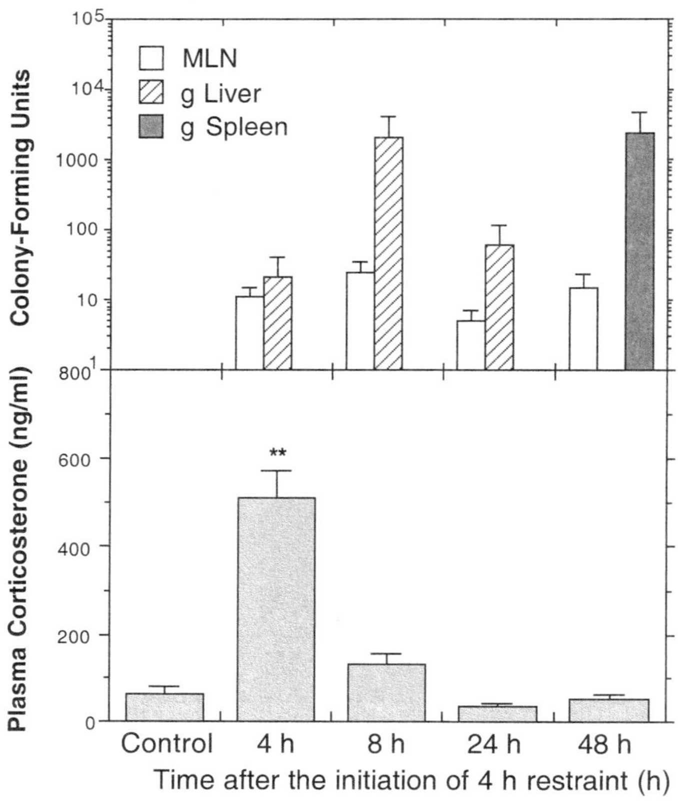

FIGURE 3. Effect of 4 hours of restraint on translocation of indigenous gastrointestinal microflora. Mice (n = 10) were restrained for 4 hours and killed immediately, 4, 8, 24, or 48 hours after initiating the restraint. (*Upper panel*) Mean number of CFUs for the whole MLN or per gram of liver or spleen. (*Lower panel*) Plasma corticosterone. **Significantly different from unrestrained control (P <0.01; Fisher's LSD test). Modified from Ando *et al.*[5]

see Ando *et al.*[5]) Results showed no translocation of gram-negative bacteria and a rather limited translocation of gram-positive bacteria, which increased as a function of the duration of the restraint (FIG. 1). By contrast, plasma corticosterone was elevated after the shortest period of restraint (30 minutes) and remained elevated after 1, 2, and 4 hours of restraint (FIG. 1). Increases paralleling those in corticosterone were observed in the ratios of 3-methoxy,4-hydroxyphenylethyleneglycol (MHPG) to norepinephrine (NE) and 5-hydroxyindoleacetic acid (5-HIAA) to 5-hydroxytryptamine (5-HT) as well as in tryptophan in the frontal cortex, hypothalamus, and

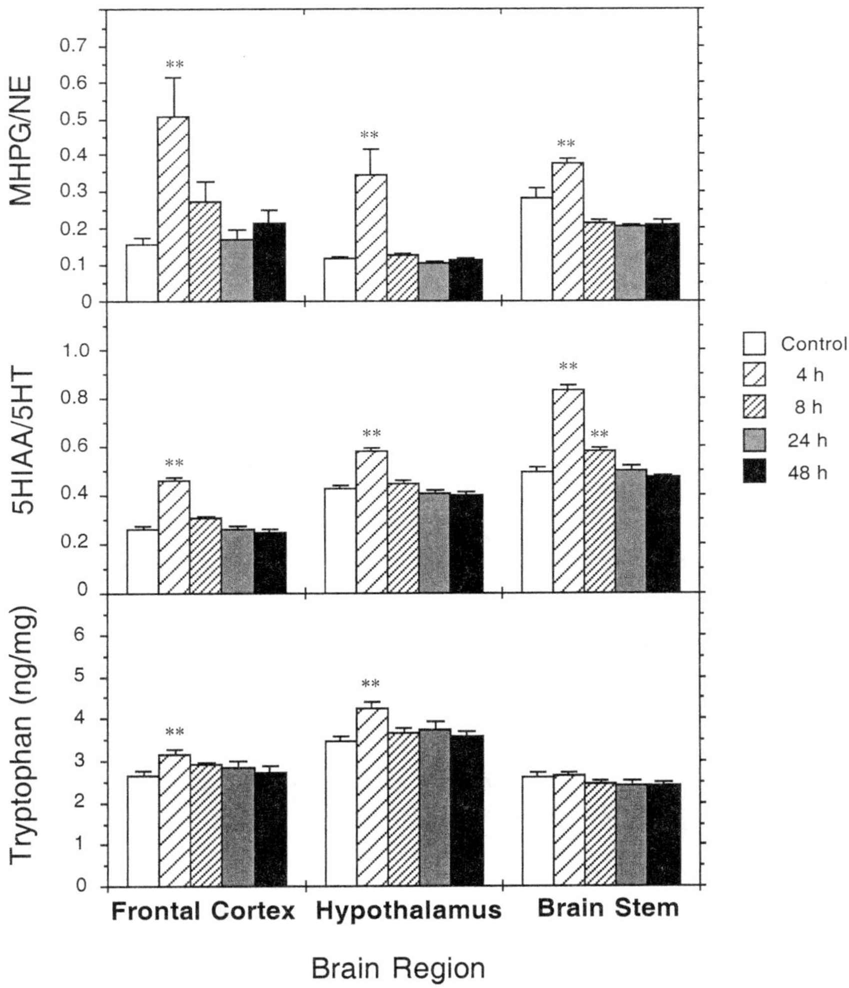

FIGURE 4. Effects of 4 hours of restraint on brain MHPG:NE, 5-HIAA:5-HT, and tryptophan 4, 8, 24, and 48 hours after initiating restraint. Same experiment as in FIGURE 3. **Significantly different from unrestrained control ($P < 0.01$; Fisher's LSD test). Modified from Ando *et al.*[5]

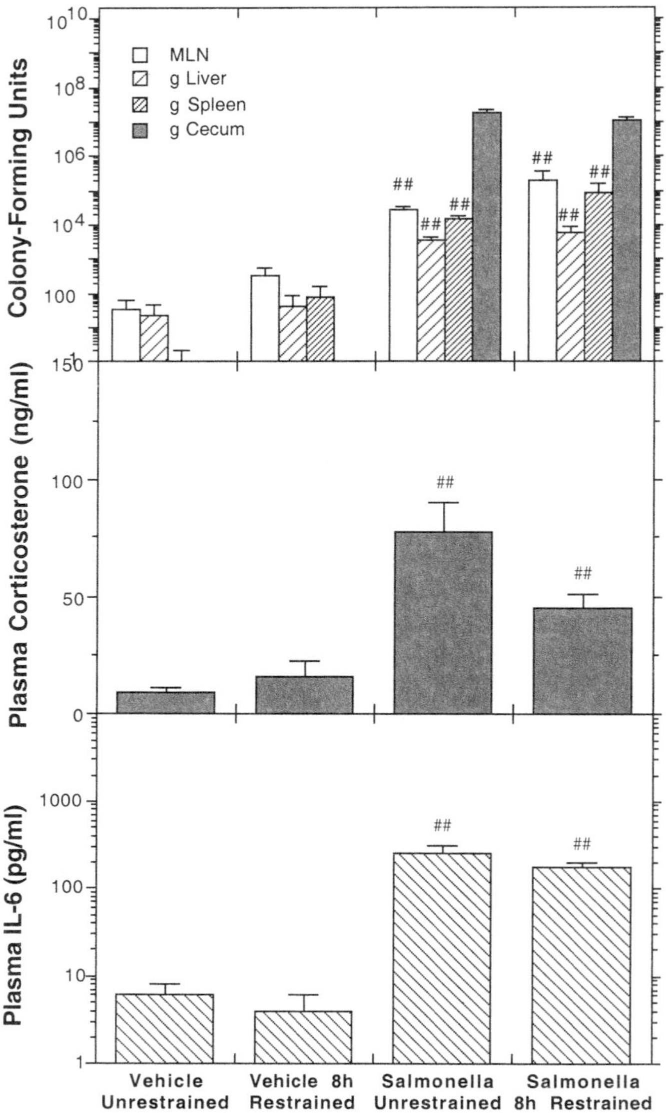

FIGURE 5. Effect of restraint on bacterial translocation of *S. typhimurium*. Mice (n = 10) were decontaminated by oral pretreatment with antibiotics for 3 days and then inoculated orally with *S. typhimurium* for 2 days. They were then restrained for 8 hours and tested 48 hours after initiating the restraint. (*Upper panel*) Mean number of CFUs for the whole MLN or per gram of liver, spleen, and cecum. There was no effect of restraint on translocation of *S. typhimurium*. (*Middle panel*) Plasma corticosterone; (*lower panel*) plasma IL-6. ##Significantly different from corresponding group not treated with *Salmonella* (P <0.01: Student's t test). Modified from Ando *et al.*[5]

brain stem (FIG. 2). In a second experiment, mice were restrained for 4 hours, and translocation, plasma corticosterone, and brain neurochemical responses were assessed 0, 4, 8, 24, and 48 hours after restraint. Translocation of gram-positive bacteria was similar to that in the first experiment, but continued to increase up to 48 hours after the period of restraint (FIG. 3).[5] However, while plasma corticosterone (FIG. 3) and MHPG:NE, 5-HIAA:5-HT ratios, and tryptophan were elevated immediately after the period of restraint, they were not statistically significantly elevated at later times (FIG. 4). Therefore, HPA and neurochemical changes dissipated while translocation of live bacteria was still increasing. Thus, no correlation existed between endocrine and neurochemical changes and the translocation of live gram-

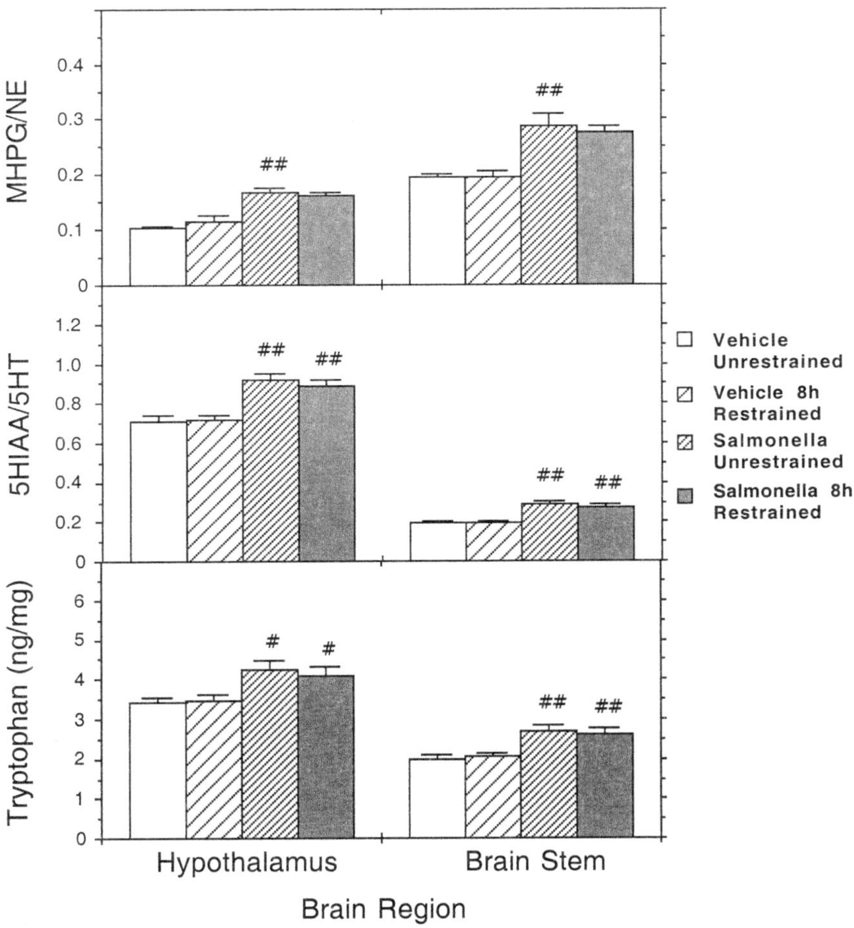

FIGURE 6. Effect of restraint on brain MHPG/NE, 5-HIAA/5-HT, and tryptophan in *S. typhimurium*-monoassociated mice. Ssame experiment as in FIGURE 5. There were no statistically significant effects of restraint on brain MHPG:NE, 5-HIAA/5-HT, and tryptophan. #Significantly different from corresponding group not treated with *Salmonella* (#P <0.05, ##P <0.01: Student's t test). Modified from Ando *et al.*[5]

positive bacteria. These results suggested that the latter changes were not related to the translocation process.

This conclusion was supported by two further observations: administration of an antibody to LPS failed to alter the responses to restraint, and restraint induced neurochemical changes in the brain of germ-free mice that were indistinguishable from those of germ-free mice that had been inoculated with intestinal microflora from normal mice.[5]

To determine whether bacterial translocation was capable of activating the HPA axis and brain noradrenergic and indoleamine systems, we studied the effects in mice that were infected with *Salmonella typhimurium,* a pathogenic bacterium that translocates in the absence of stress.[5] Mice were infected with *S. typhimurium* and restrained for 8 hours. Bacterial translocation and the endocrine and neurochemical parameters were measured 48 hours after restraint was initiated. Live gram-positive bacteria were found in the MLN, liver, and spleen of both uninfected and *S. typhimurium*-infected mice, but they were substantially more numerous in the latter (FIG. 5). Restraint had no statistically significant effect on the translocation. However, plasma corticosterone, plasma interleukin-6 (IL-6), and brain MHPG:NE, 5-HIAA:5-HT ratios and tryptophan were all increased in the mice infected with *S. typhimurium* (FIGS. 5 and 6). These results indicate that infection with *S. typhimurium* produces endocrine and neurochemical changes like those of LPS. It is likely that this occurred because of LPS production when the translocated bacteria were killed in the peritoneum or lymph nodes. Indeed, Takaki *et al.*[6] have shown that immobilization of rats rapidly increased plasma concentrations of LPS in portal blood. While translocation of gram-negative bacteria was not observed, our assays were designed to detect only live bacteria. Therefore, it is possible that gram-negative bacteria such as *S. typhimurium* did translocate, but were rapidly killed and thus not detected.

COMMENTS

The foregoing results suggest that when substantial bacterial translocation occurs, it can cause elevation of plasma IL-6, activation of the HPA axis, as well as activations of brain noradrenergic and indoleamine systems. However, in our normal male CD-1 mice, translocation of indigenous bacteria cannot account for the responses to restraint. Nevertheless, this conclusion may not apply to other species, to other strains of mice, or under other conditions. Whether or not bacterial translocation plays a role may depend on the particular indigenous bacterial flora in the specific group of animals being studied.

It is also relevant that the neurochemical responses to commonly used laboratory stressors are not identical to those observed after LPS. In particular, footshock and restraint induce pronounced increases in brain 3,4-dihydroxyphenylacetic acid (DOPAC):dopamine (DA) ratios, indicative of activation of dopaminergic neurons.[7] Such changes are rarely observed with interleukin-1, but may be observed after LPS.[4] However, after LPS, the changes in DOPAC:DA are similar in all brain regions, whereas after footshock or restraint, the DOPAC:DA increases are substantially larger in limbic areas of cortex (especially the medial prefrontal cortex) than in the striatum and other areas of the brain.[4,7] This alone suggests that the restraint-induced neurochemical changes are not attributable to generation of LPS.

REFERENCES

1. BERG, R.D. 1992. Bacterial translocation from the gastrointestinal tract. J. Med. **23:** 217–244.
2. DUNN, A.J. 1992. Endotoxin-induced activation of cerebral catecholamine and serotonin metabolism: comparison with interleukin-1. J. Pharmacol. Exp. Ther. **261:** 964–969.
3. DUNN, A.J. 1988. Stress-related changes in cerebral catecholamine and indoleamine metabolism: lack of effect of adrenalectomy and corticosterone. J. Neurochem. **51:** 406–412.
4. DUNN, A.J. 2001. Effects of cytokines and infections on brain neurochemistry. *In* Psychoneuroimmunology. R. Ader, D.L. Felten & N. Cohen, Eds. :649–666. Academic Press. New York.
5. ANDO, T., R.F. BROWN, R.D. BERG & A.J. DUNN. 2000. Bacterial translocation can increase plasma corticosterone and brain catecholamine and indoleamine metabolism. Am. J. Physiol. **279:** R2164–R2172.
6. TAKAKI, A., K. SHIODA, A. ARIMURA & T. HORI. 1996. Immobilization increases plasma LPS in the hepatic portal vein in rats. J. Endotoxin Res. **3:** 54.
7. DUNN, A.J. 1988. Stress-related activation of cerebral dopaminergic systems. Ann. N.Y. Acad. Sci. **537:** 188–205.

Pathophysiology of Cerebral Malaria

Role of Host Cells in the Modulation of Cytoadhesion

SAMUEL C. WASSMER, VALÉRY COMBES, AND GEORGES E. GRAU

Unité de Parasitologie Expérimentale, EA 3282, IFR 48, Faculties of Medicine and Pharmacy, Université de la Méditerranée, F-13 385 Marseille Cedex 05, France

ABSTRACT: Cerebral malaria (CM), one of the most serious complications of *Plasmodium falciparum* infection, is characterized by the sequestration of infected erythrocytes (IEs) in cerebral microvascular beds. The precise mechanisms involved in the onset of neuropathology remain unknown, but parasite sequestration in the brain, metabolic disturbances, and host immune responses all play a role. Studies in a murine model of CM showed a potential role for host cells, especially platelets, in the pathogenesis of CM. Indeed, urokinase plasminogen activator receptor (uPAR; CD87) deficiency attenuates the severity of CM, most likely by its important role in platelet kinetics and trapping. These results led us to evaluate whether platelets have a role in the human disease. By immunostaining of brain samples from Malawian patients, we determined that the surface of platelet accumulation and the proportion of vessels filled with platelets were significantly higher in patients who died of CM than in those who died of other causes. We then investigated the role of platelets in IE cytoadhesion *in vitro*, using CD36-binding IE (IECD36) and CD36-deficient (CD36DEF) brain microvascular endothelial cells (ECs). Coincubation studies indicated that platelets can induce strong IECD36 binding to CD36DEF ECs and, conversely, can hide constitutively expressed falciparum receptors such as chondroitin sulfate A. Thus, platelets may provide an adhesion receptor to microvascular beds originally devoid of it. This novel mechanism of cytoadhesion may reorient the sequestration of different parasite phenotypes and play an important role in the pathogenesis of severe malaria.

KEYWORDS: cerebral malaria; cytoadhesion; host cells; platelets; pathogenesis

INTRODUCTION

According to World Health Organization (WHO) estimates, between 300 and 500 million persons are infected with malaria every year. The classic clinical presentation of malaria consists of bouts of fever accompanied by other symptoms such as headache, malaise, nausea, muscular pain, or mild diarrhea, often mistaken for influenza or gastrointestinal infection. Almost all of the 1.7–2.5 million deaths worldwide from malaria each year are attributable to *Plasmodium falciparum* infection.

Address for correspondence: Dr. Georges E. Grau, Unité de Parasitologie Expérimentale, EA 3282, IFR 48, Faculties of Medicine and Pharmacy, Université de la Méditerranée, 27, Boulevard Jean Moulin, F-13 385 Marseille Cedex 05, France. Voice: +33-4-91 32 46 48; fax: + 33-4-91 32 46 34.

georges.grau@medecine.univ-mrs.fr

Ann. N.Y. Acad. Sci. 992: 30–38 (2003). © 2003 New York Academy of Sciences.

Over 90% of all cases of life-threatening malaria occur in African children, especially those in sub-Saharan Africa.[1]

Cerebral malaria (CM) and severe anemia are the most serious complications of falciparum infection and are associated with a high mortality rate. From a few months of age onwards, infected infants may develop severe disease. Some studies suggest that about one infection in one hundred progresses to cause complications.[2] It is difficult to define severe malaria because of the large number of symptoms and signs. WHO has established criteria that need to be met in order to identify rapidly the patients at high risk of developing complications.[1]

The pathogenic mechanisms underlying CM are not fully understood and remain a subject of debate. Moreover, it is not clear why only a small percentage of patients with *P. falciparum* develop CM. Apart from factors related to transmission characteristics, the virulence and drug sensitivities of the infectious agent *P. falciparum*, numerous genetic, nutritional, and immunological host factors have been implicated. Three pathogenic theories have been proposed for human CM: the theory of permeability, the mechanistic theory, and the immunological theory. However, a combination of factors from both the host and the parasite apparently contributes to the acute access of falciparum malaria and more precisely to the brain lesions of CM (reviewed in Refs. 3–5).

A characteristic feature of CM histopathology is the sequestration of *P. falciparum*-infected erythrocytes (IEs) in the microvasculature. Sequestration is observed in almost all organs, but particularly in the brain. However, several questions as to the exact involvement of IE sequestration in CM remain unanswered. For example, is sequestration the cause or the consequence of endothelial lesions? In addition to IE, histopathological analysis of brain samples from patients who died of CM recently revealed the presence of other cell types, such as platelets and monocytes.[6] Since tumor necrosis factor (TNF)-inducible adhesion molecules ICAM-1, VCAM-1, and ELAM-1 are upregulated in CM, it seems likely that endothelial cells (ECs) would also bind both IE and leukocytes.[4] In addition to the Th1 immune response exhibited in the murine CM model, platelets and monocytes also appear to be involved in CM pathogenesis (reviewed in Ref. 7).

In this paper, we review, first, the role of host cells in a mouse CM model, second, recent histopathological evidence of platelet sequestration in brain vessels from Malawian children who died from CM, and third, an *in vitro* model of the human cerebral lesion, involving brain ECs, IEs, and human platelets.

MURINE MODELS OF CEREBRAL MALARIA

Upon *Plasmodium berghei* ANKA (PbA) infection, various mouse strains exhibit a differential responsiveness to the malaria parasite. Some strains are highly susceptible to the development of cerebral malaria (CM), whereas other strains are resistant despite similar levels of parasitemia during the acute phase of the infection.[7,8] We have taken advantage of this difference to evaluate the pathogenic importance of some host factors, by comparing their expression in susceptible and resistant animals. The murine model of CM has thus allowed us to focus on host-dependent mechanisms, rather than those pertaining to the parasite.

Tumor Necrosis Factor, Lymphotoxin, and Tumor Necrosis Factor Receptors

Previous results suggesting that TNF is a key element in the pathogenesis of experimental CM have been reviewed in details elsewhere.[9] These include the observation of high serum levels of this cytokine at the time of CM, the prevention of the neurological syndrome by the *in vivo* neutralization of the cytokine, and the induction of CM-like syndrome in CM-resistant mice by infusion of TNF. Subsequently, the absence of CM in transgenic mice expressing high levels of sTNFR1[10] and in TNF/LT double knockout mice[11] supported the role of TNF, but were also compatible with a role of lymphotoxin (LT), previously called TNF-beta. Recent data in single knockout mice suggest that LT is the principal mediator of CM.[12] TNF overproduction is induced by an immune response elicited by the presence of the parasite in the blood.[13] Indeed, depletion of CD4 T lymphocytes or administration of cyclosporin A to PbA-infected mice prevents acute mortality, apparently by decreasing TNF production. This involvement of T cells is also compatible with a predominant role of LT, because this cytokine is predominantly produced by lymphocytes.

Involvement of TNF receptor-1 (TNFR-1, p55) in CM is still not clearly established, in contrast to TNF-receptor 2 (TNFR2, p75), whereas the reverse is true in most immunological and/or infectious diseases. Indeed, a significant increase in the expression of TNFR-2, but not TNFR-1, was found on brain microvessels at the time of CM in susceptible animals.[14] Moreover, mice genetically deficient in TNFR-2 (*Tnfr2*^{0}) were significantly protected from experimental CM, in contrast to TNFR-1–deficient (*Tnfr1*^{0}) mice, which were as susceptible as wild-type mice. These results led to the conclusion that the interaction between membrane TNF and TNFR-2 is crucial in the development of this neurological syndrome.[14,15] A study was more recently carried out in bone marrow chimeric mice to evaluate the cell compartment of the host responsible for mediating the TNF-dependent mortality associated with murine CM. It was demonstrated that the presence of TNFR-2 on blood leukocytes was not sufficient to make mice susceptible to CM and that the expression of TNFR-2 on endothelial cells is crucial for the brain pathology to occur.[16] Again, these results are compatible with a predominant involvement of LT over TNF in the development of murine CM, as both cytokines bind to TNFR-2. Data obtained in LT knockout mice[12] are additional evidence for a pathogenic role of this receptor in the development of CM (FIG. 1).

Monocytes

As previously described in several studies, monocyte adhesion to the cerebral endothelium (day 5–7 postinfection) is commonly associated with fatal murine CM.[17,18] The cerebral vessels of susceptible mice showed focal accumulation of packed monocytes, which may lead to the predominance of lesions in the central nervous system. Activation of pigment-phagocytosing monocytes may be a late feature, and the immune cell response to intravascular sequestration appears to be limited. This sequestration of monocytes was shown to be enhanced by the TNF-induced overexpression of adhesion molecules such as ICAM-1 or VCAM-1 on the endothelium. Immunohistochemical and electron microscopy studies have shown that murine CM is characterized by widespread cerebral EC activation, as evidenced by

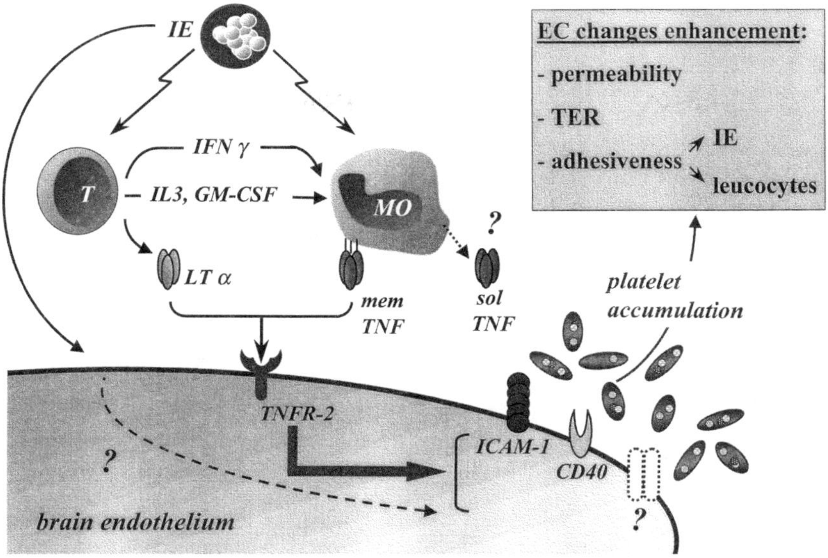

FIGURE 1. Importance of host cells in the modulation of *P. falciparum*-infected erythrocyte (IE) cytoadhesion in the pathogenesis of cerebral malaria (CM). Malaria parasites (*IE*), apart from possible direct effects on brain endothelium, stimulate the host immune response, leading to overproduction of IFN-γ, GM-CSF, and IL-3 by Th1 cells. These T-cell–derived cytokines then amplify the activation of monocytes, which express higher levels of the transmembrane form of tumor necrosis factor-alpha (*memTNF)* and produce the soluble form of the cytokine TNF (*solTNF*). Both forms and tumor necrosis factor-beta (lymphotoxin alpha, LT), released by T lymphocytes, induce, via their interaction with TNFR-2, an upregulation of various adhesion molecules on brain endothelial cells. These include at least ICAM-1 and CD40[33] (also, Wassmer *et al.*, submitted) and as yet unidentified molecules. In turn, high levels of these adhesion molecules favor platelet binding to brain endothelial cells, responsible for enhancement of endothelial changes, as reviewed in Ref. 7.

ICAM-1, VCAM-1 upregulation, and morphological changes ranging from endothelial swelling to focal EC damage and necrosis.[17–20]

Monocytes were therefore expected to play a major part in the immunopathology of CM, but a recent study in mice suggests rather the opposite.[21] This study dealt with the urokinase plasminogen activator (uPA) and urokinase plasminogen activator receptor (uPAR, CD87) system, which has been reported to modulate the function of the β_2 integrin LFA-1, one of the leukocyte ligands for endothelial ICAM-1.[22,23] Since LFA-1 has been implicated in murine CM pathogenesis,[19] we investigated the uPA-uPAR system in this syndrome. Surprisingly, in uPA and uPAR genetically deficient mice infected with PbA, the sequestration of monocytes was unchanged.[21] However, the most profound effect of uPAR deficiency was seen on platelet kinetics and accumulation in brain vessels, suggesting an important role of platelets in the development of the neurological syndrome. In uPA or uPAR-deficient mice, there was a good correlation between protection against CM and prevention of platelet sequestration in the brain.

Platelets

In addition to IE and leukocyte sequestration in the brain microvasculature, platelets also seem to contribute to the neurovascular lesions in murine CM. *In vivo* studies in the PbA model provided four lines of evidence that support the view that platelets are critical effectors of neurovascular injury. First, electron microscopic analysis at the time of CM disclosed platelets in the lumen of brain venules, between sequestered monocytes and IE.[24] Second, radiolabeled platelet distribution studies indicated that platelets are sequestered in the brain and lung vasculature during CM. Noncerebral malaria was not associated with cerebral sequestration of platelets. Third, *in vivo* treatment with a monoclonal antibody (mAb) to LFA-1 (which is expressed on platelets) selectively abrogated the cerebral sequestration of platelets, and this correlated with prevention of CM. Fourth, the role of platelets in the development of the neurovascular lesions of CM was more directly assessed by a depletion experiment. Malaria-infected animals rendered thrombocytopenic were significantly protected against CM. Thus, a CD11a-dependent interaction between platelets and EC appears pivotal to microvascular damage. These data suggest a novel mechanism of action for anti-LFA-1 mAbs *in vivo* and illustrate an unexpected role of platelets, in addition to monocytes, in vascular pathology.

As just mentioned, more recent evidence implicating platelets in microvascular lesions was provided by the response of uPA/uPAR genetically deficient mice to PbA infection.[21] Thrombocytopenia is associated with both murine and human CM, and appears to represent a risk factor, as recently demonstrated in African children.[25] This decrease in platelet counts results, at least in part, from sequestration in various organs.[24,26] Malaria-induced thrombocytopenia was markedly attenuated in $uPA^{-/-}$ and $uPAR^{-/-}$ mice, and platelet trapping in pulmonary and cerebral microvascular beds was dramatically reduced in PbA-infected $uPAR^{-/-}$ mice.

It is obvious that mouse CM cannot reproduce exactly the brain pathology of this complication in humans, but the number of similarities between several models and the human disease is growing. The accumulation of platelets, previously described in mouse brain microvessels, was recently found to be another new parallel between human and murine CM.[6] This new element represented our starting point for the following study of the potential role of platelets in human CM development.

HISTOPATHOLOGY OF HUMAN CM LESIONS: EVIDENCE FOR THE PRESENCE OF PLATELETS AND MONONUCLEAR CELLS IN ADDITION TO IE

Immunohistopathologic study of the platelet-specific glycoprotein GPIIb-IIIa was carried out on tissue from multiple brain sites in Malawian children whose fatal illness was severe malarial anemia (SMA), CM, or nonmalarial encephalopathy (NME). Analysis of these biopsy specimens allowed us to demonstrate that the degree of platelet accumulation in microvessels is significantly greater in patients with CM than in those with SMA and NME and that platelets are colocalized with malaria pigment and white cells in most CM patients.[6] Platelet accumulation was shown to occur in the microvasculature of patients with CM and may therefore play a role in the pathogenesis of the disease. Moreover, immunohistopathologic analysis of lung and placenta isolated from infected patients showed platelets intimately bound to endothelium and to IEs, suggesting that they can also act in the development of other malaria-related pathologies such as placental malaria and the acute respiratory distress syndrome (Wassmer *et al.*, submitted). These results led us to further investigate the role of platelets specifically during the development of the neurological syndrome in human malaria infection. To this end, we developed a new *in vitro* tripartite model of CM that was composed of brain endothelial cells, IEs, and platelets.

IN VITRO MODEL SYSTEM OF HUMAN CM LESION: CO-CULTURES WITH BRAIN ENDOTHELIAL CELLS

Despite sequestration in all patients infected with *P. falciparum*, the reason why only a small percentage of patients develop CM is still not fully understood. In the *Saimiri sciureus* monkey infected by *P. falciparum*, the only CM model presently recommended by the World Health Organization,[27] IE sequestration may occur not only in the brain,[28] but also in several organs such as heart, lung, kidney, liver, and spleen. Furthermore, postmortem brain histopathologic analysis in *Saimiri* monkeys showed that marked sequestration of IE in the microvasculature occurred only in animals presenting the neurologic syndrome and not in animals succumbing from overwhelming *P. falciparum* infection or nonmalarial pathologies.[28]

To explore *P. falciparum* cytoadhesion at the molecular level and to avoid excessive use of animals, brain ECs were isolated from several *Saimiri* monkeys. Five cell lines were selected[29] among these brain ECs and were shown to express at least four different IE cytoadhesion receptors (CSA, ICAM-1, CD36, and E-selectin) either alone or in different combinations. Interestingly, the adhesion molecules CD36, ICAM-1, and E-selectin have been found on cerebral microvascular ECs from patients who died of CM,[30–32] suggesting the usefulness of these cells in a new *in vitro* model. This led us to use a specific clone of these brain microvascular ECs, which was shown to be constitutively deficient in a specific *P. falciparum* receptor, CD36.

To investigate the role of platelets in IE sequestration, we used IE selected to adhere only to CD36 (IE^{CD36}). Coincubation studies indicated that platelets, which express high levels of CD36 (previously called "platelet glycoprotein IV"), can induce the binding of IE^{CD36} to CD36-deficient brain microvascular ECs. Indeed, IE cytoadhesion to the brain endothelium was significantly increased by prior stimulation with TNF and abolished by anti-CD36 mAb treatment. Overall, immunofluorescence studies performed after these coincubations showed that platelets served as a bridge between IEs^{CD36} and the surface of ECs. Furthermore, this binding of platelets to the EC surface was demonstrated to involve CD40, which is upregulated in brain ECs on TNF stimulation. However, antibodies to CD40 and to other endothelial adhesion molecules only led to partial prevention of platelet binding to brain ECs, suggesting that other undefined receptors are likely to take part in this phenomenon (Wassmer *et al.*, submitted). These inhibition data are consistent with the involvement of CD40/CD40L in murine CM.[33] To assess the relevance of these findings in physiological conditions, parallel coincubations were carried out under flow conditions, and the platelet-mediated IE cytoadhesion just described was found to be resistant to physiological shear stress.

Finally, bound platelets were shown to conceal another EC receptor, chondroitin-4-sulfate (CSA), thereby affecting parasite phenotype during sequestration: CD36-binding parasites were allowed to bind ECs via the platelet CD36, whereas CSA-binding parasites were excluded by the platelet physical overcrowding of their endothelial receptors (Wassmer *et al.*, submitted).

Platelets already have been implicated in homologous cell-cell bridging in the pathogenesis of malaria: they were found to facilitate IE clumping[34] in peripheral blood. This formation of *P. falciparum*-IE clumps also required expression of the platelet surface glycoprotein CD36, and the phenomenon was strongly associated with severe malaria. The results presented here demonstrate that in addition to their role in the clumping of identical cells, platelets may also act as a bridge between two different cell types, in this case ECs and IEs. Thus, platelets may either provide receptors for adhesion to microvascular beds that otherwise lack adhesion receptors and/or hide receptors that are present. This novel mechanism may modify sequestration target sites and may therefore be crucial in the pathogenesis of CM and other TNF-induced microvascular diseases.

CONCLUSIONS AND PERSPECTIVES

In addition to the involvement of IE cytoadhesion during brain microvessel obstruction, numerous studies have shown the pathogenic role of several host cells. In this paper, we more specifically summarized the importance of platelets in the pathogenesis of CM. The murine model of CM suggested that platelet accumulation in brain microvessels was involved in the triggering of CM lesions. This was followed by the demonstration of the presence of platelets in brain vessels from Malawian patients who died of CM. More recently, using an *in vitro* model of the endothelial lesion, we demonstrated that in addition to direct cytotoxic activity,[35] platelets may act as a bridge between IEs and ECs, thereby inducing a modulation of cytoadhesion.

REFERENCES

1. Beales, P.F., B. Brabin, E. Dorman, *et al.* 2000. Severe falciparum malaria. Trans. Roy. Soc. Trop. Med. Hyg. **94:** S1–S90.
2. Greenwood, B., K. Marsh & R. Snow. 1991. Why do some African children develop severe malaria? Parasitol. Today **7:** 277–281.
3. Clark, I.A. & K.A. Rockett. 1994. The cytokine theory of human cerebral malaria. Parasitol. Today **10:** 410–412.
4. Grau, G.E. & S. de Kossodo. 1994. Cerebral malaria: mediators, mechanical obstruction or more? Parasitol. Today **10:** 408–409.
5. Berendt, A.R., G.D.H. Turner & C.I. Newbold. 1994. Cerebral malaria: the sequestration hypothesis. Parasitol. Today **10:** 412–414.
6. Grau, G.E., C.D. MacKenzie, R.A. Carr, *et al.* 2003. Platelet accumulation in brain microvessels in fatal paediatric cerebral malaria. J. Infect. Dis. **187:** 461–466.
7. Lou, J., R. Lucas & G.E. Grau. 2001. Pathogenesis of cerebral malaria: recent experimental data and possible applications in man. Clin. Microbiol. Rev. **14:** 810–820.
8. Grau, G.E., L.F. Fajardo, P.F. Piguet, *et al.* 1987. Tumor necrosis factor (cachectin) as an essential mediator in murine cerebral malaria. Science **237:** 1210–1212.

9. GRAU, G.E. & J.N. LOU. 1994. TNF-induced microvascular pathology in the TH1-mediated lesions of mouse cerebral malaria: possible new mechanisms. *In* Cytokines: Basic Principles and Clinical Applications. S. Romagnani, G. DelPrete & A.K. Abbas, Eds. :265–279. Ares-Serono Symposia. Rome.
10. GARCIA, I., K. ARAKI, Y. MIYAZAKI, *et al.* 1995. Transgenic mice expressing soluble TNF-R1-IgG3 molecules are protected from lethal septic shock and cerebral malaria, and are highly sensitive to *Listeria monocytogenes* and *Leishmania major* infections. Eur. J. Immunol. **25:** 2401–2407.
11. RUDIN, W., H.P. EUGSTER, G. BORDMANN, *et al.* 1997. Resistance to cerebral malaria in tumor necrosis factor-alpha/beta-deficient mice is associated with a reduction of intercellular adhesion molecule-1 up-regulation and T helper type 1 response. Am. J. Pathol. **150:** 257–266.
12. ENGWERDA, C.R., T.L. MYNOTT, S. SAWHNEY, *et al.* 2002. Locally up-regulated lymphotoxin alpha, not systemic tumor necrosis factor alpha, is the principle mediator of murine cerebral malaria. J. Exp. Med. **195:** 1371–1377.
13. GRAU, G.E., P.F. PIGUET, H.D. ENGERS, *et al.* 1986. L3T4+ T lymphocytes play a major role in the pathogenesis of murine cerebral malaria. J. Immunol. **137:** 2348–2354.
14. LUCAS, R., P. JUILLARD, E. DECOSTER, *et al.* 1997. Crucial role of tumor necrosis factor (TNF) receptor 2 and membrane-bound TNF in experimental cerebral malaria. Eur. J. Immunol. **27:** 1719–1725.
15. LUCAS, R., J.N. LOU, P. JUILLARD, *et al.* 1997. Respective role of TNF receptors in the development of experimental cerebral malaria. J. Neuroimmunol. **72:** 143–148.
16. STOELCKER, B., T. HEHLGANS, K. WEIGL, *et al.* 2002. Requirement for tumor necrosis factor receptor 2 expression on vascular cells to induce experimental cerebral malaria. Infect. Immunol. **70:** 5857–5859.
17. JERUSALEM, C., T.W. POLDER, M. WIJERSROUW, *et al.* 1983. Comparative clinical and experimental study on the pathogenesis of cerebral malaria. Contrib. Microbiol. Immunol. **7:** 130–138.
18. POLDER, T.W., C.R. JERUSALEM & W.M.C. ELING. 1991. Morphological characteristics of intracerebral arterioles in clinical (*Plasmodium-falciparum*) and experimental (*Plasmodium-berghei*) cerebral malaria. J. Neurol. Sci. **101:** 35–46.
19. GRAU, G.E., P. POINTAIRE, P.F. PIGUET, *et al.* 1991. Late administration of monoclonal antibody to leukocyte function-antigen 1 abrogates incipient murine cerebral malaria. Eur. J. Immunol. **21:** 2265–2267.
20. TURNER, G. 1997. Cerebral malaria. Brain Pathol. **7:** 569–582.
21. PIGUET, P.F., C. DALAPERROUSAZ, C. VESIN, *et al.* 2000. Delayed mortality and attenuated thrombocytopenia associated with severe malaria in urokinase- and urokinase receptor-deficient mice. Infect. Immunol. **68:** 3822–3829.
22. CHAPMAN, H.A. 1997. Plasminogen activators, integrins, and the coordinated regulation of cell adhesion and migration. Curr. Opin. Cell. Biol. **9:** 714–724.
23. SITRIN, R.G., P.M. PAN, R.A. BLACKWOOD, *et al.* 2001. Cutting edge: evidence for a signaling partnership between urokinase receptors (CD87) and L-selectin (CD62L) in human polymorphonuclear neutrophils. J. Immunol. **166:** 4822–4825.
24. GRAU, G.E., F. TACCHINI-COTTIER, C. VESIN, *et al.* 1993. TNF-induced microvascular pathology: active role for platelets and importance of the LFA-1/ICAM-1 interaction. Eur. Cytokine Netw. **4:** 415–419.
25. GERARDIN, P., C. ROGIER, A.S. KA, *et al.* 2002. Prognostic value of thrombocytopenia in African children with falciparum malaria. Am. J. Trop. Med. Hyg. **66:** 686–691.
26. HO, M. & N.J. WHITE. 1999. Molecular mechanisms of cytoadherence in malaria. Am. J. Physiol. Cell. Physiol. **45:** C1231–C1242.
27. GYSIN, J. 1991. Relevance of the squirrel monkey as a model for experimental human malaria. Res. Immunol. **142:** 649–654.
28. GYSIN, J., M. AIKAWA, N. TOURNEUR & T. TEGOSHI. 1992. Experimental *Plasmodium falciparum* cerebral malaria in the squirrel monkey *Saimiri sciureus*. Exp. Parasitol. **75:** 390–398.
29. GAY, F., C. ROBERT, B. POUVELLE, *et al.* 1995. Isolation and characterization of brain microvascular endothelial cells from Saimiri monkeys: an *in vitro* model for seques-

tration of *Plasmodium falciparum*-infected erythrocytes. J. Immunol. Methods **184:** 15–28.
30. Ockenhouse, C.F., T. Tegoshi, Y. Maeno, *et al.* 1992. Human vascular endothelial cell adhesion receptors for *Plasmodium-falciparum*-infected erythrocytes: roles for endothelial leukocyte adhesion molecule-1 and vascular cell adhesion molecule-1. J. Exp. Med. **176:** 1183–1189.
31. Porta, J., A. Carota, G.P. Pizzolato, *et al.* 1993. Immunopathological changes in human cerebral malaria. Clin. Neuropathol. **12:** 142–146.
32. Turner, G.D.H., H. Morrison, M. Jones, *et al.* 1994. An immunohistochemical study of the pathology of fatal malaria: evidence for widespread endothelial activation and a potential role for intercellular adhesion molecule-1 in cerebral sequestration. Am. J. Pathol. **145:** 1057–1069.
33. Piguet, P.F., C. DaKan, C. Vesin, *et al.* 2001. Role of CD40-CD40L in mouse severe malaria. Am. J. Pathol. **159:** 733–742.
34. Pain, A., D.J.P. Ferguson, O. Kai, *et al.* 2001. Platelet-mediated clumping of *Plasmodium falciparum*-infected erythrocytes is a common adhesive phenotype and is associated with severe malaria. Proc. Natl. Acad. Sci. USA **98:** 1805–1810.
35. Lou, J., Y.R.A. Donati, P. Juillard, *et al.* 1997. Platelets play an important role in TNF-induced microvascular endothelial cell pathology. Am. J. Pathol. **151:** 1397–1405.

Interleukin-1 in the Brain

Mechanisms of Action in Acute Neurodegeneration

H.C. PATEL, H. BOUTIN,[a] AND S.M. ALLAN

School of Biological Sciences, 1.124 Stopford Building, University of Manchester, Manchester, M13 9PT, UK

ABSTRACT: Interleukin-1 (IL-1) exerts a number of diverse actions in the brain, and it is currently well accepted that it contributes to experimentally induced neurodegeneration. Much of this is based on studies using the IL-1 receptor antagonist, which inhibits cell death caused by ischemia, brain injury, or excitotoxins. Our aim is to determine how and where in the brain IL-1 acts to produce these effects. Most of the neurodegenerative effects of IL-1 are thought to be through IL-1β. However, we have data implicating IL-1α in excitotoxic cell death. Furthermore mice lacking both IL-1α and IL-1β show dramatically reduced ischemic cell death, whereas deletion of IL-1α or IL-1β alone fails to modify damage. It has also been demonstrated that IL-1 exacerbates ischemic injury in mice in the absence of the type I IL-1 receptor, suggesting the existence of novel IL-1 receptors in the brain. IL-1 also dramatically exacerbates neuronal loss in response to intrastriatal administration of the excitotoxin AMPA in the rat brain, an effect accompanied by marked increases in cytokine expression in the frontoparietal cortex, which precedes subsequent cell death in this region. Intrastriatal AMPA also results in limbic seizures that are exacerbated by IL-1, and we hypothesize, therefore, that IL-1 exacerbates cell death through increased seizure activity. Therefore, IL-1 appears to induce acute neurodegeneration through a number of mechanisms.

KEYWORDS: interleukin-1; excitotoxic cell death; cerebral ischemia; seizures

INTRODUCTION

Interleukin-1 (IL-1) is a 17-kDa polypeptide that exists as a barrel-shaped molecule composed of 12-14β strands. Although other putative IL-1 subtypes have recently been identified, IL-1 exists as two, well-characterized isoforms, IL-1α and IL-1β.[1–3] A natural, specific IL-1 receptor antagonist (IL-1ra) has also been identified and characterized.[1,2] IL-1α and IL-1β are the products of separate genes located on chromosome 2.[2] They share some structural homology and are both produced as precursors, which lack leader sequences and require enzymatic cleavage to the

[a]Present address: CEA-SHFJ-INSERM ERITM 103, 4 place du general Leclerc, 91401 Orsay cedex, France.

Address for correspondence: S.M. Allan, School of Biological Sciences, 1.124 Stopford Building, University of Manchester, Oxford Road, Manchester, M13 9PT. UK. Voice: +44 161 275 5255; fax: +44 161 275 5948.

stuart.allan@man.ac.uk

Ann. N.Y. Acad. Sci. 992: 39–47 (2003).

mature form by specific cellular proteases. Whereas pro-IL-1a is active, inactive pro-IL-1β depends on activation by IL-1 converting enzyme (ICE), otherwise known as caspase 1, which is an important executor of apoptosis.[4,5] IL-1α and IL-1β act through binding to the IL-1 receptor I (IL-1RI, 80 kDa), which requires association with an accessory protein (AcP) for cellular activation.[1,6] The other known IL-1 receptor, IL-1 RII, has no intracellular domain and is unable to transduce intracellular signals.[7,8] The IL-1 receptor antagonist (IL-1ra) has a molecular weight of 22 kDa and binds to the IL-1 receptor without inducing cellular activation.

IL-1 is not generally expressed or secreted in normal healthy tissues and plays little part in normal growth and development.[1] Its main role therefore appears to be limited to disease states, when it is expressed in a wide range of tissues.[2]

IL-1β IN ACUTE BRAIN INJURY

Elevated levels of IL-1β and IL-1ra have been noted in the cerebrospinal fluid of patients with severe head injury, or subarachnoid hemorrhage.[9,10] Furthermore, increased expression of IL-1β mRNA and protein is evident in experimental brain injury caused by excitotoxin infusion, cerebral ischemia, or traumatic brain injury in rodents.[11–17] Although IL-1β itself does not cause neuronal cell death, intrastriatal or intracerebroventricular (icv) injection of IL-1β results in a significant increase in the magnitude of cell death caused by excitotoxic, ischemic, or traumatic brain injury in rodents.[18–20] By virtue of its specific antagonism to IL-1, the greatest evidence supporting a causal role for IL-1 in brain injury comes from experiments in which IL-1ra (the naturally occurring IL-1 receptor antagonist) has been used. Injection of IL-1ra, icv, intrastriatally, or peripherally, causes a 50–60% reduction in cell death in all models of experimental brain injury in rodents.[19–22] Further evidence supporting a causal role for IL-1β in acute brain injury comes from observations in which reductions in cell death have been reported in rodents exposed to cerebral ischemia and treated with ICE inhibitors or IL-1β antibody.[23,24]

MECHANISM OF ACTION OF IL-1β IN ACUTE BRAIN INJURY: SITE-SPECIFIC THEORY

The mechanism(s) by which IL-1β exacerbates acute brain injury, however, remains unknown. One suggestion is that IL-1β exacerbates brain injury through specific sites in the brain. This hypothesis that IL-1β acts through specific sites in the brain is based on a number of observations.

When human recombinant (hr) IL-1β is coinjected into the striatum with the excitotoxin S-AMPA (a glutamate agonist), a dramatic increase in ipsilateral cortical damage is observed (FIG. 1A).[18] The damage affects the whole ipsilateral hemisphere and is at a site distant to the site of injection. As no increase in cell death is seen after coinjection of S-AMPA with hrIL-1β (vs S-AMPA) in the cortex,[18] it has been postulated that IL-1β exacerbates neurodegeneration by acting specifically in the striatum. Consistent with observations of increased cortical death induced by striatal injection of S-AMPA with hrIL-1β, increased infarct volume (70% increase) is also seen when hrIL-1β is injected into the striatum or into the cerebral ventricles

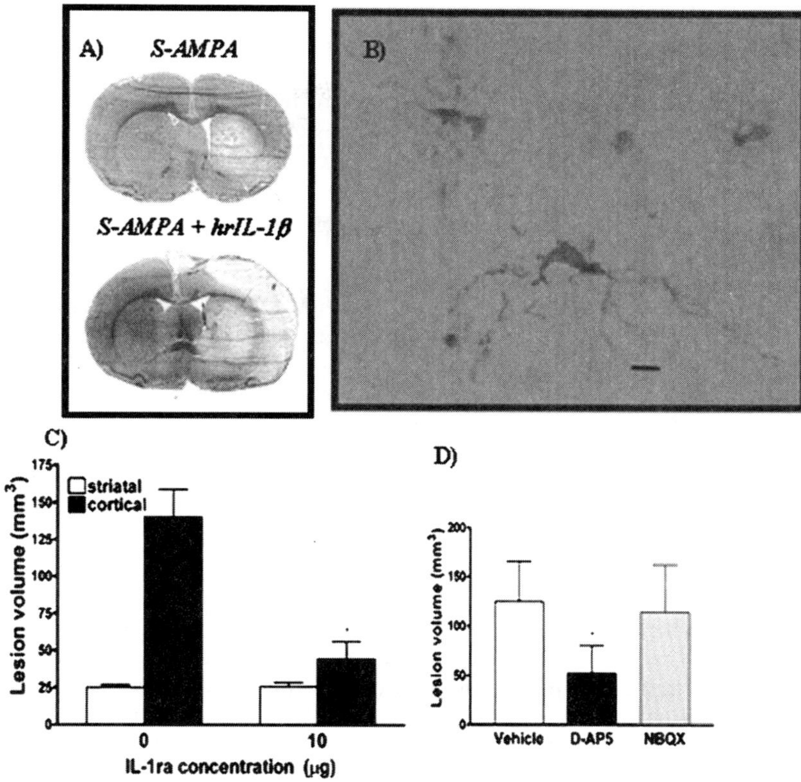

FIGURE 1. (**A**) Representative brain sections demonstrating cortical cell death observed in response to S-AMPA (7.5 nmol) or S-AMPA (7.5 nmol) + hrIL-1β (10 ng). (**B**) Photomicrographs taken at high power, showing immunoreactive IL-1β cells seen in the cortex in response to S-AMPA (7.5 nmol) + hrIL-1β (10 ng) 8 hours after striatal injections. Scale bar = 10 μm. Effect of intracortical (C) IL-1ra (10 μg) or (D) D-AP5 (25 nmol; NMDA receptor antagonist) and NBQX (25 nmol; AMPA receptor antagonist) on lesion volume induced by striatal injection of S-AMPA (7.5 nmol) + hrIL-1β (10 ng). (*P <0.01 striatal S-AMPA and hrIL-1 + IL-1ra (cortex) vs vehicle (cortex); striatal S-AMPA and hrIL-1 + D-AP5 (cortex) vs vehicle).

in rats subjected to middle cerebral artery occlusion. No increase is seen, however, when hrIL-1β is injected directly into the ischemic cortex, supporting the site-specific actions of IL-1β seen with excitotoxic injections.[25]

The observation that IL-1ra exerts its neuroprotective effects only when injected into the striatum or given icv but fails to do so when injected directly into the site of cortical damage further supports the postulate that IL-1 mediates its neurodegenerative effects through specific sites in the brain.[18,22]

Recently the hypothalamus has also been identified as a potential site through which IL-1β acts. This is based on evidence of early IL-1β mRNA and protein expression (preceding cortical cell death) after excitotoxic damage, combined with the observation that infusion of hrIL-1β into the hypothalamus enhances, whereas injection of IL-1ra significantly reduces, cortical damage induced by striatal infusion of S-AMPA and S-AMPA with hrIL-1β, respectively.[11] The ventral striatum and the nucleus accumbens are also considered to be important sites for IL-1 action, because injection of IL-1 in these areas results in greater frequency of cortical lesions than that observed with injections in other regions of the striatum.[26]

However, we recently observed that immunoreactive IL-1β is upregulated in the cortex in rats 8 hours after striatal injection of S-AMPA with hrIL-1β and precedes cortical cell death as determined by examining adjacent sections stained with fluoro-jade (FIG. 1B).

Injection of IL-1ra into the cortex reduced cortical cell death produced in response to striatal co-infusion of S-AMPA with hrIL-1β (FIG. 1C). Furthermore, cortical injection of the NMDA receptor antagonist AP-5 also reduced cell death in the cortex induced by striatal injection of S-AMPA with hrIL-1β (FIG. 1D). Moreover, IL-1 has been shown to decrease the uptake of glutamate by astrocytes,[27] and therefore this may play an important role in mediating the "neurotoxic" effects of IL-1. Altogether, these data suggest that IL-1 exacerbates brain injury through local effects that include modulation of glutamate action, release, and/or uptake.

IL-1β AND SEIZURES

S-AMPA is a glutamate antagonist that acts via AMPA/kainate receptors and has been demonstrated to induce seizures. Intrahippocampal S-AMPA results in cell death in sites "distant" to the site of injection. This distant cell death is reduced by the anticonvulsant diazepam; therefore, it has been suggested that "distant" cell death is related to seizure activity.[28] This postulate is further supported by the observation that regions of high metabolic activity consistent with seizure activity correspond to sites of excitotoxin-induced distant cell death.[29]

IL-1 was recently demonstrated to be upregulated in response to seizure activity.[30,31] Furthermore, IL-1 increases the duration of kainate-induced seizures in the rat, and overexpression of IL-1ra has been shown to reduce the duration of bicuculline-induced seizures in the mouse.[31,32] We therefore investigated the effect of striatal injection of S-AMPA versus S-AMPA with IL-1 on the number of sites of cell death.

Co-infusion of S-AMPA with hrIL-1β versus S-AMPA resulted in an increase in the number of sites of cell death. Cell death was seen in similar subcortical and allocortical regions in response to S-AMPA versus S-AMPA with hrIL-1β (sites in which cell death was seen is represented in FIGURE 2A). Co-infusion of S-AMPA with hrIL-1β resulted in a 68% increase in the number of sites in which cell death was observed in response to striatal injection of S-AMPA alone. Diazepam reduced this increase induced by co-infusion of S-AMPA with hrIL-1β versus S-AMPA alone, suggesting that the increased cell death induced by S-AMPA with hrIL-1β may be related to seizure activity (FIG. 2B).

The mechanism by which IL-1 increases seizures, however, remains unknown. Exogenous IL-1 fails to alter the latency to onset of kainic acid seizures in the rat,[31] and IL-1ra does not modify bicuculline-induced interictal spiking in the mouse hippocampus, suggesting that IL-1 does not influence focal neuronal excitability or the mechanisms of seizure generation. However, the observation that bicuculline-

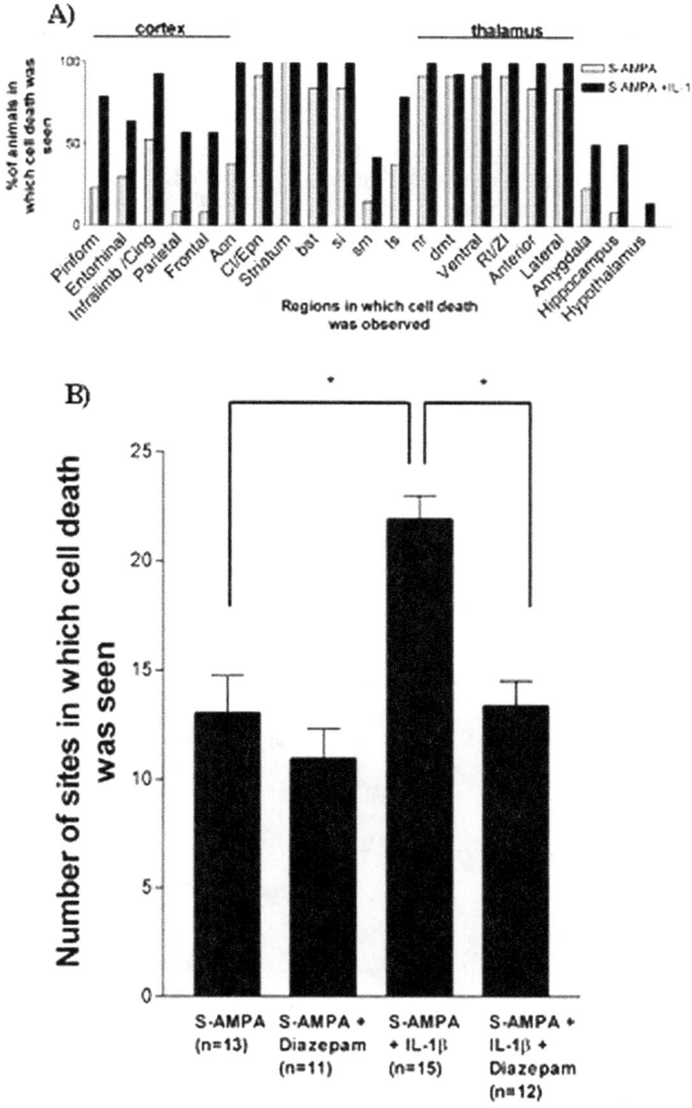

FIGURE 2. (**A**) Sites of cell death, and frequency of cell death per site, observed 24 hours after striatal injection of S-AMPA (7.5 nmol) *vs* S-AMPA (7.5 nmol) + hrIL-1β (10 ng). Data are expressed as percentage. (nr, nucleus reuniens; dmt, dorsomedial thalamus; si, substantia innominata; bst, bed nucleus of stria terminalis; rt/zi, reticular thalamus/zona incerta; cl/epn, claustrum/endopiriform nucleus; ls, lateral septum). (**B**) Number of sites in which cell death was seen in response to striatal injection of S-AMPA (7.5 nmol) ± diazepam (5 mg/kg i.p.) and S-AMPA (7.5 nmol) + hrIL-1β (10 ng) ± diazepam. $^*P < 0.001$.

induced bilateral neocortical c-fos expression is reduced or absent in mice over-expressing IL-1ra (vs wild-type mice) suggests that IL-1 may increase seizure activity by inducing seizure generalization.[32]

ROLE OF I-1α

Most data on the role of IL-1 in acute brain injury has been centered on IL-1β, and the role of IL-1α in exacerbating brain injury is limited. We have shown that IL-1α mRNA and protein are increased in the cortex in response to striatal injection of S-AMPA with hrIL-1β, although more IL-1β mRNA and protein is seen in response to the same stimulus (FIG. 3). In addition, co-injection of S-AMPA with rrIL-1α into the rat striatum also results in a significant increase in the volume of cell death versus S-AMPA alone. As with exacerbation of cell death in response to S-AMPA with hrIL-1β, the increase in cell death induced by striatal injection of S-AMPA with rrIL-1α was mainly a result of increased ipsilateral cortical cell death (TABLE 1).

Cell death in response to middle cerebral artery occlusion is also partially mediated by IL-1α. Infarct volume is not significantly different between mice lacking the IL-1β or IL-1α gene versus wild-type mice in response to cerebral ischemia induced by middle cerebral artery occlusion. However, infarct volume is reduced (by 70%)

TABLE 1. Volume of cell death in response to striatal injection of S-AMPA (7.5 nmol), S-AMPA (7.5 nmol) + recombinant rat (rr)IL-1α (100 ng) or S-AMPA (7.5 nmol) + rrIL-1β (50 ng)

	Lesion volume mm^3	
Striatal treatment	Striatal injection	Cortical injection
S-AMPA (7.5 nmol) ($n = 12$)	21.4 ± 3.1	22.5 ± 5.22
S-AMPA (7.5 nmol) + rrIL-1α (100 ng) ($n = 11$)	24.2 ± 2.73	67.7 ± 16.9*
S-AMPA (7.5 nmol) + rrIL-1β (50 ng) ($n = 13$)	28.4 ± 3.28	85.9 ± 21.3**

*$P < 0.05$; ** $P < 0.01$ vs S-AMPA alone.

TABLE 2. Cell death volume in response to transient cerebral ischemia in mice[a]

	Wild type	IL-1α KO	IL-1β KO	Il-1αβ KO
Lesion volume (mm^3)	52 ± 6	44 ± 5	54 ± 5	16 ± 2*

[a]Thirty-minute middle cerebral artery occlusion in IL-1α, IL-1β, or IL-1α/β gene knockout (KO) vs wild-type mice (WT). (IL-1α/β KO vs WT, *$P < 0.05$)

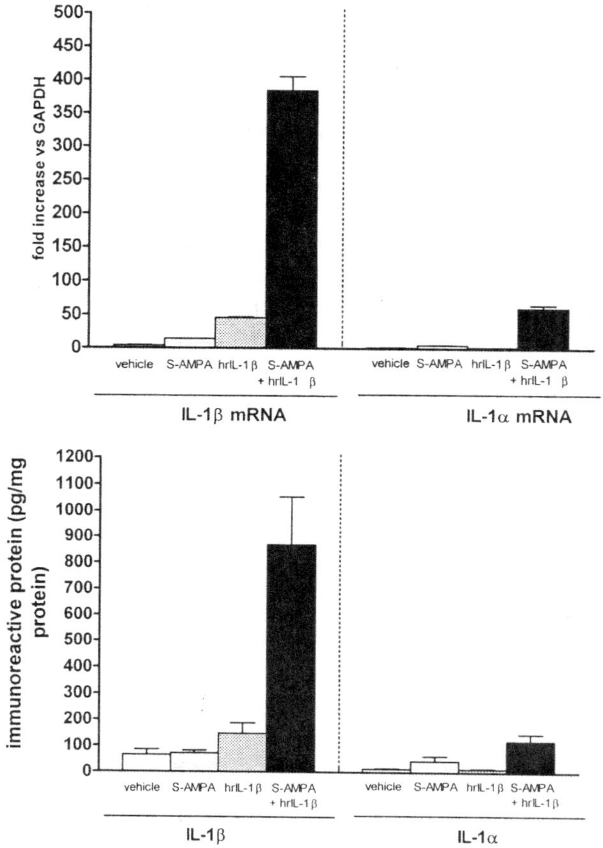

FIGURE 3. (**A**) IL-1α and IL-1β mRNA and protein observed in the cortex in response to striatal injection of vehicle, hrIL-1β (10 ng), S-AMPA (7.5 nmol), or S-AMPA (7.5 nmol) + hrIL-1β (10 ng).

in mice lacking both IL-1α and IL-1β genes versus wild-type animals, suggesting a requirement for both IL-1α and IL-1β in mediating the effects of IL-1 in acute brain injury (TABLE 2).[33]

However, IL-1β and not IL-1α mRNA was upregulated in response to middle cerebral artery occlusion in wild-type and IL-1α knockout mice, also suggesting a preferential role for IL-1β. However, IL-1ra failed to reduce infarct volume in IL-1β or IL-1α/β knockout mice, suggesting a compensatory increase in IL-1 independent mediators of cell death in IL-1β receptor knockout mice.[33] It has also been suggested that IL-1β acts independently of the IL-1 RI receptor to exacerbate brain injury, as IL-1β (administered intracerebroventricularly) exacerbated infarct volume in IL-1RI knockout mice that was not attenuated by IL-1ra.[34]

CONCLUSIONS

The deleterious role of IL-1 in acute brain injury is now firmly established and is supported by experimental evidence across species and across numerous brain injury models. Although we have suggested some of the mechanism(s) by which IL-1 exacerbates cell death, it would seem that IL-1 mediates cell death through many different ways, some of which have yet to be studied (effects on brain temperature, effects on blood brain barrier breakdown, effects on neutrophil accumulation, etc). These features have the potential to affect many different pathways of cell death and may see IL-1 emerge as a more clinically efficacious therapeutic target than others targeting one specific cell death pathway that have largely failed.

REFERENCES

1. Dinarello, C.A. & R.C. Thompson. 1991. Blocking IL-1: interleukin-1 receptor antagonist *in vivo* and *in vitro*. Immunol. Today **12:** 404–410.
2. Dinarello, C.A. 1994. The interleukin-1 family: 10 years of discovery. FASEB J. **8:** 1314–1325.
3. Rothwell, J. & G. Luheshi. 2000. Interleukin-1 in the brain: biology, pathology and therapeutic targets. TINS **23:** 618–625.
4. Alnemri, E.S., T. Fernandes-Alnemri & G. Litwack. 1995. Cloning and expression of four novel isoforms of human interleukin-1 beta converting enzyme with different apoptotic activities. J. Biol. Chem. **270:** 4312–4317.
5. Enari, M., H. Hug & S. Nagata. 1995. Involvement of an ICE-like protease in Fas-mediated apoptosis. Nature **375:** 78–81.
6. Dinarello, C.A. 1997. Blocking interleukin-1 and tumor necrosis factor in disease. Eur. Cytokine Netw. **8:** 294–296.
7. Greenfeder, S.A., P. Nunes, L. Kwee, *et al.* 1995. Molecular cloning and characterization of a second subunit of the interleukin 1 receptor complex. J. Biol. Chem. **270:** 13757–13765.
8. Loddick, S.A., C. Liu, T. Takao, *et al.* 1998. Interleukin-1 receptors: cloning studies and role in central nervous system disorders. Brain Res.-Brain Res. Rev. **26:** 306–319.
9. McClain, C.J., D. Cohen, L. Ott, *et al.* 1987. Ventricular fluid interleukin-1 activity in patients with head injury. J. Lab. Clin. Med. **110:** 48–54.
10. Mathiesen, T., G. Edner, E. Ulfarsson & B. Andersson. 1997. Cerebrospinal fluid interleukin-1 receptor antagonist and tumor necrosis factor-α following subarachnoid hemorrhage. J. Neurosurg. **87:** 215–220.
11. Allan, S.M., L.C. Parker, B. Collins, *et al.* 2000. Cortical cell death induced by IL-1 is mediated via actions in the hypothalamus of the rat. Proc. Natl. Acad. Sci. USA **97:** 5580–5585.
12. Buttini, M., A. Sauter & H.W. Boddeke. 1994. Induction of interleukin-1 beta mRNA after focal cerebral ischaemia in the rat. Brain Res.-Mol. Brain Res. **23:** 126–134.
13. Davies, C.A., S.A. Loddick, S. Toulmound, *et al.* 1999. The progression and topographic distribution of interleukin-1beta expression after permanent middle cerebral artery occlusion in the rat. J. Cerebr. Blood Flow Metab. **19:** 87–98.
14. Iannotti, F., S. Kida, R. Weller, *et al.* 1993. Interleukin 1b in focal cerebral ischaemia in rats. J. Cereb. Blood Flow Metab. **13:** S125.
15. Minami, M., Y. Kuraishi, K. Yabuuchi, *et al.* 1992. Induction of interleukin-1β mRNA in rat brain after transient forebrain ischemia. J. Neurochem. **58:** 390–392.
16. Pearson, V.L., N.J. Rothwell & S. Toulmound. 1999. Excitotoxic brain damage in the rat induces interleukin-1beta protein in microglia and astrocytes: correlation with the progression of cell death. Glia **25:** 311–323.

17. YABUUCHI, K., M. MINAMI, S. KATSUMATA & M. SATOH. 1993. In situ hybridization study of interleukin-1 beta mRNA induced by kainic acid in the rat brain. Brain Res.-Mol. Brain Res. **20:** 153–161.
18. LAWRENCE, C.B., S.M. ALLAN & N.J. ROTHWELL. 1998. Interleukin-1beta and the interleukin-1 receptor antagonist act in the striatum to modify excitotoxic brain damage in the rat. Eur. J. Neurosci. **10:** 1188–1195.
19. LODDICK, S.A. & N.J. ROTHWELL. 1996. Neuroprotective effects of human recombinant interleukin-1 receptor antagonist in focal cerebral ischaemia in the rat. J. Cereb. Blood Flow Metab. **16:** 932–940.
20. RELTON, J.K. & N.J. ROTHWELL. 1992. Interleukin-1 receptor antagonist inhibits ischaemic and excitotoxic neuronal damage in the rat. Brain Res. Bull. **29:** 243–246.
21. BETZ, A.L., G.P. SCHIELKE & G.-Y. YANG. 1996. Interleukin-1 in cerebral ischemia. Keio J. Med. 45: 230–238.
22. STROEMER, R.P. & N.J. ROTHWELL. 1997. Cortical protection by localized striatal injection of IL-1ra following cerebral ischemia in the rat. J. Cereb. Blood Flow Metab. **17:** 597–604.
23. LODDICK, S.A., A. MACKENZIE & N.J. ROTHWELL. 1996. An ICE inhibitor, z-VAD-DCB attenuates ischaemic brain damage in the rat. Neuroreport **7:** 1465–1468.
24. YAMASAKI, Y. & K. KOGUIRE. 1997. Cytokines, growth factors, adhesion molecules, and inflammation after ischemia. *In* Primer on Cerebrovascular Diseases. K.M.A. Welch, L.R. Kaplan, D.J. Reis, B.K. Siesjo & B. Weir, Eds. :265. Academic Press Inc. San Diego.
25. STROEMER, R.P. & N.J. ROTHWELL. 1998. Exacerbation of ischemic brain damage by localized striatal injection of interleukin-1beta in the rat. J. Cerebr. Blood Flow Metab. **18:** 833–839.
26. GRUNDY, R.I., N.J. ROTHWELL & S.M. ALLAN. 2002. Site-specific actions of interleukin-1 on excitotoxic cell death in the rat striatum. Brain Res. **926:** 142–148.
27. YE, Z.C. & H. SONTHEIMER. 1996. Cytokine modulation of glial glutamate uptake: a possible involvement of nitric oxide. Neuroreport **7:** 2181–2185.
28. LEES, G.J. & W. LEONG. 2001. In vivo, the direct and seizure-induced neuronal cytotoxicity of kainate and AMPA is modified by the non-competitive antagonist, GYKI 52466. Brain Res. **890:** 66–77.
29. BEN-ARI, Y., E. TREMBLAY, O.P. OTTERSEN & B.S. MELDRUM. 1980. The role of epileptic activity in hippocampal and "remote" cerebral lesions induced by kainic acid. Brain Res. **191:** 79–97.
30. DE SIMONI, M.G., C. PEREGO, T. RAVIZZA, *et al.* 2000. Inflammatory cytokines and related genes are induced in the rat hippocampus by limbic status epilepticus. Eur. J. Neurosci. **12:** 2623–2633.
31. VEZZANI, A., M. CONTI, A. DE LUIGI, *et al.* 1999. Interleukin-1beta immunoreactivity and microglia are enhanced in the rat hippocampus by focal kainate application: functional evidence for enhancement of electrographic seizures. J. Neurosci. **19:** 5054–5065.
32. VEZZANI, A., D. MONETA, M. CONTI, *et al.* 2000. Powerful anticonvulsant action of IL-1 receptor antagonist on intracerebral injection and astrocytic overexpression in mice. Proc. Natl. Acad. Sci USA **97:** 11534–11539.
33. BOUTIN, H., R.A. LEFEUVRE, R. HORAI, *et al.* 2001. Role of IL-1alpha and IL-1beta in ischemic brain damage. J. Neurosci. **21:** 5528–5534.
34. TOUZANI, O., H. BOUTIN, R. LEFEUVRE, *et al.* 2002. Interleukin-1 influences ischemic brain damage in the mouse independently of the interleukin-1 type I receptor. J. Neurosci. **22:** 38–43.

Antibodies to Neuronal Targets in Neurological and Psychiatric Diseases

ANGELA VINCENT, PAOLA DALTON, LINDA CLOVER,
JACKIE PALACE, AND BETHAN LANG

Neurosciences Group, Weatherall Institute of Molecular Medicine, John Radcliffe Hospital, Oxford, UK

ABSTRACT: The role of antibodies to specific neuronal and muscle ion channels in the etiology of neuromuscular transmission disorders is now well accepted. In addition, maternal antibodies can cross the placenta and cause neonatal disease or even alter the development of the infant, raising the possibility that some neurodevelopmental conditions could be caused by maternal antibodies. Voltage-gated ion channels are expressed in the brain as well as at the neuromuscular junction, and in recent years it has become clear that antibodies to some central nervous system (CNS) channels can be associated with CNS disease. This review highlights features of these conditions, preliminary investigations into neurodevelopmental disorders, and areas for further study.

KEYWORDS: myasthenia gravis; arthrogryposis multiplex congenita; fetal acetylcholine receptor; Lambert-Eaton myasthenic syndrome; neuromyotonia; limbic syndromes; autism

MYASTHENIA GRAVIS AS A PARADIGM FOR ANTIBODY-MEDIATED DISEASE

Myasthenia gravis (MG) is still the best example of an antibody-mediated neurological disease. The patients complain of muscle weakness and fatigue, frequently involving the ocular muscles initially but spreading to bulbar or limb muscles. In younger patients, often females, the thymus gland is hyperplastic with germinal centers, and plasma cells within the gland synthesize acetylcholine receptor (AChR) antibodies. In about 10% of patients, a thymic tumor, thymoma, is found, but in many older patients the thymus is apparently normal for age. MG is reviewed in Refs. 1 and 2.

Antibodies to the muscle form of the nicotinic AChR are found in the serum of 85% of patients with MG.[3] The antibodies are directed against extracellular determinants of the AChR and can be detected by an immunoprecipitation assay. This uses muscle AChR radioactively tagged by the binding of ^{125}I-bungarotoxin, a neurotoxin from the venom of *Bungarus multicinctus*, that binds specifically and irre-

Address for correspondence: Dr. A. Vincent, Neurosciences Group, Weatherall Institute of Molecular Medicine, John Radcliffe Hospital, Oxford OX3 9DS, UK. Voice: 44-1865 222321; fax: 44 1865 222402.

Angela.Vincent@imm.ox.ac.uk

Ann. N.Y. Acad. Sci. 992: 48–55 (2003).

versibly to the AChR.[3] The levels of antibodies to the AChR differ considerably between patients, with values in MG patients ranging from 0.5 nM to over 1,000 nM; healthy individuals or patients with other diseases have serum levels less than 0.5 nM.

The pathogenic importance of these antibodies was clearly demonstrated by several observations. MG patients improve when their plasma is exchanged,[4] and the level of AChR antibody in an individual correlates well with its clinical severity over time. Injection of plasma or purified IgG into mice reproduces the electrophysiological characteristics, and some clinical characteristics, of the condition.[5] IgG and complement components are present at the neuromuscular junctions of human patients, colocalizing with reduced amounts of AChRs.[6] In addition, active immunization against purified AChR induces an experimental form of MG, experimental autoimmune myasthenia gravis.[7]

These features of the disease have been important in defining a condition as being antibody mediated: the presence of antibodies to the extracellular surface of a functional protein, clinical response to plasma exchange or other immunotherapies, transfer of disease to mice by IgG, and presence of antibodies on the target tissue. These issues are discussed in Ref. 8.

The study of MG has also taught us much about the nature of autoantigens. The AChR is a multimeric membrane protein consisting of five subunits (two alpha subunits and one each of the beta, delta, and epsilon subunits), each of which spans the plasma membrane around a central ion channel or pore.[9] Each of the subunits contains an N-terminal 200-amino acid extracellular domain. When ACh binds to the two alpha subunits, the ion channel opens transiently, leading to transient membrane depolarization. In myasthenia gravis, the number of AChRs is reduced, due to antibody-mediated mechanisms, and therefore the amount of depolarization at the neuromuscular junction may be insufficient to trigger muscle activity.[1,2] This can be reversed, to some extent, by inhibiting enzyme acetylcholine esterase. Therapeutic levels of acetylcholinesterase inhibitors increase the amount of ACh, increase AChR channel openings, and improve neuromuscular transmission. In patients who do not have AChR antibodies, other antibodies are present that cause the disease. Recently, the receptor tyrosine kinase MuSK was shown to be a target for antibodies in about 40% of patients without AChR antibodies.[10] This is one of the first conditions to be associated with antibodies to a receptor tyrosine kinase, and the mechanisms by which these antibodies cause the disease remain to be elucidated.

During development and following denervation, the epsilon replaces a gamma subunit. This means that both functionally and antigenically, subtle differences exist between AChRs present on developing neuromuscular junctions and those in adult muscle.[9]

ANTIBODY-MEDIATED ARTHROGRYPOSIS

The existence of two forms of AChR is relevant to maternal myasthenia and the developing baby. It is well known that a proportion of mothers with MG have babies with a transient neonatal form of MG.[1,2] This condition usually lasts a few weeks and is responsive to treatment of the baby with cholinesterase inhibitors. Many of the AChR antibodies in MG patients bind to a site on the two alpha subunits, called the main immunogenic region,[9] but mothers of infants with neonatal MG appear to have higher levels of antibodies that bind specifically to the fetal isoform.[9] In humans, the fetal isoform is expressed throughout pregnancy and is replaced by the adult isoform during the last few weeks of gestation.

Another situation occurs if the mother's antibodies are highly specific for the fetal isoform. Several cases have been reported of women with myasthenia giving birth to infants with arthrogryposis multiplex congenital (AMC).[11] This is a severe developmental condition that results from a lack of fetal movement. The infant is born with fixed joint contractures and often other deformities. In most cases, the cause is genetic or environmental,[12] but in a few instances the mother has MG. Antibodies that specifically inhibit the function of the fetal isoform and have little or no effect on the function of the adult isoform have been detected in seven mothers of AMC infants.[13,14] In most cases, the mother had had several consecutive babies affected, consistent with a maternal rather than a genetic basis for the condition.[11]

To prove that maternal antibodies were capable of causing the condition, maternal serum or IgG was injected into pregnant mice.[15] A large proportion of mouse offspring were born with fixed joint contractures, and some had other developmental abnormalities. Thus, antibody-mediated AMC can be transferred to mice by injection of serum or IgG. In addition, two women whose infants had AMC have given birth to normal infants after plasma exchange and other immunosuppressive treatments of their associated MG.[15]

Antibodies to other fetal antigens could also cause AMC, and a study of 200 serum samples from mothers of AMC infants revealed evidence of antibodies to muscle and nerve antigens in around 10%. However, it has yet to be demonstrated that these antibodies are directly responsible for the AMC, rather than an epiphenomenon (P. Dalton and A. Vincent, unpublished observations, 2002).

ANTIBODIES TO VOLTAGE-GATED ION CHANNELS AND PERIPHERAL NEUROLOGICAL DISEASE

The AChRs are not the only targets of antibody-mediated disease at the neuromuscular junction. The voltage-gated calcium channels (VGCC) that are present on the presynpatic nerve terminal (FIG. 1) are the target for antibodies in the Lambert Eaton myasthenic syndrome (LEMS).[16] In this condition, the antibodies cause a reduction in the number of VGCCs, but they do not act via complement-mediated lysis. Indeed, they appear to act only by cross-linking the VGCCs on the motor nerve terminal surface and causing their clustering and internalization.[17] The resulting loss of VGCCs causes a reduction in the calcium-induced release of ACh and thus reduced AChR activation. About 50% of the patients have small cell lung cancer. These tumors express VGCCs on their surface, and the development of VGCC antibodies is probably part of the normal immune response of the patient towards tumor antigens. Interestingly, these patients often have autonomic disturbance, presumably due to reduced ACh release at parasympathetic nerve endings.[18]

Another peripheral ion channel disorder is neuromyotonia (NMT).[19] Antibodies to voltage-gated potassium channels (VGKCs) are found in about 40% of patients and appear to act by reducing the number of VGKCs at the motor nerve terminal and along the motor nerve itself. As a result, the nerve membrane potential becomes

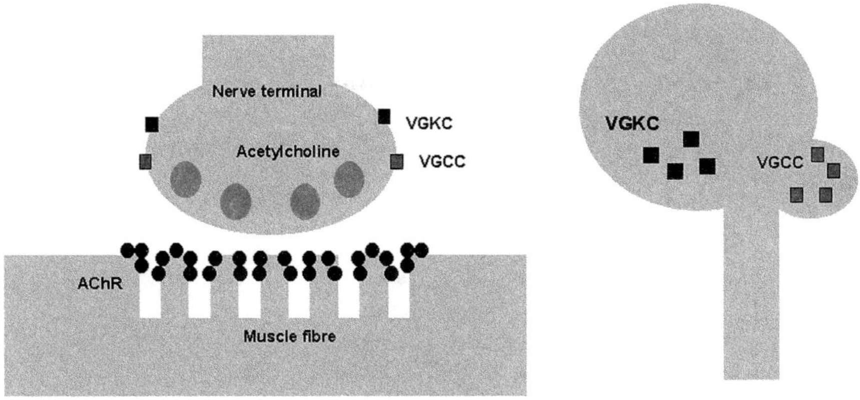

FIGURE 1. The neuromuscular junction and CNS. A simple scheme to draw attention to the presence of voltage-gated calcium channels (VGCCs) and voltage-gated potassium channels (VGKCs) shared between peripheral and central nervous systems. Antibodies to these channels predominantly affect the neuromuscular junction, but they are beginning to be found also in some CNS disorders involving the cerebellum (VGCC) and the limbic system (VGKC).

unstable and the nerve hyperexcitable.[20] This leads to increased ACh release with increased activation of AChRs and repetitive and spontaneous muscle activity. The patient complains of cramps and muscle twitching. About 20% of patients have a thymoma, but it is not yet clear how strongly this tumor expresses VGKCs. Some of the patients with thymoma also have MG.[19]

Both LEMS and NMT are antibody-mediated conditions, because the patients improve with plasma exchange and the antibodies can be measured by *in vitro* tests using the ion channels labeled with specific neurotoxins. Transfer of disease to mice has been studied extensively in LEMS,[16] but the data for NMT are much less complete.

ANTIBODIES TO ION CHANNELS IN THE CNS

A small proportion of patients with LEMS and small cell lung cancer also have cerebellar ataxia, suggesting that the immune response against the tumor is also directed against the VGCCs or other antigens in the cerebellum.[21,22] Similarly, some patients with acquired neuromyotonia develop CNS symptoms, such as anxiety and sleep problems,[23] and rarely full-blown Morvan's syndrome.[24] This condition is thought to be very rare. The patients have a combination of peripheral muscle hyperexcitability, autonomic disturbance, and insomnia, memory loss, confusion, and hallucinations. They can be very disturbed, and the condition can be life-threatening, although it sometimes improves spontaneously. VGKC antibodies are present in most cases that we have had the opportunity to test, and they appear to be closely linked to the disease (A. Vincent, unpublished observations). The few patients treated so far have improved following plasma exchange.

Moreover, patients with similar "limbic" symptoms (memory loss, seizures, confusion, anxiety, and disorientation), but without peripheral muscle involvement may also have VGKC antibodies and respond clinically to plasma exchange.[23] Some of these individuals have first presented with psychiatric or behavioral disorders (J. Palace, unpublished observations, 2002). These observations are defining for the first time a relatively common, but clinically diverse, form of CNS disorder that appears to be antibody mediated.

CAN MATERNAL ANTIBODIES CAUSE NEURODEVELOPMENTAL CONDITIONS?

Antibodies to VGKCs appear to be involved in mediating CNS disorders (see above), and maternal antibodies to the fetal form of an ion channel have been shown to cause a peripheral developmental condition, AMC. Bringing together these two observations, we can speculate that some neurodevelopmental conditions could be due to maternal antibodies directed at functional CNS membrane proteins or other accessible targets. Moreover, the ability to transfer AMC to mice[15] raised the possibility of investigating the role of maternal antibodies in neurodevelopmental disorders.

We first tested the hypothesis, and the feasibility of performing the experiments, by looking at five mothers who had had two of more children with dyslexia and injecting the maternal serum samples into pregnant mice. One of the maternal serum samples produced subtle changes in the behavior of the mouse offspring.[25] We then turned to autism. Although the cause of autism is unknown,[26] some workers have suggested that maternal antibodies may play a role in developmental conditions,[27] and antibodies to lymphocyte antigens, which are often shared with neuronal antigens, were reported in the serum of mothers of autistic children.[28] We asked if antibodies to neurons may be present in serum samples from mothers of children with autism or autistic spectrum disorders (ASD) and if the sera could passively transfer behavioral disturbances in the mouse "maternal-to-fetal" transfer model.

Five serum samples from women who have had two or more children with neurodevelopmental problems, including autism and specific language disorders, were tested. Two serum samples contained detectable levels of antibodies binding to adult rat brain neurons, particularly cerebellar Purkinje cells, but also to other large neurons. The antibodies also bound to neurons in developing, neonatal mouse cerebellum. Such antibodies were not found in serum samples from mothers of healthy children. An important feature was that the antibodies in one mother also bound to the extracellular surface of a neuronal cell line, indicating that they could potentially be pathogenic *in vivo*.[29]

In one case, sufficient serum was available for further experiments. One milliliter of serum was injected daily into pregnant mice from E11-E17 (where E0 is the day at which the vaginal plug is detected). The mice were born at term and developed normally, but they were relatively poor in open-field exploration (FIG. 2, top).[30] Moreover, when tested on a multiple static rods test that assesses motor coordination, they performed very poorly (FIG. 2, bottom), taking longer to turn 180 degrees on the rods. (For methods see Refs. 31 and 32.) The results were significantly different from those of mice treated similarly with serum from mothers of healthy children.[29]

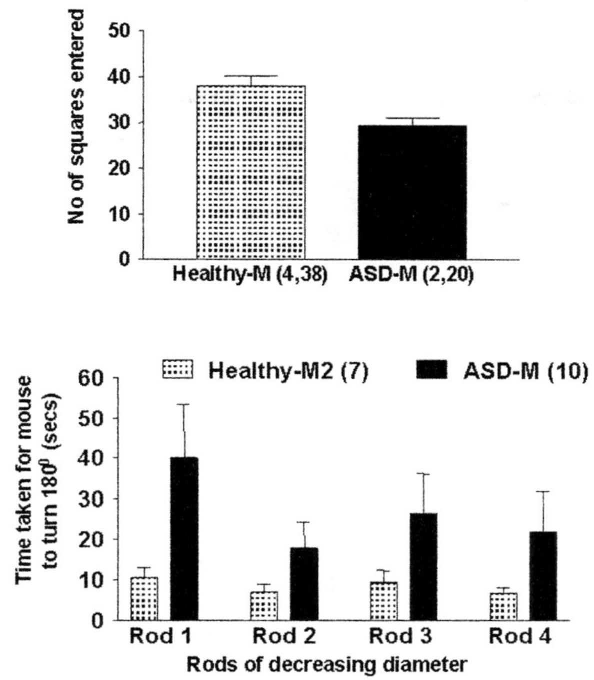

FIGURE 2. Results of behavioral testing of mice born to mothers injected with serum from mothers of healthy infants (Healthy-M) or mothers of children who developed autism spectrum disorders (ASD). (***Top)*** Number of squares entered by mice in an open-field exploration experiment. Offspring of mice injected with serum from the mother of children with ASD were significantly less active ($P = 0.008$) than those of mice injected with serum from mothers of healthy children. (***Below)*** Time taken to turn around on rods of decreasing diameters. The ASD offspring performed poorly on this test, taking much longer to turn. Complete results of these experiments can be found in Ref. 29.

Cerebellar abnormalities have previously been demonstrated in children with ASDs.[26] To determine if cerebellar abnormalities were present in the mice, magnetic resonance spectroscopy was performed. The results showed reduced levels of choline and creatine, with normal levels of N acetyl aspartate. The interpretation of these findings is difficult, but they are consistent with altered cerebellar structure or cellular components.[29] Detailed morphological studies on the mouse brain have not yet been done.

Although preliminary, the results of these experiments are consistent with a role for maternal antibodies in some cases of ASD and other neurodevelopmental disorders. It is not expected that many mothers will transmit pathogenic antibodies to their infants, but to assess the proportion, a much wider screen of maternal serum samples is planned. One surprising feature of these findings is that maternal IgG appears to affect the development of the brain. Although the blood-brain barrier is present during fetal development, the choroid plexus is relatively leaky, and large amounts of IgG can gain access to the ventricles (A. Vincent and L. Clover, in preparation). It may be that this provides sufficient levels of antibodies in the brain parenchyma to affect development. Alternatively, the blood-brain barrier may be more leaky at an earlier stage of development. Further studies are needed to measure the extent of diffusion of IgG into the brain of fetal animals and to confirm that maternal antibodies can reach the CNS and alter development.

CONCLUSIONS

Antibody-mediated diseases of the peripheral nervous system are well defined and can cause a variety of symptoms. Antibodies affecting the CNS are still not well established, but growing evidence indicates that antibodies to voltage-gated potassium and calsium channels are involved in limbic syndromes, and in some cases studied, the symptoms are predominantly psychiatric or behavioral. Thus, the role of antibodies in some psychiatric disorders should be investigated further. In addition, maternal antibodies specific for a fetal muscle antigen can cause a peripheral developmental condition, arthrogryposis, and a role for maternal antibodies in causing neurodevelopmental conditions is possible.

ACKNOWLEDGMENTS

We are grateful to Dr. M. Pike for the maternal sera and to Dr. Rob Deacon for help with the behavioral studies.

REFERENCES

1. DRACHMAN, D.B. 1994. Myasthenia gravis. N. Engl. J. Med. **330:** 1797–1810.
2. VINCENT, A., J. PALACE & D. HILTON-JONES. 2001. Myasthenia gravis. Semin. Lancet **357:** 2122–2128.
3. LINDSTROM, J.M., M.E. SEYBOLD, V.A. LENNON, *et al.* 1976. Antibody to acetylcholine receptor in myasthenia gravis. Prevalence, clinical correlates, and diagnostic value. Neurology **26:** 1054–1059.
4. NEWSOM-DAVIS, J., A.J. PINCHING, A. VINCENT & S.G. WILSON. 1978. Function of circulating antibody to acetylcholine receptor in myasthenia gravis: investigation by plasma exchange. Neurology **28:** 266-272.
5. TOYKA, K.V., D.B. DRACHMAN, D.E. GRIFFIN, *et al.* 1977. Myasthenia gravis: study of humoral immune mechanisms by passive transfer to mice. N. Engl. J. Med. **296:** 25-131.
6. ENGEL, A.G. 1984. Myasthenia gravis and myasthenic syndromes. Ann. Neurol. **16:** 519-534.
7. PATRICK, J. & J. LINDSTROM. 1973. Autoimmune response to acetylcholine receptor. Science **180:** 871-872.
8. VINCENT, A. 2002. Measuring and evaluating the significance of autoantibodies in neurological disorders. Clin. Allergy Immunol. Rev. **3:** 127–151.
9. TZARTOS, S.J., T. BARKAS, M.T. CUNG, *et al.* 1998. Anatomy of the antigenic structure of a large membrane autoantigen, the muscle-type nicotinic acetylcholine receptor. Immunol Rev. **163:** 89–120.
10. HOCH, W., J. MCCONVILLE, S. HELMS, *et al.* 2001. Autoantibodies to the receptor tyrosine kinase MuSK in patients with myasthenia gravis without acetylcholine receptor antibodies. Nat. Med. **7:** 365–368.

11. POLIZZI, A., S.M. HUSON & A. VINCENT. 2000. Teratogen update: maternal myasthenia gravis as a cause of congenital arthrogryposis. Teratology **62:** 332–341.
12. HALL, J. & A. VINCENT. 2001. Arthrogryposis. *In* Handbook of Muscle Diseases of Childhood. R. Jones & B. Darras, Eds. Elsevier Science (USA). Burlington, MA.
13. VINCENT, A., C. NEWLAND, L. BRUETON, *et al.* 1995. Arthrogryposis multiplex congenita with maternal autoantibodies specific for a fetal antigen. Lancet **346:** 24-25.
14. BRUETON, L.A. *et al.* 2000 Asymptomatic maternal myasthenia as a cause of the Pena-Shokeir phenotype. Am. J. Med. Genet. **92:** 1–6.
15. JACOBSON, L., A. POLIZZI, G.M. MORRISS-KAY & A. VINCENT. 1999. An animal model of antibody-mediated neurodevelopmental disease: arythrogryposis multiplex congenita caused by antibodies to fetal acetylcholine receptor. J. Clin. Invest. **103:** 1031–1038.
16. LANG, B., J. NEWSOM-DAVIS, C. PRIOR & D. WRAY. 1983. Antibodies to motor nerve terminals: an electrophysiological study of a human myasthenic syndrome transferred to mouse. J. Physiol. **344:** 335–345.
17. VINCENT, A., B. LANG & J. NEWSOM-DAVIS. 1989. Autoimmunity to the voltage-gated calcium channel underlies the Lambert-Eaton myasthenic syndrome, a paraneoplastic disorder. Trends Neurosci. **12:** 496–502.
18. WATERMAN, S.A., B. LANG & J. NEWSOM-DAVIS. 1997. Effect of Lambert-Eaton myasthenic syndrome antibodies on autonomic neurons in the mouse. Ann. Neurol. **42:** 147–156.
19. NEWSOM-DAVIS, J. & K.R. MILLS. 1993. Immunological associations of acquired neuromyotonia (Isaacs' syndrome). Report of five cases and literature review. Brain **116:** 453–469.
20. SHILLITO, P., P.C. MOLENAAR, A. VINCENT, *et al.* 1995. Acquired neuromyotonia: evidence for autoantibodies against K+ channels of peripheral nerves. Ann. Neurol. **38:** 714–722.
21. LENNON, V.A., T.J. KRYZER, G.E. GRIESMANN, *et al.* 1995. Calcium-channel antibodies in the Lambert-Eaton syndrome and other paraneolastic syndromes. N. Engl. J. Med. **332:** 1467–1474.
22. GRAUS, F., B. LANG, P. POZO-ROSICH, *et al.* 2002. P/Q type calcium channel antibodies in paraneoplastic cerebellar degeneration with lung cancer. Neurology **59:** 764–766.
23. BUCKLEY, C., J. OGER, L. CLOVER, *et al.* 2001. Potassium channel antibodies in two patients with reversible limbic encephalitis. Ann. Neurol. **50:** 74–79.
24. LIGUORI, R., A. VINCENT, L. CLOVER, *et al.* 2001 Morvan's syndrome: peripheral and central nervous system and cardiac involvement with antibodies to voltage-gated potassium channels. Brain **124:** 2417–2426.
25. VINCENT, A., R. DEACON, P. DALTON, *et al.* 2002. Maternal antibody-mediated dyslexia? Evidence for a pathogenic serum factor in a mother of two dyslexic children shown by transfer to mice using behavioural studies and magnetic resonance spectroscopy. J. NeuroImmunol. **130:** 243–247.
26. POUSTKA, F. 1998. Neurobiology of autism. *In* Autism and Pervasive Developmental Disorders. F.R. Volkmar, Ed. :130–168. Cambridge Monographs in Child and Adolescent Psychiatry. Cambridge, UK.
27. ADINOLFI, M. 1993 Fetal exposure to maternal brain antibodies and neurological handicap. *In* Dyslexia and Development. A.M. Galaburda, Ed. :155–167. Harvard University Press. Cambridge, MA
28. WARREN, R.P., P. COLE, J.D. ODELL, *et al.* 1990. Detection of maternal antibodies in infantile autism. J. Am. Acad. Child Adolesc. Psychiatry **29:** 873–877.
29. DALTON, P., R. DEACON, A.M. BLAMIRE, *et al.* 2003. Experimental evidence for a fetopathogenic antibody in the mother of children with autism and a severe speech disorder. Ann. Neurol. **53:** 533–537.
30. CRAWLEY, J.N. 2000. What's Wrong with My Mouse? Behavioral Phenotyping of Transgenic and Knockout Mice. Wiley-Liss. New York.
31. GUENTHER, K., R.M. DEACON, V.H. PERRY & J.N. RAWLINS. 2001. Early behavioural changes in scrapie-affected mice and the influence of dapsone. Eur. J. Neurosci. **14:** 401–409.
32. DEACON, R.M.J., D.M. BANNERMAN, B.P. KIRBY, *et al.* 2002. Effects of cytotoxic hippocampal lesions in mice on a cognitive test battery. Behav. Brain Res. **133:** 57–68.

Activation of Complement in the Central Nervous System

Roles in Neurodegeneration and Neuroprotection

JOHAN VAN BEEK, KRISTINA ELWARD, AND PHILIPPE GASQUE

Brain Inflammation and Immunity Group (BIIG), Department of Medical Biochemistry and Immunology, University of Wales College of Medicine, Cardiff, UK

ABSTRACT: The complement system is an essential effector of the humoral and cellular immunity involved in cytolysis and immune/inflammatory responses. Complement participates in host defense against pathogens by triggering the formation of the membrane attack complex. Complement opsonins (C1q, C3b, and iC3b) interact with surface complement receptors to promote phagocytosis, whereas complement anaphylatoxins C3a and C5a initiate local inflammatory responses that ultimately contribute to the protection and healing of the host. However, activation of complement to an inappropriate extent has been proposed to promote tissue injury. There is now compelling evidence that complement activation in the brain is a double-edged sword in that it can exert beneficial or detrimental effects depending on the pathophysiological context. This review focuses on the roles of the complement system in the pathogenesis of acute brain injury (cerebral ischemia and trauma) and chronic neurodegeneration (Alzheimer's disease). Because many effects of the complement appear to promote neuronal survival and tissue remodeling, directing activation of the complement system in the brain may provide a better therapeutic rationale than inhibiting it.

KEYWORDS: complement; central nervous system; inflammation; ischemia; trauma; Alzheimer's disease

THE COMPLEMENT SYSTEM, A PIVOTAL EFFECTOR ARM OF THE INNATE IMMUNE RESPONSE

Functions of the complement system include the recognition and killing of invading pathogens (e.g., bacteria, virus-infected cells, and parasites) while preserving normal "self" cells. The complement system through its activation products also contributes to the release of inflammatory mediators, promoting tissue injury at sites of inflammation.[1] Having preceded the emergence of adaptive immunity, the complement system has maintained a high degree of phylogenic conservation among both invertebrates and mammals, underlying the critical role of complement in tissue homeostasis.[2]

Address for correspondence: Dr. Johan van Beek, Department of Medical Biochemistry and Immunology, Tenovus Building 3rd Floor, University of Wales College of Medicine, Cardiff CF14 4XX, United Kingdom. Voice: +44 2920 745254; fax: +44 2920 744305.
van_beek@hotmail.com

Ann. N.Y. Acad. Sci. 992: 56–71 (2003).

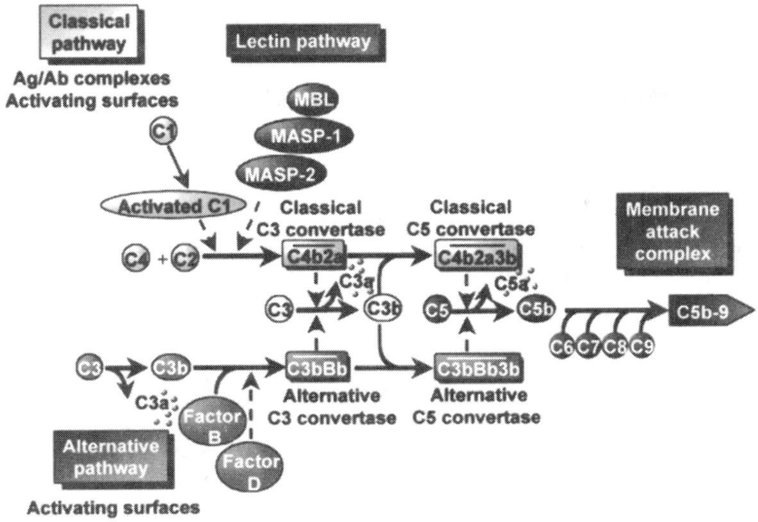

FIGURE 1. Schematic representation of the complement cascade. The complement system can be activated through the classical, the alternative, or the lectin pathway, leading to a common terminal pathway: the cytolytic membrane attack complex. Proteolytic cleavage of components C3 and C5 leads to the release of pro-inflammatory anaphylatoxins C3a and C5a, respectively. MBL, mannose-binding lectin; MASP, MBL-associated serine protease. Ag, antigen; Ab, antibody.

The complement system consists of some 30 fluid-phase and cell-membrane associated proteins. Complement can be activated by three distinct routes (FIG. 1). The classical pathway (involving C1q, C1r, C1s, C4, C2, and C3 components) is activated primarily by the interaction of C1q with immune complexes (antibody-antigen), but activation can also be achieved after interaction of C1q with non-immune molecules such as DNA, RNA, C-reactive protein, serum amyloid P, bacterial lipopolysaccharides, and some fungal and virus membranes. The initiation of the alternative pathway (involving C3, factor B, factor D, and properdin) does not require the presence of immune complexes and leads to the deposition of C3 fragments on target cells. Mannose-binding lectin (MBL), a lectin homologous to C1q, can recognize carbohydrates such as mannose and *N*-acetylglucosamine on pathogens and initiate the complement pathway independently of both the classical and the alternative activation pathways. MBL is associated with two serine proteases, mannose-binding lectin-associated serine proteases (MASP)-1 and -2 that, like the C1 complex in the classical pathway, cleave C4 and C2 components, leading to the formation of the classical C3 convertase.

COMPLEMENT RECEPTORS INVOLVED IN PHAGOCYTOSIS

The target pathogen coated with complement opsonins (the C1q and C3 activation by-products C3b and iC3b) is specifically recognized and phagocytosed by macrophages expressing complement C1q and receptors for C3 fragments (complement receptor [CR] type 1, CR3, and CR4). In addition to its role in pathogen clearance, C1q plays an important role in the clearance of apoptotic cells. C1q binds directly to surface blebs of apoptotic keratinocytes and T cells and there can initiate complement opsonization.[3,4] These observations support the hypothesis that C1q serves as an opsonin in the recognition and clearance of apoptotic cells. The transmembrane glycoprotein termed "C1q receptor that enhances phagocytosis" (C1qRp), recently shown to be identical to CD93, has emerged as a possible defense collagen receptor.[5] Monocytes that have adhered on C1q-coated surfaces display a 4- to 10-fold enhancement of phagocytosis of targets coated with IgG or complement.[6] However, the alleged binding of C1q to CD93 has been challenged, and the cellular and molecular properties of the multicomplex receptor CD93 are yet to be elucidated.[5]

C3, when activated on a cell surface, binds covalently (opsonization) as C3b and is subsequently cleaved into a very stable fragment, iC3b. CR3 (CD11b/CD18) and CR4 (CD11c/CD18) are involved in the phagocytosis process of targets opsonized with C3b and iC3b fragments.[7] CR1 (CD35) is also a multifunctional receptor, binding to C4b, C3b, iC3b, and C1q, and as such has been implicated in phagocytic and complement regulatory activities.[8]

THE LYTIC TERMINAL COMPLEX AND COMPLEMENT REGULATORS

Ultimately, activation of the complement system, through the complement terminal pathway (involving C5, C6, C7, C8, and C9 components), leads to the formation of the membrane attack complex (MAC), which forms a pore in the phospholipid bilayer to lyse the target cell (i.e., bacteria or virally infected cells). However, activation of the complement system at inappropriate sites and/or to an inappropriate extent can lead to host tissue damage.

To protect "self" cells against bystander lysis, host cells express a battery of regulatory proteins (complement inhibitors) that inhibit either assembly of the C3-cleaving enzymes or the formation of the MAC (FIG. 2).[9] C1 inhibitor (C1-INH), C4 binding protein (C4bp), factor H, factor I, S-protein, and clusterin are soluble inhibitors that are secreted and released in the fluid phase. Membrane-associated complement inhibitors include membrane cofactor protein (MCP, CD46), decay-accelerating factor (DAF, CD55), and CD59. Of note, an inhibitor of complement activation, termed "complement receptor-related protein y" (Crry), is expressed on rodent, but not human, cell membranes. Crry is broadly distributed and is a functional and structural analog of human DAF and MCP.

COMPLEMENT EXPRESSION BY BRAIN CELLS

In mammals, the liver is the major source of most complement proteins with the exception of C1q, C7, and FD. The brain is separated from the plasma by the blood-brain barrier (BBB), formed by endothelial cells of microvessels, smooth muscle cells (also called pericytes), and astrocytes. The BBB acts as a molecular sieve and

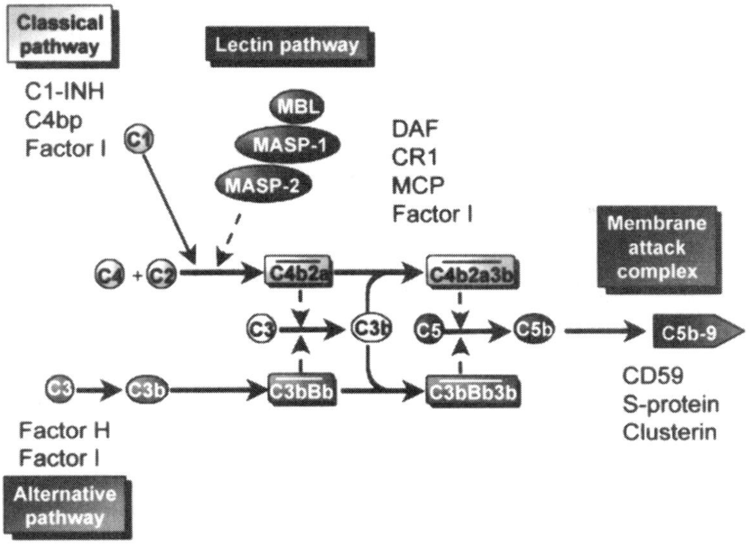

FIGURE 2. Regulation of the complement cascade. The different pathways of the complement cascade are tightly regulated by membrane-associated (DAF, MCP, CD59, and CR1) or soluble (C1-INH, C4bp, Factor I, Factor H, S-protein, and clusterin) inhibitors. C1-INH, C1 inhibitor; C4bp, C4 binding protein; DAF, decay-accelerating factor; MCP, membrane cofactor protein; CR1, complement receptor 1.

isolates the brain parenchyma from plasma proteins, including complement components, as well as circulating immunocompetent cells such as lymphocytes, macrophages, and natural killer cells. However, transudation of plasma proteins through a damaged BBB can contribute to the deposition of potentially cytotoxic and cytolytic complement components in the brain parenchyma.

In addition, we and others have proposed that brain cells can produce complement proteins to recognize and kill pathogens locally, while preserving normal cells in the central nervous system (CNS).[10] Levi-Strauss and Mallat[11] were the first to demonstrate that brain cells can synthesize complement components. They showed that cultured rodent astrocyte cell lines and primary cultures of mouse astrocytes produced C3 and FB and that the expression of complement was increased upon stimulation with lipopolysaccharide. In the last decade, this observation has been extended to include astrocytes, microglia, neurons, and oligodendrocytes.[12,13] Cell lines and primary cultures of human origin were used to show that glial and neuronal cells could produce most complement proteins, particularly after stimulation with inflammatory cytokines.[14–17] Complement mRNAs were also found to be expressed, albeit at a low level, in normal human brain tissue.[18–23] From these studies, it was proposed that brain cells, appropriately stimulated with cytokines, can assemble a full complement system to exert toxic and lytic activities against pathogens.

In addition, considerable evidence now indicates that local expression of complement by resident cells can be dramatically increased following brain infection.

Increased levels of complement mRNAs have been reported in experimental models of brain infection (meningitis, scrapie, and encephalomyelitis) in rodents.[24–27]

COMPLEMENT IN ACUTE BRAIN INFLAMMATION: CEREBRAL ISCHEMIA AND TRAUMA

After an acute brain insult, such as stroke or traumatic brain injury, local inflammation within the brain parenchyma can contribute to the exacerbation of neuronal loss. The concept that complement activation may contribute to the pathogenesis of acute brain injury developed from observations using experimental models of stroke and trauma. Systemic complement depletion using cobra venom factor, which functions as an unregulated C3 convertase, thus activating and depleting C3 and C5 via the alternative pathway, improved blood flow and neurological function after transient cerebral ischemia in the rat.[28] More recently, Huang and colleagues[29] demonstrated that a bifunctional molecule designed to inhibit both complement activation and selectin-mediated adhesive events can inhibit neutrophil and platelet accumulation and reduce cerebral infarct size in the mouse. Furthermore, treatment with soluble CR1 was found to reduce neutrophil accumulation after traumatic brain injury in rats.[30]

The presence of complement components within the brain parenchyma following experimental cerebral ischemia has previously beeen documented. Intracerebral complement levels following acute brain injury might increase after BBB breakdown, leading to passive leakage of serum-derived complement into the brain parenchyma. In 1994, Czurko and Nishino[31] reported the presence of C3, along with the infiltration of immunoglobulins, within both the striatum and the cortex following transient focal cerebral ischemia in the rat. Additionally, potential cellular sources of complement within the injured brain have been identified. Using in situ hybridization, widespread increased synthesis of C1q was found in microglial cells in response to transient global cerebral ischemia in rats.[32] Intracerebral expression of complement following focal cerebral ischemia was mainly associated with the glial cell response, but neurons can also be a source of complement.[33] Local complement production has also been described in experimental models of trauma. For instance, expression of mRNA for C1q was found in the peritrauma region after a cortical aspiration lesion in rats.[34] Deposition of the complement activation product C3d and C9, an indicator of MAC deposition, was observed on neurons after experimental cerebral contusion in the rat.[35]

In line with these findings in experimental models, observations reported intrathecal synthesis of complement, as assessed by the presence of several activation products of the cytotoxic/cytolytic complement system in the cerebrospinal fluid (CSF) of head trauma or stroke patients. In these studies, elevated levels of complement components C3 and factor B were found in the ventricular CSF of patients with traumatic brain injury.[27] Interestingly, intrathecal levels of complement-derived soluble MAC correlate with BBB dysfunction, implicating the complement system in the pathogenesis of clinical trauma, with regard to posttraumatic BBB dysfunction.[36] Complement activation in CSF and plasma following cerebral ischemia or hemorrhage has also been reported.[37,38]

Strikingly, complement activation products have been localized within the CNS parenchyma of head trauma[39] and stroke patients,[38] providing a strong body of evidence that complement-mediated cell death is prominent in areas of brain damage. Using immunohistochemistry, we found that neurons surrounding the ischemic core are strongly stained for complement components C1q, C3, and C4 as well as the activation product C3b, indicating that complement activation is taking place on neurons (J. van Beek, C.L. Harris, J.W. Neal, and P. Gasque, unpublished observations). In support of these findings, using an antibody against a neo-epitope exposed on activated MAC, Bellander and colleagues[39] demonstrated that neurons in the penumbra are target cells for the complement cascade following head trauma.

NEURONS ARE SUSCEPTIBLE TO COMPLEMENT ATTACK

Brain cells such as astrocytes and microglia express complement inhibitors to control complement activation on their membranes and seem to be relatively well protected from complement-mediated damage. This finding is in sharp contrast to neurons, which are extremely susceptible to complement attack. Indeed, human neuroblastoma cells as well as embryonic neurons *in vitro* have the propensity to activate spontaneously the complement system and, consequently, they are susceptible to complement-mediated lysis.[40,41] C1q binds specifically to the membrane of neurons, leading to activation of the classical pathway in an antibody-independent manner. The poor capacity of neurons to control complement activation has been attributed to the fact that these cells express low levels of complement regulators.[42,43] Overall, considerable evidence now indicates that increased intracerebral complement biosynthesis and uncontrolled complement activation in the CNS contribute to the development of tissue damage. However, further data on complement activation in stroke and trauma patients are needed before suggesting the possibility of a pharmacological manipulation of the complement system in acute brain injury.[44,45]

COMPLEMENT ANAPHYLATOXINS AND THEIR RECEPTORS

The most potent inflammatory molecules generated on complement activation are the anaphylatoxins C3a and C5a. C3a and C5a are small polypeptides (~9–10 kDa) that are highly pleiotropic in function and exert their effect at picomolar to nanomolar concentrations.[46] C3a and C5a derive from the enzymatic cleavage of C3 and C5, respectively, and are involved in the stimulation and chemotaxis of myeloid cells. The functional responses induced by C3a and C5a are mediated through their binding to specific receptors, C3a and C5a receptors (C3aR and C5aR), respectively.[46] These receptors are members of the rhodopsin family of seven transmembrane G-protein–coupled receptors.[47–51]

C5a is an important chemoattractant molecule that stimulates cells to express increased levels of cytokines, chemokines, adhesion molecules, and complement components.[46] In contrast to the broad proinflammatory effects of C5a, the effects of C3a appear to be more selective and rather anti-inflammatory. C3a is chemoattractant, but only for mast cells and eosinophils and not for either macrophages or microglia. Recent data indicate that C3a can decrease the production of proinflammatory cytokines by lipopolysaccharide-stimulated macrophage. on the one hand, and can induce the production of immunosuppressive cytokines, such as IL-10, on the other.[46] Furthermore, mice with targeted disruption of C3aR exhibited enhanced lethality when subjected to endotoxin shock, underlying the potential anti-inflammatory properties of anaphylatoxin C3a.[52]

The expression of C3aR and C5aR was thought to be restricted largely to cells of the myeloid lineage such as macrophages, eosinophils, basophils, and mast cells.[53–55] However, in recent years, studies have reported widespread expression of these receptors throughout many tissues and cell types outside the immune system, supporting the view that anaphylatoxins might exert effects unrelated to inflammation.[56–58] If the presence of C3aR and C5aR on microglia was expected given the monocytic origin of these cells, their expression on astrocytes and neurons was not anticipated. The functional significance of the presence of anaphylatoxin receptors on neurons remains ill-defined, but preliminary work suggess that anaphylatoxins might be involved in the modulation of neuronal functions.[59]

Upregulated expression of anaphylatoxin receptors by brain cells has been described in experimental models of focal cerebral ischemia[60,61] and trauma,[62,63] suggesting a role for anaphylatoxins in these pathologies. Human astrocyte cell lines stimulated with C5a produce increased amounts of IL-6, while the levels of IL-1, TNF-α, and TGF-β remain unchanged.[64] Unexpectedly, C5a has been shown to induce apoptosis of the human neuroblastoma cell line TGW.[65,66] Taken together, these data suggest that C5a release during CNS inflammation could contribute to the exacerbation of tissue damage. However, protective roles of C5a cannot be excluded, because anaphylatoxin C5a has been shown to protect neurons against excitotoxicity.[67–69] Interestingly, Heese and colleagues have shown that a human microglial cell line exposed to C3a expressed de novo nerve growth factor (NGF), a molecule involved in neuronal growth and survival.[70] These data would support the view that C3a, in contrast to C5a, acts as an anti-inflammatory signal promoting the resolution of the inflammatory process. Unlike C5a, C3a failed to display any effect on apoptosis-mediated neuronal cell death; however, C3a was shown to protect neurons against *N*-methyl-D-aspartate toxicity, extending its role beyond immune functions.[71] Further studies to investigate the role of complement anaphylatoxins in the modulation of neuroprotective/neurotoxic pathways are warranted.

SUBLYTIC EFFECTS OF MEMBRANE ATTACK COMPLEX

Assembly of the MAC, by definition, is involved in cytolytic activities. However, when the number of MAC molecules is limited, cells can escape cell death by rapidly eliminating membrane-inserted MAC by endocytosis and membrane shedding.[72] When it does not cause death, the MAC is involved in cell stimulation.[72,73] Sublytic levels of MAC have been shown to increase Ca^{2+} influx, to activate phospholipases and protein kinases, and to induce the generation of arachidonic acid-derived inflammatory mediator.[74–79] The MAC at sublytic levels has also been shown to stimulate endothelial cells to express complement regulatory proteins and to protect against secondary damage.[80] Taken together, these data indicate that the MAC at sublytic levels could act as a stress signal to activate cells to express increased levels of complement inhibitors and to protect against subsequent damage.

As an example of the protective role of the MAC, postmitotic oligodendrocytes exposed to sublytic effects of the MAC have been shown to enter the cell cycle.[81,82] Moreover, exposure to sublytic effects of the MAC can protect oligodendrocytes from apoptosis induced by serum deprivation[81] or exposure to tumor necrosis factor-α.[83] The question of whether sublytic assembly of the MAC could also modulate the outcome of damage during the course of demyelinating disease was addressed recently using experimental allergic encephalomyelitis. C5-sufficient mice with EAE were found to develop less pronounced levels of inflammation when compared to C5-deficient mice unable to form the MAC.[84] In addition, active remyelination with restoration of tissue integrity was observed in chronic lesions only in C5-sufficient mice.[84] Taken together, these data suggest a possible role for the sublytic assembly of the MAC in the modulation of tissue inflammation and the initiation of tissue repair. Complement has long been considered an inflammatory mediator in many diseases. However, recent observations implicate complement in novel, non-inflammatory functions and provide the basis for further study of complement-mediated effects on cell survival and proliferation in the CNS.

COMPLEMENT IN CHRONIC BRAIN INFLAMMATION: ALZHEIMER'S DISEASE

Intracerebral levels of complement are increased during the course of several chronic neurodegenerative disorders such as Alzheimer's disease (AD),[85–87] Parkinson's disease,[88] Pick's disease,[89] and Huntington's disease.[43] There is clear indication that the BBB remains intact during the course of AD, excluding the possibility of transudation of serum complement from the plasma into the brain parenchyma. Accordingly, studies using RT-PCR have shown locally upregulated complement mRNA in AD brain, particularly in areas of primary pathology (entorhinal cortex, hippocampus, and midtemporal gyrus).[22,23] C1q mRNA was increased 11- to 80-fold over control levels, and C9 mRNA 10- to 27-fold, indicating that complement components are produced in affected areas of the AD brain and that full activation of the classical complement pathway may be contributing significantly to AD pathology.[23] In situ hybridization and immunohistochemical experiments showed that not only reactive glial cells but also neurons were sources of complement.[19,90] Increased expression of receptors for complement anaphylatoxins C3a and C5a has also been documented in AD, suggesting that anaphylatoxins, released during intracerebral complement activation, drive inflammation in this pathology.[91,92] However, protective effects of anaphylatoxins in the pathogenesis of AD cannot be ruled out because C5a has been shown to be mitogenic for undifferentiated human neuroblastoma cells and also appears to protect terminally differentiated human neuroblastoma cells against toxicity mediated by the β-amyloid (Aβ) peptide.[93]

Eikelenboom and Stam[86] were the first to demonstrate the presence of complement proteins in senile amyloid plaques and neurofibrillary tangles. Subsequently, numerous groups reported the association of complement proteins of the classical pathway in AD brains.[20,23,85,94-96] More recently, the MAC has been found to co-localize with amyloid plaques and to be associated with neurofibrillary tangles containing neurons.[97] C1q has been shown to bind to fibrillar but not soluble Aβ, resulting in the activation of the classical pathway as seen in AD brains.[98,99] However, there are conflicting reports as to whether C1q binding to Aβ fibrils occurs through its collagen stalk[100,101] or by its globular head.[102] In addition, several other molecules associated with AD lesions such as serum amyloid protein and C-reactive protein are known to interact with C1q and therefore could also contribute to activation of the complement cascade during the course of AD.[103–105] Although, as mentioned before, neurofibrillary tangles were also immunopositive for complement components such as C1q, C3, and C4, the mechanism involved in complement activation on neurofibrillary tangles remains unknown.

THE ROLE OF COMPLEMENT IN THE CLEARANCE OF AMYLOID PLAQUES

Based on their ability to release inflammatory mediators, glial cells have been implicated in the progression of AD.[106] However, professional phagocytes such as microglia can exhibit scavenger cell activity and, as such, can provide beneficial functions by clearing the pathogenic peptide Aβ. Amyloid fibrils have been detected in microglial cells of AD brains as a possible attempt to clear abnormal protein deposits.[107,108] Interestingly, injection of amyloid cores isolated from AD brains into the cortex and hippocampus of rats elicited a phagocytic cell response.[109] A recent study by Schenk *et al.*[110] showed that Aβ deposition in a transgenic mouse model overexpressing the gene for a mutant form of the human amyloid precursor protein was dramatically diminished by prior immunization of the animals with synthetic Aβ peptide. Moreover, a single application of anti-Aβ antibodies to the cortical surface of these mice results in the clearance of existing senile plaques.[111] It has been proposed that this clearance process by microglial cells involves both Fc-dependent and non-Fc–mediated mechanisms.[111,112] Studies of mutant mice lacking complement proteins suggest that impaired phagocytosis can result in immune-mediated tissue damage and inflammation.[3,4] Mice lacking C1q display impairment in the clearance of apoptotic cells in the kidney, leading to severe glomerulonephritis with immune deposits.[3] Taken together, these data emphasize the critical role of complement in clearance processes. Recently, Wyss-Coray and colleagues[113] demonstrated for the first time that complement activation can protect against Aβ-induced toxicity and may reduce the accumulation or promote the clearance of senile plaques. AD mice expressing a soluble form of the complement inhibitor Crry under the control of the glial fibrillary acidic protein promotor displayed higher Aβ deposition and more prominent neurodegeneration than that in age-matched mice. This important observation underlines the critical role of intracerebral complement activation in mechanisms underlying brain repair and tissue remodeling.

CONCLUSION

Given the multiple functions of the complement system, it has been difficult so far to identify their specific roles in the pathogenesis of CNS disorders. Although a wealth of data implicates the complement system in the propagation of brain inflam-

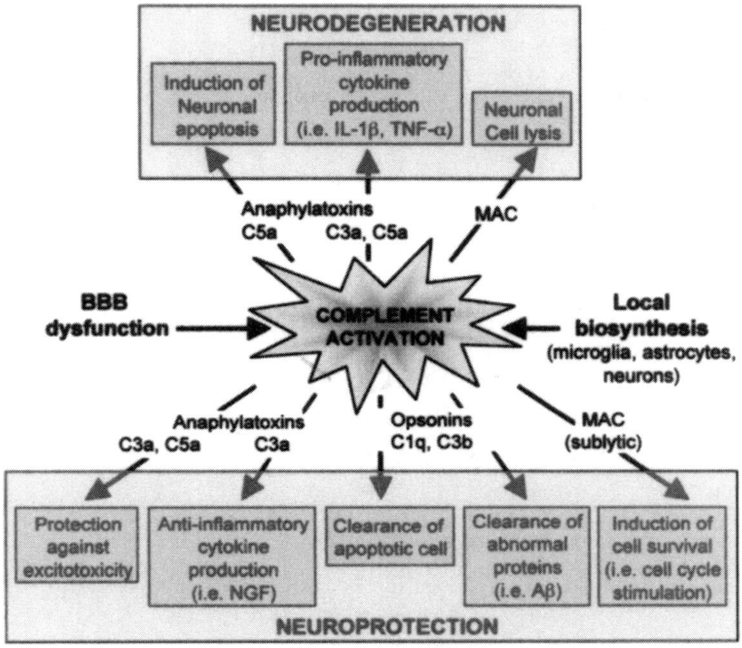

FIGURE 3. Complement activation within the CNS: a double-edged sword. Complement components found in the brain parenchyma under pathological conditions can originate either from the plasma after blood-brain barrier (BBB) dysfunction or from local biosynthesis by actvated brain cells. Intracerebral complement activation may promote tissue damage by inducing neuronal cell death (anaphylatoxins and membrane attack complex, MAC) and by promoting the release of pro-inflammatory cytokines by activated glial cells. On the other hand, complement activation can exert beneficial effects on the brain by promoting neuroprotection (anaphylatoxins and sublytic MAC) and tissue remodeling (opsonins and anaphylatoxins).

mation and tissue injury, the possibility that complement is involved in neuroprotective and repair activities is emerging. These double-edged sword activities of the local innate complement system in the CNS are summarized in FIGURE 3.

The case for an important role of complement in the initiation and/or exacerbation of brain inflammation has implications for therapeutic strategies to prevent secondary tissue injury. Complement therapeutics have undergone a mini-revolution over the last decade with the development of agents, based on the naturally occurring regulators of complement, that efficiently inhibit complement when administered to animal or man.[114] As noted earlier, some of these agents (e.g., complement inhibitor sCR1) have been shown to markedly reduce brain inflammation and tissue damage.[29] However, none of the current crop of complement therapeutics is suited to treatment of a chronic disease. All are large molecules, active only when administered systemically and have relatively short half-lives. These shortcomings effectively restrict use to acute disorders. Furthermore, to be used in CNS diseases, the next generation of complement inhibitors will have to be designed so they can be specifically delivered to the brain (by the use of specific targeting moieties) or expressed in the brain (by gene therapy). Because many of the responses mediated by the complement system can lead to beneficial effects, directing activation of the complement system, rather than inhibiting it, might inaugurate the basis for the development of new complement therapeutics.

ACKNOWLEDGMENTS

We thank Professor B. Paul Morgan for helpful comments on the manuscript. This work was supported by the Wellcome Trust (grant to J.v.B.) and the Medical Research Council (grant to P.G.).

REFERENCES

1. FRANK, M.M. & L.F. FRIES. 1991. The role of complement in inflammation and phagocytosis. Immunol. Today **12:** 322–326.
2. SUNYER, J.O., I.K. ZARKADIS & J.D. LAMBRIS. 1998. Complement diversity: a mechanism for generating immune diversity? Immunol. Today **19:** 519–523.
3. BOTTO, M., C. DELL'AGNOLA, A.E. BYGRAVE, *et al.* 1998. Homozygous C1q deficiency causes glomerulonephritis associated with multiple apoptotic bodies. Nat. Genet. **19:** 56–59.
4. TAYLOR, P.R., A. CARUGATI, V.A. FADOK, *et al.* 2000. A hierarchical role for classical pathway complement proteins in the clearance of apoptotic cells in vivo. J. Exp. Med. **192:** 359–366.
5. MCGREAL, E.P., N. IKEWAKI, H. AKATSU, *et al.* 2002. Human C1qRp is identical with CD93 and the mNI-11 antigen but does not bind C1q. J. Immunol. **168:** 5222–5232.
6. GUAN, E., S.L. ROBINSON, E.B. GOODMAN & A.J. TENNER. 1994. Cell-surface protein identified on phagocytic cells modulates the C1q-mediated enhancement of phagocytosis. J. Immunol. **152:** 4005–4016.
7. EHLERS, M.R. 2000. CR3: a general purpose adhesion-recognition receptor essential for innate immunity. Microbes Infect. **2:** 289–294.
8. KRYCH-GOLDBERG, M. & J.P. ATKINSON. 2001. Structure-function relationships of complement receptor type 1. Immunol. Rev. **180:** 112–122.
9. MORGAN, B.P. & C.L. HARRIS. 1999. Complement Regulatory Proteins. B.P. Morgan & C.L. Harris, Eds. Academic Press. San Diego.
10. MORGAN, B.P. & P. GASQUE. 1996. Expression of complement in the brain: role in health and disease. Immunol. Today **17:** 461–466.
11. LEVI-STRAUSS, M. & M. MALLAT. 1987. Primary cultures of murine astrocytes produce C3 and factor B, two components of the alternative pathway of complement activation. J. Immunol. **139:** 2361–2366.
12. GASQUE, P., Y.D. DEAN, E.P. MCGREAL, *et al.* 2000. Complement components of the innate immune system in health and disease in the CNS. Immunopharmacology **49:** 171–186.
13. BARNUM, S.R. 1995. Complement biosynthesis in the central nervous system. Crit. Rev. Oral Biol. Med. **6:** 132–146.
14. GASQUE, P., M. FONTAINE & B.P. MORGAN. 1995. Complement expression in human brain. Biosynthesis of terminal pathway components and regulators in human glial cells and cell lines. J. Immunol. **154:** 4726–4733.
15. GASQUE, P., A. ISCHENKO, J. LEGOEDEC, *et al.* 1993. Expression of the complement classical pathway by human glioma in culture. A model for complement expression by nerve cells. J. Biol. Chem. **268:** 25068–25074.
16. GASQUE, P., N. JULEN, A.M. ISCHENKO, *et al.* 1992. Expression of complement components of the alternative pathway by glioma cell lines. J. Immunol. **149:** 1381–1387.

17. THOMAS, A., P. GASQUE, D. VAUDRY, *et al.* 2000. Expression of a complete and functional complement system by human neuronal cells in vitro. Int. Immunol. **12:** 1015–1023.
18. FISCHER, B., H. SCHMOLL, P. RIEDERER, *et al.* 1995. Complement C1q and C3 mRNA expression in the frontal cortex of Alzheimer's patients. J. Mol. Med. **73:** 465–471.
19. SHEN, Y., R. LI, E.G. MCGEER & P.L. MCGEER. 1997. Neuronal expression of mRNAs for complement proteins of the classical pathway in Alzheimer brain. Brain Res. **769:** 391–395.
20. WALKER, D.G. & P.L. MCGEER. 1992. Complement gene expression in human brain: comparison between normal and Alzheimer disease cases. Brain Res. Mol. Brain Res. **14:** 109–116.
21. WITTE, D.P., T.R. WELCH & L.S. BEISCHEL. 1991. Detection and cellular localization of human C4 gene expression in the renal tubular epithelial cells and other extrahepatic epithelial sources. Am. J. Pathol. **139:** 717–724.
22. YASOJIMA, K., E.G. MCGEER & P.L. MCGEER. 1999. Complement regulators C1 inhibitor and CD59 do not significantly inhibit complement activation in Alzheimer disease. Brain Res. **833:** 297–301.
23. YASOJIMA, K., C. SCHWAB, E.G. MCGEER & P.L. MCGEER. 1999. Up-regulated production and activation of the complement system in Alzheimer's disease brain. Am. J. Pathol. **154:** 927–936.
24. DANDOY-DRON, F., F. GUILLO, L. BENBOUDJEMA, *et al.* 1998. Gene expression in scrapie. Cloning of a new scrapie-responsive gene and the identification of increased levels of seven other mRNA transcripts. J. Biol. Chem. **273:** 7691–7697.
25. DIETZSCHOLD, B., W. SCHWAEBLE, M.K. SCHAFER, *et al.* 1995. Expression of C1q, a subcomponent of the rat complement system, is dramatically enhanced in brains of rats with either Borna disease or experimental allergic encephalomyelitis. J. Neurol. Sci. **130:** 11–16.
26. STAHEL, P.F., K. FREI, A. FONTANA, *et al.* 1997. Evidence for intrathecal synthesis of alternative pathway complement activation proteins in experimental meningitis. Am. J. Pathol. **151:** 897–904.
27. STAHEL, P.F., D. NADAL, H.W. PFISTER, *et al.* 1997. Complement C3 and factor B cerebrospinal fluid concentrations in bacterial and aseptic meningitis. Lancet **349:** 1886–1887.
28. VASTHARE, U.S., F.C. BARONE, H.M. SARAU, *et al.* 1998. Complement depletion improves neurological function in cerebral ischemia. Brain Res. Bull. **45:** 413–419.
29. HUANG, J., L.J. KIM, R. MEALEY, *et al.* 1999. Neuronal protection in stroke by an sLex-glycosylated complement inhibitory protein. Science **285:** 595–599.
30. KACZOROWSKI, S.L., J.K. SCHIDING, C.A. TOTH & P.M. KOCHANEK. 1995. Effect of soluble complement receptor-1 on neutrophil accumulation after traumatic brain injury in rats. J. Cereb. Blood Flow Metab. **15:** 860–864.
31. CZURKO, A. & H. NISHINO. 1994. Appearance of immunoglobulin G and complement factor C3 in the striatum after transient focal ischemia in the rat. Neurosci. Lett. **166:** 51–54.
32. SCHAFER, M.K., W.J. SCHWAEBLE, C. POST, *et al.* 2000. Complement C1q is dramatically up-regulated in brain microglia in response to transient global cerebral ischemia. J. Immunol. **164:** 5446–5452.
33. VAN BEEK, J., P. CHAN, M. BERNAUDIN, *et al.* 2000. Glial responses, clusterin, and complement in permanent focal cerebral ischemia in the mouse. Glia **31:** 39–50.
34. PASINETTI, G.M., S.A. JOHNSON, I. ROZOVSKY, *et al.* 1992. Complement C1qB and C4 mRNAs responses to lesioning in rat brain. Exp. Neurol. **118:** 117–125.
35. BELLANDER, B.M., H. VON HOLST, P. FREDMAN & M. SVENSSON. 1996. Activation of the complement cascade and increase of clusterin in the brain following a cortical contusion in the adult rat. J. Neurosurg. **85:** 468–475.
36. STAHEL, P.F., M.C. MORGANTI-KOSSMANN, D. PEREZ, *et al.* 2001. Intrathecal levels of complement-derived soluble membrane attack complex (sC5b-9) correlate with blood-brain barrier dysfunction in patients with traumatic brain injury. J. Neurotrauma **18:** 773–781.

37. KASUYA, H. & T. SHIMIZU. 1989. Activated complement components C3a and C4a in cerebrospinal fluid and plasma following subarachnoid hemorrhage. J. Neurosurg. **71:** 741–746.
38. LINDSBERG, P.J., J. OHMAN, T. LEHTO, *et al.* 1996. Complement activation in the central nervous system following blood-brain barrier damage in man. Ann. Neurol. **40:** 587–596.
39. BELLANDER, B.M., S.K. SINGHRAO, M. OHLSSON, *et al.* 2001. Complement activation in the human brain after traumatic head injury. J. Neurotrauma **18:** 1295–1311.
40. SINGHRAO, S.K., J.W. NEAL, N.K. RUSHMERE, *et al.* 2000. Spontaneous classical pathway activation and deficiency of membrane regulators render human neurons susceptible to complement lysis. Am. J. Pathol. **157:** 905–918.
41. GASQUE, P., A. THOMAS, M. FONTAINE & B.P. MORGAN. 1996. Complement activation on human neuroblastoma cell lines in vitro: route of activation and expression of functional complement regulatory proteins. J. Neuroimmunol. **66:** 29–40.
42. SINGHRAO, S.K., J.W. NEAL, N.K. RUSHMERE, *et al.* 1999. Differential expression of individual complement regulators in the brain and choroid plexus. Lab. Invest. **79:** 1247–1259.
43. SINGHRAO, S.K., J.W. NEAL, B.P. MORGAN & P. GASQUE. 1999. Increased complement biosynthesis by microglia and complement activation on neurons in Huntington's disease. Exp. Neurol. **159:** 362–376.
44. DI NAPOLI, M. 2001. Systemic complement activation in ischemic stroke. Stroke **32:** 1443–1448.
45. DEL ZOPPO, G.J. 1999. In stroke, complement will get you nowhere. Nat. Med. **5:** 995–996.
46. EMBER, J.A., M.A. JAGELS & T.E. HUGLI. 1998. Characterization of complement anaphylatoxins and biological responses. *In* The Human Complement System in Health and Disease. J.E. Volanakis & M.M. Frank, Eds. :241. Marcel Dekker. New York.
47. AMES, R.S., Y. LI, H.M. SARAU, *et al.* 1996. Molecular cloning and characterization of the human anaphylatoxin C3a receptor. J. Biol. Chem. **271:** 20231–20234.
48. CRASS, T., U. RAFFETSEDER, U. MARTIN, *et al.* 1996. Expression cloning of the human C3a anaphylatoxin receptor (C3aR) from differentiated U-937 cells. Eur. J. Immunol. **26:** 1944–1950.
49. GERARD, N.P. & C. GERARD. 1991. The chemotactic receptor for human C5a anaphylatoxin. Nature **349:** 614–617.
50. BOULAY, F., L. MERY, M. TARDIF, *et al.* 1991. Expression cloning of a receptor for C5a anaphylatoxin on differentiated HL-60 cells. Biochemistry **30:** 2993–2999.
51. ROGLIC, A., E.R. PROSSNITZ, S.L. CAVANAGH, *et al.* 1996. cDNA cloning of a novel G protein-coupled receptor with a large extracellular loop structure. Biochim. Biophys. Acta **1305:** 39–43.
52. KILDSGAARD, J., T.J. HOLLMANN, K.W. MATTHEWS, *et al.* 2000. Cutting edge: targeted disruption of the C3a receptor gene demonstrates a novel protective anti-inflammatory role for C3a in endotoxin-shock. J. Immunol. **165:** 5406–5409.
53. ZWIRNER, J., O. GOTZE, G. BEGEMANN, *et al.* 1999. Evaluation of C3a receptor expression on human leucocytes by the use of novel monoclonal antibodies. Immunology **97:** 166–172.
54. MARTIN, U., D. BOCK, L. ARSENIEV, *et al.* 1997. The human C3a receptor is expressed on neutrophils and monocytes, but not on B or T lymphocytes. J. Exp. Med. **186:** 199–207.
55. DAFFERN, P.J., P.H. PFEIFER, J.A. EMBER & T.E. HUGLI. 1995. C3a is a chemotaxin for human eosinophils but not for neutrophils. I. C3a stimulation of neutrophils is secondary to eosinophil activation. J. Exp. Med. **181:** 2119–2127.
56. EMBER, J.A. & T.E. HUGLI. 1997. Complement factors and their receptors. Immunopharmacology **38:** 3–15.
57. ZWIRNER, J., A. FAYYAZI & O. GOTZE. 1999. Expression of the anaphylatoxin C5a receptor in non-myeloid cells. Mol. Immunol. **36:** 877–884.
58. WETSEL, R.A. 1995. Structure, function and cellular expression of complement anaphylatoxin receptors. Curr. Opin. Immunol. **7:** 48–53.

59. NATAF, S., P.F. STAHEL, N. DAVOUST & S.R. BARNUM. 1999. Complement anaphylatoxin receptors on neurons: new tricks for old receptors? Trends Neurosci. **22:** 397–402.
60. VAN BEEK, J., M. BERNAUDIN, E. PETIT, *et al.* 2000. Expression of receptors for complement anaphylatoxins C3a and C5a following permanent focal cerebral ischemia in the mouse. Exp. Neurol. **161:** 373–382.
61. BARNUM, S.R., R.S. AMES, P.R. MAYCOX, *et al.* 2002. Expression of the complement C3a and C5a receptors after permanent focal ischemia: an alternative interpretation. Glia **38:** 169–173.
62. STAHEL, P.F., K. KARIYA, E. SHOHAMI, *et al.* 2000. Intracerebral complement C5a receptor (CD88) expression is regulated by TNF and lymphotoxin-alpha following closed head injury in mice. J. Neuroimmunol. **109:** 164–172.
63. STAHEL, P.F., T. KOSSMANN, M.C. MORGANTI-KOSSMANN, *et al.* 1997. Experimental diffuse axonal injury induces enhanced neuronal C5a receptor mRNA expression in rats. Brain Res. Mol. Brain Res. **50:** 205–212.
64. SAYAH, S., A.M. ISCHENKO, A. ZHAKHOV, *et al.* 1999. Expression of cytokines by human astrocytomas following stimulation by C3a and C5a anaphylatoxins: specific increase in interleukin-6 mRNA expression. J. Neurochem. **72:** 2426–2436.
65. FARKAS, I., L. BARANYI, M. TAKAHASHI, *et al.* 1998. A neuronal C5a receptor and an associated apoptotic signal transduction pathway. J. Physiol. **507:** 679–687.
66. FARKAS, I., L. BARANYI, Z.S. LIPOSITS, *et al.* 1998. Complement C5a anaphylatoxin fragment causes apoptosis in TGW neuroblastoma cells. Neuroscience **86:** 903–911.
67. MUKHERJEE, P. & G.M. PASINETTI. 2001. Complement anaphylatoxin C5a neuroprotects through mitogen-activated protein kinase-dependent inhibition of caspase 3. J. Neurochem. **77:** 43–49.
68. OSAKA, H., A. MCGINTY, U.E. HOEPKEN, *et al.* 1999. Expression of C5a receptor in mouse brain: role in signal transduction and neurodegeneration. Neuroscience **88:** 1073–1082.
69. OSAKA, H., P. MUKHERJEE, P.S. AISEN & G.M. PASINETTI. 1999. Complement-derived anaphylatoxin C5a protects against glutamate-mediated neurotoxicity. J. Cell. Biochem. **73:** 303–311.
70. HEESE, K., C. HOCK & U. OTTEN. 1998. Inflammatory signals induce neurotrophin expression in human microglial cells. J. Neurochem. **70:** 699–707.
71. VAN BEEK, J., O. NICOLE, C. ALI, *et al.* 2001. Complement anaphylatoxin C3a is selectively protective against NMDA-induced neuronal cell death. Neuroreport **12:** 289–293.
72. MORGAN, B.P. 1989. Complement membrane attack on nucleated cells: resistance, recovery and non-lethal effects. Biochem. J. **264:** 1–14.
73. RUS, H.G., F.I. NICULESCU & M.L. SHIN. 2001. Role of the C5b-9 complement complex in cell cycle and apoptosis. Immunol. Rev. **180:** 49–55.
74. WIEDMER, T., B. ANDO & P.J. SIMS. 1987. Complement C5b-9-stimulated platelet secretion is associated with a Ca^{2+}-initiated activation of cellular protein kinases. J. Biol. Chem. **262:** 13674–13681.
75. NICULESCU, F., H. RUS, S. SHIN, *et al.* 1993. Generation of diacylglycerol and ceramide during homologous complement activation. J. Immunol. **150:** 214–224.
76. IMAGAWA, D.K., N.E. OSIFCHIN, W.A. PAZNEKAS, *et al.* 1983. Consequences of cell membrane attack by complement: release of arachidonate and formation of inflammatory derivatives. Proc. Natl. Acad. Sci. USA **80:** 6647–6651.
77. SHIRAZI, Y., F.A. MCMORRIS & M.L. SHIN. 1989. Arachidonic acid mobilization and phosphoinositide turnover by the terminal complement complex, C5b-9, in rat oligodendrocyte x C6 glioma cell hybrids. J. Immunol. **142:** 4385–4391.
78. SHIRAZI, Y., D.K. IMAGAWA & M.L. SHIN. 1987. Release of leukotriene B4 from sublethally injured oligodendrocytes by terminal complement complexes. J. Neurochem. **48:** 271–278.
79. CARNEY, D.F., T.J. LANG & M.L. SHIN. 1990. Multiple signal messengers generated by terminal complement complexes and their role in terminal complement complex elimination. J. Immunol. **145:** 623–629.

80. MASON, J.C., H. YARWOOD, K. SUGARS, *et al.* 1999. Induction of decay-accelerating factor by cytokines or the membrane-attack complex protects vascular endothelial cells against complement deposition. Blood **94:** 1673–1682.
81. RUS, H.G., F. NICULESCU & M.L. SHIN. 1996. Sublytic complement attack induces cell cycle in oligodendrocytes. J. Immunol. **156:** 4892–4900.
82. RUS, H., F. NICULESCU, T. BADEA & M.L. SHIN. 1997. Terminal complement complexes induce cell cycle entry in oligodendrocytes through mitogen activated protein kinase pathway. Immunopharmacology **38:** 177–187.
83. SOANE, L., H. RUS, F. NICULESCU & M.L. SHIN. 1999. Inhibition of oligodendrocyte apoptosis by sublytic C5b-9 is associated with enhanced synthesis of bcl-2 and mediated by inhibition of caspase-3 activation. J. Immunol. **163:** 6132–6138.
84. RUS, H., S. WEERTH, L. SOANE, *et al.* 2002. The effect of terminal complement complex on apoptosis gene expression in experimental autoimmune encephalomyelitis. Int. Immunol. **2:** 1248.
85. MCGEER, P.L., H. AKIYAMA, S. ITAGAKI & E.G. MCGEER. 1989. Activation of the classical complement pathway in brain tissue of Alzheimer patients. Neurosci. Lett. **107:** 341–346.
86. EIKELENBOOM, P. & F.C. STAM. 1982. Immunoglobulins and complement factors in senile plaques. An immunoperoxidase study. Acta Neuropathol. (Berl.) **57:** 239–242.
87. EIKELENBOOM, P. & F.C. STAM. 1984. An immunohistochemical study on cerebral vascular and senile plaque amyloid in Alzheimer's dementia. Virchow's Arch. B Cell. Pathol. Incl. Mol. Pathol. **47:** 17–25.
88. YAMADA, T., P.L. MCGEER & E.G. MCGEER. 1992. Lewy bodies in Parkinson's disease are recognized by antibodies to complement proteins. Acta Neuropathol. (Berl.) **84:** 100–104.
89. SINGHRAO, S.K., J.W. NEAL, P. GASQUE, *et al.* 1996. Role of complement in the aetiology of Pick's disease? J. Neuropathol. Exp. Neurol. **55:** 578–593.
90. TERAI, K., D.G. WALKER, E.G. MCGEER & P.L. MCGEER. 1997. Neurons express proteins of the classical complement pathway in Alzheimer disease. Brain Res. **769:** 385–390.
91. GASQUE, P., S.K. SINGHRAO, J.W. NEAL, *et al.* 1997. Expression of the receptor for complement C5a (CD88) is up-regulated on reactive astrocytes, microglia, and endothelial cells in the inflamed human central nervous system. Am. J. Pathol. **150:** 31–41.
92. GASQUE, P., S.K. SINGHRAO, J.W. NEAL, *et al.* 1998. The receptor for complement anaphylatoxin C3a is expressed by myeloid cells and nonmyeloid cells in inflamed human central nervous system: analysis in multiple sclerosis and bacterial meningitis. J. Immunol. **160:** 3543–3554.
93. O'BARR, S.A., J. CAGUIOA, D. GRUOL, *et al.* 2001. Neuronal expression of a functional receptor for the C5a complement activation fragment. J. Immunol. **166:** 4154–4162.
94. STOLTZNER, S.E., T.J. GRENFELL, C. MORI, *et al.* 2000. Temporal accrual of complement proteins in amyloid plaques in Down's syndrome with Alzheimer's disease. Am. J. Pathol. **156:** 489–499.
95. JOHNSON, S.A., M. LAMPERT-ETCHELLS, G.M. PASINETTI, *et al.* 1992. Complement mRNA in the mammalian brain: responses to Alzheimer's disease and experimental brain lesioning. Neurobiol. Aging **13:** 641–648.
96. AKIYAMA, H., T. YAMADA, T. KAWAMATA & P.L. MCGEER. 1991. Association of amyloid P component with complement proteins in neurologically diseased brain tissue. Brain Res. **548:** 349–352.
97. WEBSTER, S., L.F. LUE, L. BRACHOVA, *et al.* 1997. Molecular and cellular characterization of the membrane attack complex, C5b-9, in Alzheimer's disease. Neurobiol. Aging **18:** 415–421.
98. ROGERS, J., N.R. COOPER, S. WEBSTER, *et al.* 1992. Complement activation by beta-amyloid in Alzheimer disease. Proc. Natl. Acad. Sci. USA **89:** 10016–10020.
99. SNYDER, S.W., G.T. WANG, L. BARRETT, *et al.* 1994. Complement C1q does not bind monomeric beta-amyloid. Exp. Neurol. **128:** 136–142.

100. JIANG, H., D. BURDICK, C.G. GLABE, *et al.* 1994. beta-Amyloid activates complement by binding to a specific region of the collagen-like domain of the C1q A chain. J. Immunol. **152:** 5050–5059.
101. VELAZQUEZ, P., D.H. CRIBBS, T.L. POULOS & A.J. TENNER. 1997. Aspartate residue 7 in amyloid beta-protein is critical for classical complement pathway activation: implications for Alzheimer's disease pathogenesis. Nat. Med. **3:** 77–79.
102. TACNET-DELORME, P., S. CHEVALLIER & G.J. ARLAUD. 2001. Beta-amyloid fibrils activate the C1 complex of complement under physiological conditions: evidence for a binding site for A beta on the C1q globular regions. J. Immunol. **167:** 6374–6381.
103. YING, S.C., A.T. GEWURZ, H. JIANG & H. GEWURZ. 1993. Human serum amyloid P component oligomers bind and activate the classical complement pathway via residues 14-26 and 76-92 of the A chain collagen-like region of C1q. J. Immunol. **150:** 169–176.
104. AGRAWAL, A., A.K. SHRIVE, T.J. GREENHOUGH & J.E. VOLANAKIS. 2001. Topology and structure of the C1q-binding site on C-reactive protein. J. Immunol. **166:** 3998–4004.
105. VOLANAKIS, J.E. 1982. Complement activation by C-reactive protein complexes. Ann. N. Y. Acad. Sci. **389:** 235–250.
106. AKIYAMA, H., S. BARGER, S. BARNUM, *et al.* 2000. Inflammation and Alzheimer's disease. Neurobiol. Aging **21:** 383–421.
107. WEGIEL, J. & H.M. WISNIEWSKI. 1990. The complex of microglial cells and amyloid star in three-dimensional reconstruction. Acta Neuropathol. (Berl.) **81:** 116–124.
108. FRACKOWIAK, J., H.M. WISNIEWSKI, J. WEGIEL, *et al.* 1992. Ultrastructure of the microglia that phagocytose amyloid and the microglia that produce beta-amyloid fibrils. Acta Neuropathol. (Berl.) **84:** 225–233.
109. FRAUTSCHY, S.A., G.M. COLE & A. BAIRD. 1992. Phagocytosis and deposition of vascular beta-amyloid in rat brains injected with Alzheimer beta-amyloid. Am. J. Pathol. **140:** 1389–1399.
110. SCHENK, D., R. BARBOUR, W. DUNN, *et al.* 1999. Immunization with amyloid-beta attenuates Alzheimer-disease-like pathology in the PDAPP mouse. Nature **400:** 173–177.
111. BACSKAI, B.J., S.T. KAJDASZ, R.H. CHRISTIE, *et al.* 2001. Imaging of amyloid-beta deposits in brains of living mice permits direct observation of clearance of plaques with immunotherapy. Nat. Med. **7:** 369–372.
112. BARD, F., C. CANNON, R. BARBOUR, *et al.* 2000. Peripherally administered antibodies against amyloid beta-peptide enter the central nervous system and reduce pathology in a mouse model of Alzheimer disease. Nat. Med. **6:** 916–919.
113. WYSS-CORAY, T., F. YAN, A.H. LIN, *et al.* 2002. Prominent neurodegeneration and increased plaque formation in complement-inhibited Alzheimer's mice. Proc. Natl. Acad. Sci. USA **99:** 10837–10842.
114. MORGAN, B.P. 1996. Intervention in the complement system: a therapeutic strategy in inflammation. Biochem. Soc. Trans. **24:** 224–229.

Role of Nitric Oxide in Regulating the Rat Hypothalamic-Pituitary-Adrenal Axis Response to Endotoxemia

CATHERINE RIVIER

The Clayton Foundation Laboratories for Peptide Biology, The Salk Institute, La Jolla, California 92037, USA

ABSTRACT: This work examines the role of nitric oxide (NO) in the periphery (i.e., on the pituitary) and the brain (particularly on corticotropin-releasing factor [CRF] and vasopressin [VP] neurons in the paraventricular nucleus [PVN] of the hypothalamus) as a modulator of the ACTH response to lipopolysaccharide. We previously showed that NO restricted the pituitary response to VP while it facilitated the synthesis of PVN CRF and VP. In our experience, only relatively high doses of lipopolysaccharide (>50 μg/kg, injected intravenously [iv]) cause detectable increases in PVN neuronal activation. Our hypothesis, therefore, was that pituitary NO-VP interactions would predominate in rats injected with a low dose of lipopolysaccharide (0.5 μg/kg, iv) while the stimulatory influence of the gas on PVN neuronal activity would play an important role following iv injection of a large dose of lipopolysaccharide (50 μg/kg, iv). We observed that the ability of 0.5 μg/kg lipopolysaccharide to release ACTH was significantly enhanced by the subcutaneous (sc), but not the intracerebroventricular (icv) injection of L-NAME, an arginine derivative that blocks NO synthesis. The effect of sc L-NAME was reversed by immunoneutralization of endogenous VP, which indicated that in this model, the ability of lipopolysaccharide to release ACTH depended, at least in part, on the influence exerted by NO on the pituitary response to VP. In rats injected with the high lipopolysaccharide dose, the sc injection of L-NAME decreased plasma ACTH levels compared to those in rats pretreated with the vehicle. The effect of sc L-NAME was not significantly altered by VP antibodies. These results indicate that in this model, the primary influence of NO was exerted in the PVN and/or its afferents and that it did not depend on a peripheral, VP-mediated effect of the gas. On the one hand, these data are at odds with our finding that the icv injection of L-NAME only marginally altered the ACTH response to the large dose of lipopolysaccharide. As icv injected L-NAME should have primarily decreased hypothalamic, but not pituitary NOS, its only modest influence on ACTH release may have been due to a balance between stimulating and inhibiting effects of NO within the brain. As high doses of lipopolysaccharide increase brain levels of prostaglandin, monoamine, and proinflammatory cytokines, it will be important to investigate the influence exerted by NO on these secretagogues and on their interactions with PVN CRF and VP neurons, which may help us resolve the issues raised by our results. Collectively, these data support our hypothesis that the mechanisms mediating the ACTH

Address for correspondence: Catherine Rivier, Ph.D., The Salk Institute, 10010 N. Torrey Pines Road, La Jolla, CA 92037. Voice: 858-453-4100; fax: 858-552-1546.
crivier@salk.edu

Ann. N.Y. Acad. Sci. 992: 72–85 (2003). © 2003 New York Academy of Sciences.

response to a low lipopolysaccharide concentration involve the inhibitory VP-mediated influence of NO on pituitary activity. By contrast, the stimulatory effect of high doses of lipopolysaccharide on ACTH release depends, at least in part, on the ability of NO to upregulate PVN neuronal activity.

KEYWORDS: ACTH; nitric oxide; lipopolysaccharide (LPS); endotoxemia; rats; HPA axis

INTRODUCTION

Nitric oxide (NO) in an unstable gas that acts as a diffusible messenger in the brain, where it mediates critical processes such as neurotransmission, immune defense, vasodilatation, and endocrine signaling.[1–8] NO has also been reported to modulate a variety of neuroendocrine activities, including the response of the hypothalamic-pituitary-adrenal (HPA) axis to homeostatic threats ("stressors").[9,10] Our interest in the putative role of NO in regulating the HPA axis was based on the observation that NO synthase (NOS), the enzymes responsible for NO formation, was present in hypothalamic neurons known to produce two peptides that regulate ACTH release, namely, corticotropin-releasing factor (CRF) and vasopressin (VP).[11–17] Our studies aimed at investigating the role of NO in regulating ACTH secretion showed that blockade of NO formation with arginine derivatives such as L-N_{ω}nitro-L-arginine-methylester (L-NAME) significantly augmented the ACTH response to VP (but interestingly not CRF) and circulating proinflammatory cytokines.[10,18–21] These results indicated an inhibitory influence of NO on the pituitary response to secretagogues such as VP. On the other hand, we also reported that L-NAME blunted the HPA axis response to physico-emotional stresses.[22,23] On the basis of these experiments, we concluded that NO stimulated CRF- and VP-containing neurons in the paraventricular nucleus (PVN) of the hypothalamus, a hypothesis recently supported by our finding that the intracerebroventricular (icv) injection of the NO donor 3-morpholino-sydnonimine (SIN-1) significantly upregulated the neuronal activity of PVN CRF and VP cell bodies.[24]

Collectively, our studies have therefore suggested that in the intact rodent, endogenous NO exerts opposite effects in the periphery (where it is inhibitory) and in brain regions protected by the blood-brain barrier (BBB, where it is stimulatory). This has greatly complicated interpretation of experiments in which NO formation was blocked with arginine derivatives injected systemically, because the ability of these reagents to readily cross the BBB does not allow the investigator to distinguish between the peripheral and central roles of this gas. On the other hand, it might provide at least a partial explanation for some puzzling results that we accumulated over the years and that indicated that the consequences of blocking NO formation in rats injected with endotoxin (lipopolysaccharide [LPS]) were variable and seemingly dependent on the dose of LPS administered.

The mechanisms mediating the ability of peripheral LPS administration to activate the HPA axis are complex and still not fully understood. LPS mimics many of the events of the acute phase response,[25] which include the release in the general circulation of proinflammatory cytokines such as tumor necrosis factor-α (TNF-α), interleukin-1β (IL-1β), and interleukin-6 (IL-6).[26–30] These cytokines can act within the median eminence where they release CRF and VP from nerve terminals, an event that comes under the inhibitory influence exerted by NO in this region.[18] As even low doses of LPS increase circulating proinflammatory levels, it is likely that the ACTH response elicited in this model depends at least in part on the peripheral influence of NO. At high doses, LPS also upregulates the neuronal activity of PVN neurons that express the CRF, CRF receptors type 1 and VP genes,[31–33] an effect that may involve brain production of secretagogues such as prostaglandins[34,35] and catecholamines.[36,37] The extent to which the influence of LPS on the HPA axis, including those on PVN neurons, depends on brain cytokines remains debated and has been extensively discussed elsewhere (ref. in Ref. 38). Regardless, however, if one accepts the concept that LPS stimulates the HPA axis through mechanisms that involve both increased CRF and VP release from nerve terminals and increased activity of their cell bodies in the PVN, a reasonable question pertains to the net influence exerted by NO: will it be dominated by the inhibitory effect of this gas on the pituitary response to VP or by its stimulatory effect on CRF/VP neurons? On the basis of recent results indicating that relatively large (≥50 μg/kg), but not more modest (≤5 μg/kg), doses of intravenously injected LPS significantly upregulate the expression of immediate early genes in the PVN (Lee and Rivier, unpublished), we propose that the early ACTH response to mild endotoxemia may primarily be dependent on an effect of the endotoxin on nerve terminals and/or the pituitary, rather than a direct influence on PVN cell bodies.

If our hypothesis is correct, systemic L-NAME should enhance ACTH release because NO inhibits the pituitary response to VP.[18] By contrast, ACTH released by large doses of LPS should also involve increased PVN neuronal activity even during the early phase of pituitary activation, a response that results from a direct, possibly vagally mediated[39] effect of endotoxin on the hypothalamus, in addition to a putative subsequent compensatory response to peptide depletion. In this case, the inhibitory effect of peripheral NO on the pituitary response to VP would probably be counterbalanced by the stimulatory influence of the gas on PVN neurons, and systemic L-NAME should either not alter or slightly inhibit ACTH release. In addition to addressing these questions, we also investigated the role of peripheral and central NO in mediating the ability of LPS to release ACTH by comparing the ability of the sc and icv injection of L-NAME to alter LPS-induced ACTH secretion. In parallel, we used another model of stress, namely, exposure to mild electrofootshocks, which releases ACTH without significantly increasing levels of circulating proinflammatory cytokines while stimulating PVN neuronal activation.[40] Finally, we injected L-NAME concomitantly with VP antibodies to eliminate the contribution of endogenous VP, which primarily reflects the peripheral influence of NO.[18,20] Collectively, these results provide additional information regarding the mechanisms through which NO modulates HPA axis activity.

MATERIALS AND METHODS

Animals

Adult male Sprague-Dawley (250–270 g) rats were acclimated to standard laboratory conditions (12 h light/12 h dark cycle, lights on from 0600) with free access to rat chow (Harlan-Teklad, Madison, WI) and water.

Experimental Procedures

When warranted, icv cannulas were inserted in the right brain ventricle, a surgery performed under anesthesia with ketamine (100 mg/kg)/acepromazine (4 mg/kg)/ xylazine (10 mg/kg).[41] Seven days later, the rats underwent ascetic insertion of a right jugular venous catheter.[18] The experiments were carried out 48–72 hours later. The iv cannulas, which were connected to syringes through about 50-cm long, PE-50 tubing filled with heparinized saline solution, served both to deliver LPS or its vehicle (0.5 ml) and to remove blood samples. The icv cannulas contained the treatments prepared in a 5 μl volume, which were infused at a rate of 1 μl/10 seconds. L-NAME or its vehicle was injected sc 3 hours icv 30 minutes prior to the start of the experiment, and treatments were timed so that each animal was individually treated according to this time schedule. VP antibodies, when used, were injected iv 15 minutes prior to L-NAME or at a corresponding time in vehicle-treated rats. Blood samples (0.3 ml/bleed) were obtained immediately prior to LPS/vehicle or shocks as well as sequentially thereafter, as indicated on the figures.

The assays were performed in awake, freely moving animals that were placed in individual buckets 3 hours prior to the start of each experiment and kept in a noise-free environment thereafter. All procedures were approved by the Salk Institute IACUC.

Shocks

Mild, inescapable footshocks (0.5 mA, 1-sec duration, 2 shocks/min) were delivered to the rats' paws using a Coulbourn HO2-08 grid floor shocker controlled by a Macintosh computer (Coulbourn Instruments, Allentown, PA).[42]

Reagents

LPS (*E. coli* serotype O26:B6, code L-3755, Lot 37H4095) and L-NAME were purchased from Sigma Corp. (St. Louis, MO). LPS and L-NAME for sc injections were diluted in apyrogenic saline solution. L-NAME for icv injection was prepared in apyrogenic water. VP antibodies, raised in rabbits in our laboratory and generously provided by Joan Vaughan and Dr. Wylie Vale (Salk Institute, La Jolla, CA), were injected iv at 1.0 ml/kg, a dose that totally blocks the ACTH response to even large concentrations of exogenously administered VP.[22] VP and rat/human CRF, synthesized by solid phase methodology[43] and generously provided by Dr. Jean Rivier (Salk Institute, La Jolla, CA), were diluted in apyrogenic phosphate-buffered saline solution containing 0.1% BSA and 0.01% ascorbic acid, and injected iv at a dose previously shown appropriate for study of its interaction with NO.[18,19] The CRF antagonist α-helCRF$_{9\text{-}41}$, also synthesized by solid phase methodology, was injected icv at a dose (10 μg) shown to significantly block centrally mediated biological responses that depend on endogenous CRF.[44,45] Control animals received the appropriate vehicles.

ACTH Assay

ACTH concentrations were determined by a two-site immunoradiometric assay (IRMA, Allegro, Nichols Institute, San Juan Capistrano, CA) using 50 μl plasma. This assay was previously validated for use in the rat.[18]

Statistical Analysis

All of the results are expressed as mean ± SEM. They were analyzed by factorial analysis of variance (ANOVA). When the analysis of variance was significant ($P < 0.05$), posthoc comparisons (Duncan New Multiple Range) were made to determine the statistical levels of differences between groups.

RESULTS

Effect of L-NAME on the ACTH Response to Vasopressin

To investigate the role of NO in brain areas protected by the BBB, L-NAME was injected icv. We first established that this icv treatment did not lead to leakage of the arginine derivative to the periphery,[46,47] which would compromise the interpretation of the results. In view of the ability of systemic L-NAME to augment the ACTH response to VP,[18] we reasoned that if icv injected L-NAME could reach the pituitary, it would alter the ACTH response to this peptide. Our previous results had indicated that 50 μg L-NAME significantly blocked hypothalamic, but not pituitary NOS activity, whereas 250 μg blocked both.[42] These data had suggested that 250 μg reached the pituitary, and the present experiment therefore focused on the 50-μg dose. As illustrated in FIGURE 1, the icv injection of this dose of L-NAME did not alter the ACTH response to VP, whereas systemic injection of the arginine derivative, at a dose (50 mg /kg, sc, 3 hours) that we previously found effective in blocking NO synthesis,[46, 47] produced the expected enhanced ACTH response.

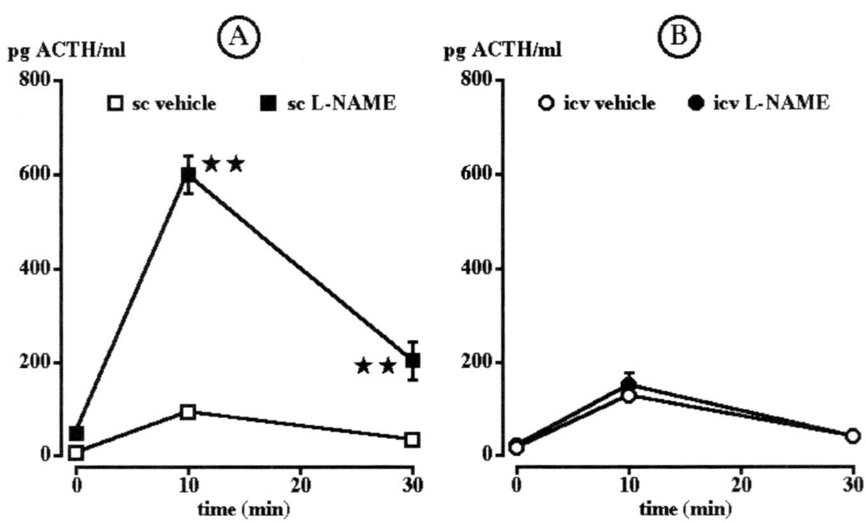

FIGURE 1. Effect of the sc (**A**, 50 mg/kg, –3 h) or icv (**B**, 50 μg, –30 min) injection of L-NAME on the ACTH response to vasopressin (VP, 0.2 μg/kg, iv). Each point represents the mean ± SEM of 5–6 intact male rats. $^{**}P < 0.01$.

Role of PVN CRF in the ACTH Response to LPS

As indicated in the Introduction, we had observed that high (>50 μg/kg), but not low (<5 μg/kg) doses of LPS upregulated PVN neuronal activity (Lee and Rivier, unpublished). These results suggested that PVN CRF might mediate, at least in part, the ACTH response to 50, but not to 0.5 μg/kg LPS. To test this hypothesis, we injected the CRF antagonist α-helCRF$_{9\text{-}41}$ icv prior to LPS. First, we showed that this model did not lead to leakage of the antagonist to the pituitary, by measuring the ACTH response to exogenous CRF injection in the presence or absence of the antagonist. As illustrated in FIGURE 2, CRF released comparable amounts of ACTH in rats pretreated with the vehicle or α-helCRF$_{9\text{-}41}$. This antagonist did not alter the ACTH response to 0.5 μg/kg LPS, but significantly (P <0.01) decreased it after injection of 50 μg/kg LPS (FIG. 3).

Effect of L-NAME on the ACTH Response to 0.5 μg or 50 μg Lipopolysaccharide/kg

These experiments were designed to determine if the mechanisms responsible for the ACTH response to a low dose of LPS primarily involved the inhibitory effect exerted by NO in the periphery, whereas those involved after injection of a high dose of LPS did not. We show here that ACTH levels of rats injected with 0.5 μg LPS/kg were significantly (P <0.01) increased by the sc injection of L-NAME (FIG. 4A), a treatment known to augment the ACTH response to VP.[18,20] By contrast, the icv injection of the arginine derivative was without effect (FIG. 4B). Sc administered L-

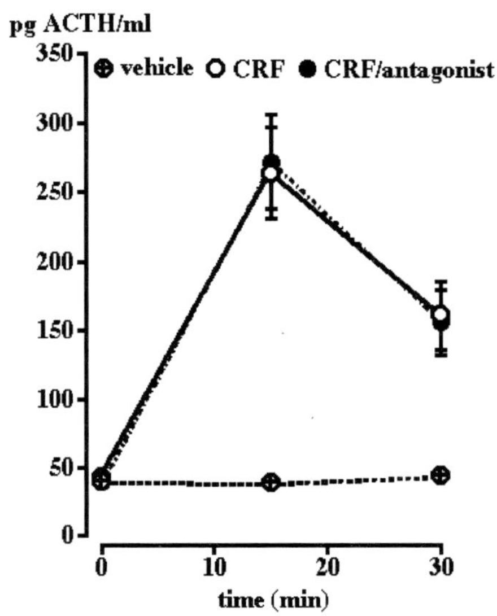

FIGURE 2. Effect of α-helCRF$_{9\text{-}41}$ (10 μg, icv, −30 min) on the ACTH response to corticotropin-releasing factor (CRF, 1 mg/kg, iv). Each point represents the mean ± SEM of 5–6 intact male rats.

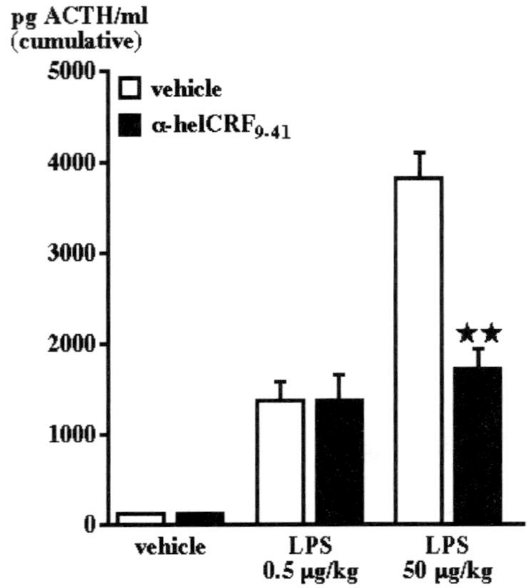

FIGURE 3. Effect of α-helCRF$_{9\text{-}41}$ (10 μg, icv, –30 min) on the ACTH response to lipopolysaccharide (LPS, 0.5 or 50 μg/kg, iv). Each point represents the mean ± SEM of 5–7 intact male rats. $^{**}P < 0.01$.

NAME significantly ($P < 0.01$) decreased the effect of 50 μg LPS/kg, whereas again L-NAME administered icv did not alter ACTH levels in endotoxemic animals (FIG. 5A and B).

Role of Vasopressin in the ACTH Response to Lipopolysaccharide

As peripheral NO inhibits the ACTH response to VP, these experiments were designed to examine the role of NO in the absence of this peptide. The ACTH response to 0.5 μg LPS/kg was significantly ($P < 0.01$) enhanced by L-NAME, administered sc (FIG. 6). These results correspond to those illustrated in FIGURE 1A. Immunoneutralization of endogenous VP decreased ($P < 0.05$) the effect of LPS, whereas concomitant removal of NO and VP yielded ACTH levels that were statistically comparable to those of rats injected with the vehicle. Both the sc and iv injection of L-NAME and VP antibodies, respectively, significantly ($P < 0.05$–0.01) decreased ACTH levels in rats injected with 50 μg LPS/kg, and concomitant injection of L-NAME and VP antibodies restored ACTH concentrations to those measured following administration of the arginine derivative alone (FIG. 7).

Role of Nitric Oxide and Vasopressin in Rats Exposed to Shocks

Shocks produced the expected rise in plasma ACTH levels (FIG. 6). Both the sc (FIG. 8A) and icv (FIG. 8B) injection of L-NAME significantly ($P < 0.01$) decreased this response. As previously reported,[22] VP antibodies also interfered with shock-induced ACTH release but did not alter the influence of NO (FIG. 9).

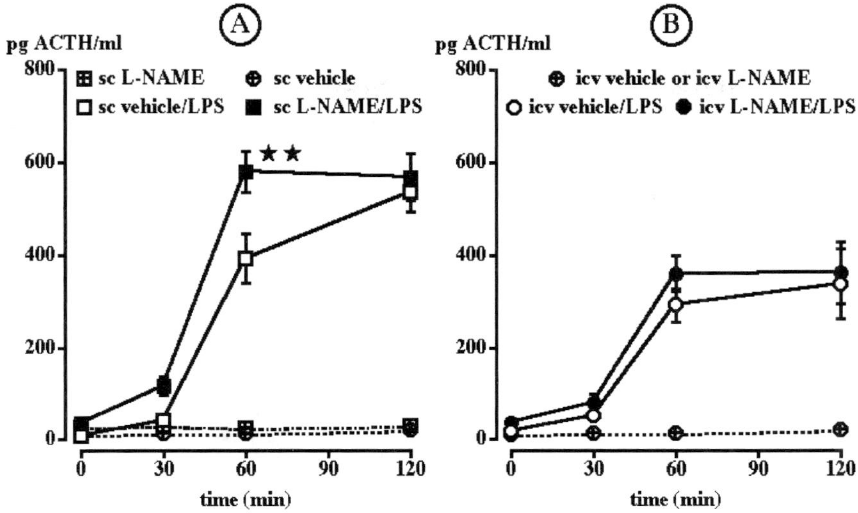

FIGURE 4. Effect of the sc (**A**, 50 mg/kg, –3 h) or icv (**B**, 50 μg, –30 min) injection of L-NAME on the ACTH response to lipopolysaccharide (LPS, 0.5 μg/kg, iv). Each point represents the mean ± SEM of 5–6 intact male rats. ***P* <0.01 vs vehicle/LPS.

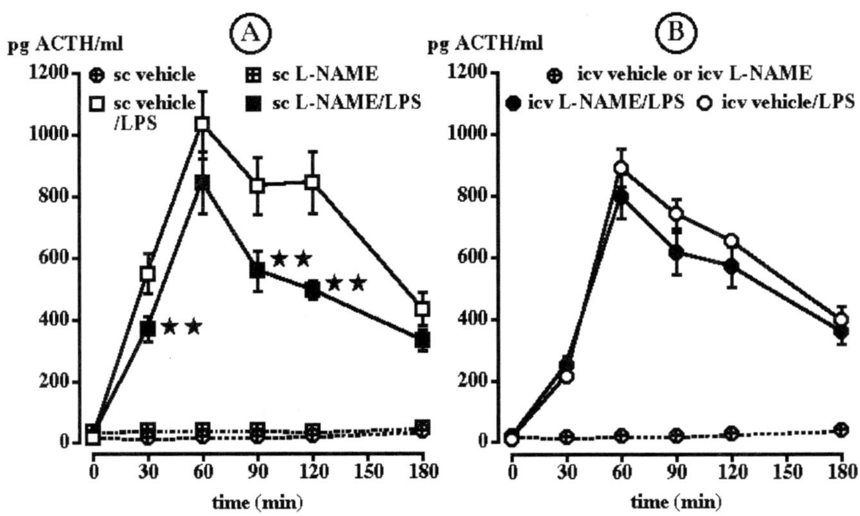

FIGURE 5. Effect of the sc (**A**, 50 mg/kg, –3 h) or icv (**B**, 50 μg, –30 min) injection of L-NAME on the ACTH response to lipopolysaccharide (LPS, 50 μg/kg, iv). Each point represents the mean ± SEM of 5–6 intact male rats. ***P* <0.01 vs vehicle/LPS.

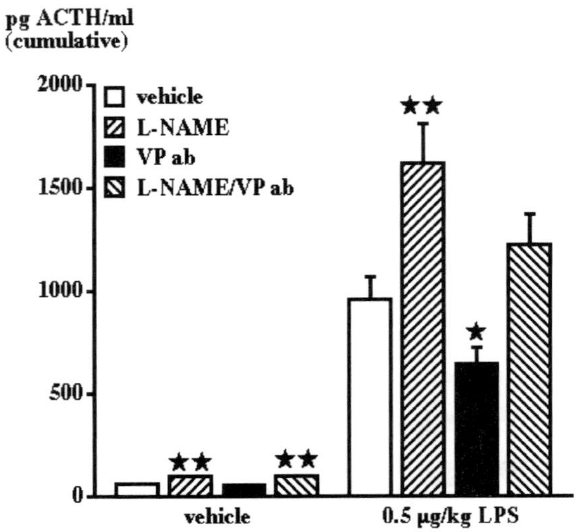

FIGURE 6. Effect of the injection of the vehicle, L-NAME (50 mg/kg, sc, –3 h), vasopressin (VP) antibodies (ab, 1.0 ml/kg, iv, –15 min) or both on the ACTH response to lipopolysaccharide (LPS, 0.5 µg/kg, iv). Data are presented as cumulative ACTH levels over 90 minutes after LPS injection. Each bar represents mean ± SEM of 5–6 intact male rats. *P <0.05 and **P <0.01 vs corresponding vehicle.

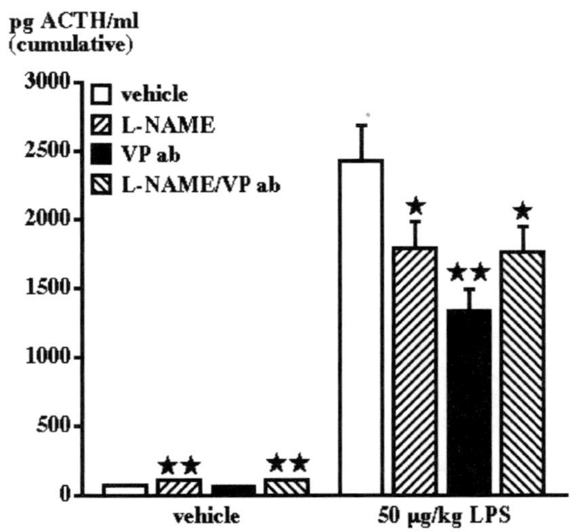

FIGURE 7. Effect of the injection of the vehicle, L-NAME (50 mg/kg, sc, –3 h), vasopressin (VP) antibodies (ab, 1.0 ml/kg, iv, –15 min), or both on the ACTH response to lipopolysaccharide (LPS, 50 µg/kg, iv). Data are presented as cumulative ACTH levels over 90 minutes after LPS injection. Each bar represents mean ± SEM of 5–6 intact male rats. *P <0.05 and **P <0.01 vs corresponding vehicle.

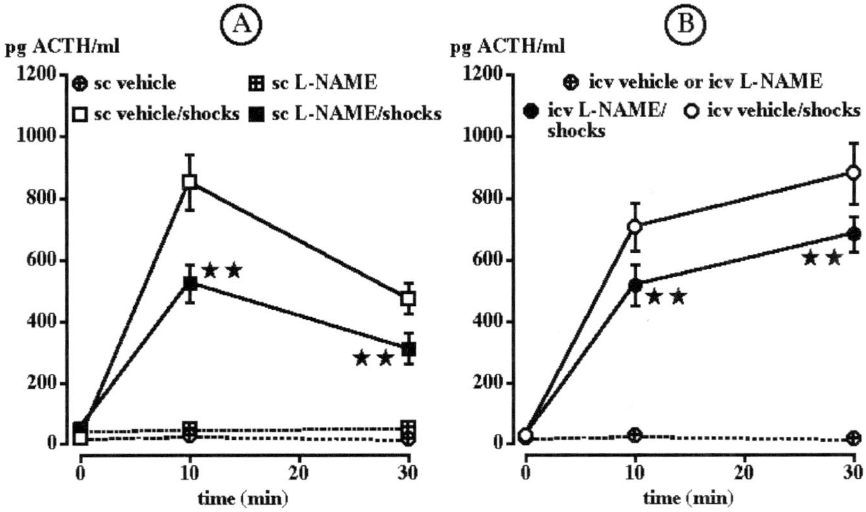

FIGURE 8. Effect of the sc (50 mg/kg, –3 h) or icv (50 µg, –30 min) injection of the L-NAME on the ACTH response to shocks. Each point represents the mean ± SEM of 6–7 intact male rats rats. $^{**}P < 0.01$ vs vehicle/shocks.

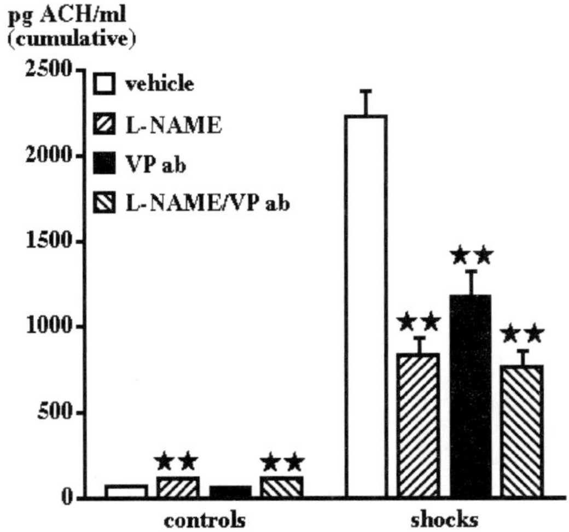

FIGURE 9. Effect of the injection of the vehicle L-NAME (50 mg/kg, sc, –3 h), vasopressin (VP) antibodies (1.0 ml/kg, iv, –15 min) or both on the ACTH response to shocks. Data are presented as cumulative ACTH levels over 45 minutes of exposure to shocks. Each bar represents mean ± SEM of 7–8 intact male rats. $^{**}P < 0.01$ vs corresponding vehicle.

DISCUSSION

The present work was designed to examine and compare the influence of NO exerted in the periphery (i.e., on peptide release from nerve terminals and/or the influence of these peptides on the corticotrophs) and that exerted in brain areas protected by the BBB, specifically, CRF and VP neurons in the PVN. We had predicted that in rats administered low LPS doses, in which PVN neuronal activation remains very modest (Lee and Rivier, unpublished) and blockade of PVN CRF receptors does not alter ACTH release, the sc injection of L-NAME would exert a stimulatory effect because the primary influence of NO would be to inhibit the pituitary response to VP.[18,20] By contrast, the icv injection of L-NAME would exert little effect, which reflected the lack of increased PVN neuronal activity. These hypotheses were confirmed by our results. Additionally, if the influence of peripheral NO was primarily mediated by its ability to inhibit VP-induced ACTH release, we expected that removing endogenous VP would interfere with it. This hypothesis was also supported by our data. In rats injected with a large dose of LPS, which exhibit significant PVN neuronal activation and in which blockade of PVN CRF receptors blunts ACTH release, we had predicted that the influence of L-NAME would be inhibitory because the dominant influence of NO would be to facilitate synthesis and release of CRF and VP from the PVN. We found that, indeed, sc L-NAME decreased the ACTH response to 50 μg/kg LPS, but surprisingly the icv administration of this reagent only had a marginal effect. As a comparable dose of icv L-NAME interfered with the ability of shocks to release ACTH, and as we previously showed that this treatment markedly reduced hypothalamic NOS activity,[42] it is unlikely that the lack of effect of the arginine derivative in endotoxemic rats was due to a faulty protocol. In trying to explain these unexpected results, it may be relevant to note that VP antibodies did not alter the influence of sc injected L-NAME in rats administered 50 μg/kg LPS. This latter observation suggests that the influence of peripheral NO in this model did not involve, as we had predicted, its inhibition of VP-induced ACTH release. As mentioned above, large doses of LPS increase brain levels of prostaglandins, monoamines, and proinflammatory cytokines.[34–37,48] At present, we do not know how NO interacts with these signals and whether it alters their net influence on PVN neuronal activity. It is therefore possible that the modest influence of icv L-NAME in rats injected with 50 μg LPS/kg reflects the balance between the stimulatory effect of NO on PVN CRF and VP neurons[49] and putative inhibitory effects on circuits that impinge on these neurons. With regard to the shock model, the ability of both sc and icv injected L-NAME to inhibit ACTH secretion emphasizes the fact that NO primarily acted on PVN neurons. Our finding that VP antibodies did not alter the consequences of blocking peripheral NO formation further supports this concept. However, these results are somewhat difficult to reconcile with the fact that by themselves, VP antibodies reduced the ACTH response to shocks. Indeed, this latter observation indicates that VP was released during shocks and participated in the ensuing activation of pituitary corticotrophs, an observation that confirms our previous work.[22,50] One possibility is that the contribution of peripheral NO may have been obscured by the role played by the gas within the hypothalamus. In other words, the ability of sc L-NAME to augment VP-induced ACTH release, and thus the ACTH response to shocks, may have been quantatively smaller than the inhibition exerted by this arginine derivative within the PVN and/or its afferents.

In conclusion, we have shown that the ACTH response to the injection of a low (0.5 μg/kg) dose of LPS is mediated in part by the ability of peripheral NO to inhibit VP-induced ACTH release. By contrast, the influence of NO in rats injected with 50 μg/kg LPS or in animals exposed to shocks does not involve VP.

ACKNOWLEDGMENTS

The excellent technical assistance of Elaine Law, Melissa Herman, and Yaira Haas is gratefully acknowledged. Research was supported by National Institutes of Health Grant MH-51774 and the Foundation for Research.

REFERENCES

1. Moncada, S., R.M.J. Palmer & E.A. Higgs. 1991. Nitric oxide: physiology, pathophysiology, and pharmacology. Pharmacol. Rev. **43:** 109–142.
2. Bredt, D.S. & S.H. Snyder. 1994. Nitric oxide: a physiologic messenger molecule. Annu. Rev. Biochem. **63:** 175–195.
3. Amir, S. 1995. Nitric oxide signalling in the hypothalamus. *In* Nitric Oxide in the Nervous System. :151–162. Academic Press Limited. San Diego.
4. Brann, D. *et al.* 1997. Gaseous transmitters and neuroendocrine regulation. Neuroendocrinology **65:** 385–395.
5. Dawson, T. & S. Snyder. 1994. Gases as biological messengers: nitric oxide and carbon monoxide in the brain. J. Neurosci. **14:** 5147–5159.
6. Schuman, E. & D. Madison. 1994. Nitric oxide and synaptic functions. Ann. Rev. Neurosci. **17:** 153–183.
7. Moilanen, E. & H. Vapaatalo. 1995. Nitric oxide in inflammation and immune responses. Ann. Med. **27:** 359–367.
8. Snyder, S.H. & T.M. Dawson. 1995. Nitric oxide and related substances as neural messengers. *In* Psychopharmacology: The Fourth Generation of Progress. F.E. Bloom & D.J. Kupfer, Eds. :609–618. Raven Press, Ltd. New York.
9. Rivier, C. 1998. Role of nitric oxide and carbon monoxide in modulating the ACTH response to immune and non-immune signals. Neuroimmunomodulation **5:** 203–213.
10. Turnbull, A. *et al.* 1998. Influence of carbon monoxide, and its interaction with nitric oxide, on the ACTH response of the intact rat to a physico-emotional stress. J. Neuroendocrinol. **10:** 793–802.
11. Rodrigo, J. *et al.* 1994. Localization of nitric oxide synthase in the adult rat brain. Phil. Trans. Roy. Soc. Lond. Ser. B - Biol. Sci. **345:** 175–221.
12. Hökfelt, T. *et al.* 1994. Plasticity of NO synthase expression in the nervous and endocrine systems. Neuropharmacology **33:** 1221–1227.
13. Torres, G., S. Lee & C. Rivier. 1993. Ontogeny of the rat hypothalamic nitric oxide synthase and colocalization with neuropeptides. Mol. Cell. Neurosci. **4:** 155–163.
14. Siaud, P. *et al.* 1994. A subpopulation of corticotropin-releasing hormone neurosecretory cells in the paraventricular nucleus of the hypothalamus also contain NADPH-diaphorase. Neurosci. Lett. **170:** 51–54.
15. Arevalo, A. *et al.* 1992. NADPH-diaphorase activity in the hypothalamic magnocellular neurosecretory nuclei of the rat. Brain Res. Bull. **28:** 599–603.
16. Sanchez, F. *et al.* 1994. Coexistence of NADPH-diaphorase with vasopressin and oxytocin in the hypothalamic magnocellular neurosecretory nuclei of the rat. Cell Tissue Res. **276:** 31–34.
17. Vincent, S.R. 1995. Localization of nitric oxide neurons in the central nervous system. *In* Nitric Oxide in the Nervous System. S.R. Vincent, Ed. :83–102. Academic Press Ltd.
18. Rivier, C. & G. Shen. 1994. In the rat, endogenous nitric oxide modulates the response of the hypothalamic-pituitary-adrenal axis to interleukin-1β, vasopressin and oxytocin. J. Neurosci. **14:** 1985–1993.

19. RIVIER, C. 1995. Blockade of nitric oxide formation augments adrenocorticotropin released by blood-borne interleukin-1β: role of vasopressin, prostaglandins, and α1-adrenergic receptors. Endocrinology **136:** 3597–3603.
20. TURNBULL, A.V. & C. RIVIER. 1996. Corticotropin-releasing factor, vasopressin and prostaglandins mediate, and nitric oxide restrains, the hypothalamic-pituitary-adrenal response to acute local inflammation in the rat. Endocrinology **137:** 455–463.
21. KIM, C.K. & C. RIVIER. 1998. Influence of nitric oxide synthase inhibitors on the ACTH and cytokine responses to peripheral immune signals. J. Neuroendocrinol. **10:** 353–362.
22. RIVIER, C. 1994. Endogenous nitric oxide participates in the activation of the hypothalamic-pituitary-adrenal axis by noxious stimuli. Endocr. J. **2:** 367–373.
23. LEE, S. & C. RIVIER. 1998. Interaction between corticotropin-releasing factor and nitric oxide in mediating the response of the rat hypothalamus to immune and non-immune stimuli. Mol. Brain Res. **57:** 54–62.
24. LEE, S. & C. RIVIER. 1998. The intracerebroventricular injection of the nitric oxide donor 3-morpholinosydnonimine (SIN-1) activates the rat hypothalamic-pituitary-adrenal axis [abstr.]. 28th Annual Meeting of the Society for Neuroscience.
25. BAUMANN, H. & J. GAULDIE. 1994. The acute phase response. Immunol. Today **15:** 74–80.
26. SHALABY, M.R. *et al.* 1989. Endotoxin, tumor necrosis factor-α and interleukin 1 induce interleukin 6 production *in vivo*. Clin. Immunol. Immunopathol. **53:** 488–498.
27. TAKAO, T. *et al.* 1997. Endotoxin induced increases in rat plasma pituitary-adreno-cortical hormones are better reflected by alterations in tumor necrosis factor α than interleukin-1β. Life Sci. **61:** PL263–PL268.
28. GIVALOIS, L. *et al.* 1994. Temporal cascade of plasma level surges in ACTH, corticosterone, and cytokines in endotoxin-challenged rats. Am. J. Physiol. **267:** R164–R170.
29. BESEDOVSKY, H.O. & A. DELREY. 1992. Immuno-neuroendocrine circuits: integrative role of cytokines. Front. Neuroendocrinol. **13:** 61–94.
30. DELREY, A. & H.O. BESEDOVSKY. 1992. Metabolic and neuroendocrine effects of pro-inflammatory cytokines. Eur. J. Clin. Invest. (Suppl.) **22:** 10–15.
31. KAKUCSKA, I. *et al.* 1993. Endotoxin-induced corticotropin-releasing hormone gene expression in the hypothalamic paraventricular nucleus is mediated centrally by interleukin-1. Endocrinology **133:** 815–821.
32. RIVEST, S., N. LAFLAMME & R. NAPPI. 1995. Immune challenge and immobilization stress induce transcription of the gene encoding the CRF receptor in selective nuclei of the rat hypothalamus. J. Neurosci. **15:** 2680–2695.
33. LACROIX, S. & S. RIVEST. 1996. Role of cyclo-oxygenase pathways in the stimulatory influence of immune challenge on the transcription of a specific CRF receptor subtype in the rat brain. J. Chem. Neuroanat. **10:** 53–71.
34. LACROIX, S. & S. RIVEST. 1997. Functional circuitry in the brain of immune-challenged rats: partial involvement of prostaglandins. J. Comp. Neurol. **387:** 307–324.
35. LACROIX, S. & S. RIVEST. 1998. Effect of acute systemic inflammatory response and cytokines on the transcription of the genes encoding cyclooxygenase enzymes (COX-1 and COX-2) in the rat brain. Neurochemistry **70:** 452–466.
36. DUNN, A. 1995. Interactions between the nervous system and the immune system: implications for psychopharmacology. *In* Psychopharmacology. F.E. Bloom & D.J. Kupfer, Eds. :719–731. Raven Press. New York.
37. LAVICKY, J. & A.J. DUNN. 1995. Endotoxin administration stimulates cerebral catecholamine release in freely moving rats as assessed by microdialysis. J. Neurosci. Res. **40:** 407–413.
38. TURNBULL, A.V.T. & C.L. RIVIER. 1999. Regulation of the hypothalamo-pituitary-adrenal (HPA) axis by cytokines: actions and mechanisms of action. Physiol. Rev. **79:** 1–71.
39. WAN, W.H. *et al.* 1994. Neural and biochemical mediators of endotoxin and stress-induced *c-fos* expression in the rat brain. Brain Res. Bull. **34:** 7–14.
40. LI, H.-Y. & P.E. SAWCHENKO. 1998. Hypothalamic effector neurons and extended circuitries activated in "neurogenic" stress: a comparison of footshock effects exerted

acutely, chronically, and in animals with controlled glucocorticoid levels. J. Comp. Neurol. **393:** 244–266.
41. LEE, S. & C. RIVIER. 1994. Hypophysiotropic role and hypothalamic gene expression of corticotropin-releasing factor and vasopressin in rats injected with interleukin-1β systemically or into the brain ventricles. J. Neuroendocrinol. **6:** 217–224.
42. KIM, C. & C. RIVIER. 2000. Nitric oxide and carbon monoxide have a stimulatory role in the hypothalamic-pituitary-adrenal response to physico-emotional stressors in rats. Endocrinology **141:** 2244–2253.
43. KORNREICH, W.D. *et al.* 1992. Alanine series of ovine corticotropin releasing factor (oCRF): a structure-activity relationship study. J. Med. Chem. **35:** 1870–1876.
44. KOOB, G.F. *et al.* 1993. The role of corticotropin-releasing factor in behavioural responses to stress. Ciba Foundation Symposium, No. 172. *In* Corticotropin-Releasing Factor. D.J. Chadwick, J. Marsh & K. Ackrill, Eds. :277–295. John Wiley & Sons. New York, NY.
45. KOOB, G.F. & S.C. HEINRICHS. 1999. A role for corticotropin releasing factor and urocortin in behavioral responses to stressors. Brain Res. **848:** 141–152.
46. TURNBULL, A. & C. RIVIER. 1998. Intracerebroventricular passive immunization. I. The effect of intracerebroventricular administration of an antiserum to tumor necrosis factor-α on the plasma adrenocorticotropin response to lipopolysaccharide in rats. Endocrinology **139:** 119–127.
47. TURNBULL, A. & C. RIVIER. 1998. Intracerebroventricular passive immunization. II. Intracerebroventricular infusion of neuropeptide antisera can inhibit neuropeptide signaling in peripheral tissues. Endocrinology **139:** 128–136.
48. VALLIÈRES, L. & S. RIVEST. 1997. Regulation of the genes encoding interleukin-6, its receptor, and gp130 in the rat brain in response to the immune activator lipopolysaccharide and the proinflammatory cytokine interleukin-1β. J. Neurochem. **69:** 1668–1683.
49. LEE, S., C. KIM & C. RIVIER. 1999. Nitric oxide stimulates ACTH secretion and the transcription of the genes encoding for NGFI–B, corticotropin-releasing factor, corticotropin-releasing factor receptor type 1 and vasopressin in the hypothalamus of the intact rat. J. Neurosci. **19:** 7640–7647.
50. RIVIER, C. 1999. Gender, sex steroids, corticotropin-releasing factor, nitric oxide and the HPA response to stress. Pharmacol. Biochem. Behav. **64:** 739–751.

Effect of Neurogenic Stress and Ethanol on Nitric Oxide Synthase and Cyclooxygenase Activities in Rat Adrenals

VALERIA RETTORI,[a] CLAUDIA MOHN,[a] CAMILA SCORTICATI,[a] PAULA VISSIO,[a] MAXIMILIANO CELLA,[a] MARIANA FARINA,[a] ANA FRANCHI,[a] AND SAMUEL M. MCCANN[b]

[a]*Centro de Estudios Farmacologicos y Botanicos (CEFYBO-CONICET), Serrano 669, 1414 Buenos Aires, Argentina*

[b]*Pennington Biomedical Research Center (LSU), Baton Rouge, Louisiana 70808-4124, USA*

ABSTRACT: Repeated restraint stress (RRS) in male rats activated the pituitary adrenal system, as indicated by increases in adrenal weight and plasma corticosterone concentration that were accompanied by a decrease in constitutive nitric oxide synthase (cNOS), but not inducible NOS (iNOS). iNOS activated cyclooxgenase, causing elevated prostaglandin E_2 (PGE_2) and $F_{2\alpha}$ in the adrenals, but had no effect on lipoxygenase. Administration of ethanol (ETOH) was also associated with elevated adrenal weight and a slight increase in corticosterone coupled with a decrease in both cNOS and iNOS and PGs in the adrenal. When ETOH was administered together with RRS, a decrease in iNOS and PGE release was noted consequent to a reduction in iNOS. Thus, ETOH probably reduced RRS-induced adrenocorticotropic hormone release. Adrenals were incubated *in vitro* to further evaluate the role of NO in these processes. Results indicated that NO released by sodium nitroprusside increased corticosterone release presumably by activating guanylyl cyclase with production of cyclic guanosine monophosphate (cGMP), because although NO also increased PGE release, PGE_2 (10^{-5}–10^{-9} M) decreased corticosterone release, an effect that was highly significant at a concentration of 10^{-7} M PGE_2. ETOH (100 mM) had no effect on corticosterone release and did not block the increase in corticosterone caused by NO; however, ETOH reduced PGE release into the medium and blocked PGE_2 release induced by NO. Consequently, NO activated corticosterone release not by PGs, but by activation of guanylyl cyclase and release of cGMP. PGs have a negative feedback to suppress corticosterone release.

KEYWORDS: restraint stress; ethanol; plasma corticosterone; constitutive and inducible nitric oxide synthase; cyclooxygenase; lipoxygenase

Address for correspondence: S.M. McCann, Pennington Biomedical Research Center (LSU), 6400 Perkins Road, Baton Rouge, LA 70808-4124, USA. Voice: 225-763-3042; fax: 225-763-3030.

mccannsm@pbrc.edu

Ann. N.Y. Acad. Sci. 992: 86–98 (2003).

INTRODUCTION

The stress syndrome was discovered by Hans Selye, who showed that various noxious stimuli would induce adrenal enlargement and involution of the thymus and lymph nodes.[1] Stress is defined today as a state of threatened homeostasis, to which the organism responds by adaptive responses of the stress system. The stress system is extremely complex; it receives and integrates a great diversity of signals and responds to them by adaptive changes. The main component of the stress system is the hypothalamic-pituitary-adrenal axis. Although there have been marked advances in stress research, many questions still remain to be answered.[2,3]

Stress increases the consumption of alcohol in humans[4] and also in animals.[5] Some investigators consider that alcohol can trigger the stress response as indicated by increased plasma corticoids,[6] whereas others suggest that alcohol can reduce the stress response.[7]

In the adaptive response to stress, many mediators are involved. Among them nitric oxide (NO) and prostaglandins (PGs) are considered to play important roles. NO is formed in the body by NO synthase (NOS), an enzyme that converts arginine in the presence of oxygen and several cofactors into equimolar quantities of citrulline and NO. The half-life of NO in aqueous solutions is 5–10 seconds. However, the half-life of the soluble gas in living systems is prolonged by combination with other substances to form nitroso compounds that slowly release the gas.[8] There are at least three isoforms of the enzyme. One, termed inducible NOS (iNOS), is formed principally by immune cells such as macrophages, but also by other cells such as vascular endothelial cells. Bacterial infection leads to release of products of their cell walls, such as bacterial lipopolysacchride (LPS), which combine with receptors on the surface of macrophages and many other cell types. The LPS-receptor combination acts in the nucleus to induce synthesis of iNOS messenger ribonucleic acid (mRNA), which then synthesizes iNOS. The induction of iNOS mRNA occurs within an hour. The large quantities of NO produced then interact with the bacteria or viruses and cause cell death by inactivating metabolic enzymes. NO is also toxic to neighboring cells and can cause apoptosis and cell death in the region of its production.[8,9]

Endothelial NOS (eNOS) is formed in vascular endothelial cells following cholinergic stimulation. It is a constitutive enzyme that requires an increase in intracellular free calcium (Ca^{2+}) stimulated by the activated muscarinic-type cholinergic receptors on the endothelial cells. The increased Ca^{2+} interacts with calmodulin and activates the enzyme. The activated enzyme produces NO, which diffuses to overlying smooth muscle, and activates soluble guanylyl cyclase, which converts guanosine triphosphate to cyclic guanosine monophosphate (cGMP). This relaxes the vascular smooth muscle. NO plays an important role in control of vascular tone.[8]

Neural NOS (nNOS) is found in the cerebellum and various regions of the cerebral cortex and also in various ganglion cells of the autonomic nervous system. Large numbers of nNOS-containing neurons are also found in the hypothalamus, particularly in the paraventricular and supraoptic nuclei, with axons projecting to the median eminence and neural lobe, which also contains large amounts of nNOS. These findings indicate that the enzyme is synthesized at all levels of the neuron from perikaryon to axon terminals.[10]

Recently, a new form of NOS was described in mitochondria of brain and liver that is localized mostly in the mitochondrial inner membranes. This form cross-reacts with some antibodies to nNOS and iNOS.[11] The production of NO by mitochondrial NOS may affect energy metabolism, O_2 consumption, and O_2 free radical formation.[12] Thus, NO is the first gaseous transmitter that, instead of acting on cell surface receptors, diffuses into the cell and activates or inhibits intracellular enzymes.

Prostaglandins are formed by cyclooxygenase (COX), which converts arachidonic acid (AA) into various PGs.[13] In addition, lipoxygenase converts AA into leukotrienes. AA is formed by phospholipase A_2 (PLA_2) in the plasma membrane and can also be derived by phospholipase C cleavage of diacylglycerol.[14] The initial step in the formation of eicosanoids, the products of both the COX and the lipoxygenase (LOX) pathways, involves the cleavage of AA from phospholipid by PLA_2 in the plasma membrane of cells. Free AA also can be derived by phospholipase C cleavage of diacylglycerol. COX or LOX enzymatic pathways can then oxygenate free AA to form the final products. COX products, PGE_2, $PGF_{2\alpha}$, PGD_2, TXA_2, and PGI_2 (prostacyclin), are synthesized in response to immediate need and are not stored in significant amounts for later release. They all exert broad physiological effects. 5-LOX products are leukotrienes and HETES. Two isoforms of COX are described; COX-1 is the classical COX, and COX-2 is highly inducible by cytokines, growth factors, hormones, and oncogenes in many cells, such as macrophages, endothelial cells, fibroblasts, and smooth muscle cells. COX-1 is constitutively expressed, but it can also be induced and plays an important role in homeostatic functions, because it catalyzes the production of protective eicosanoids.[15,16]

We initially showed that NO donors, such as sodium nitroprusside (NP), stimulate the release of PGE_2 from hypothalamic explants of normal adult male rats *in vitro,*[17] a finding confirmed later by others,[18] an action caused by activation of COX by NO interacting with a ferrous iron-heme group of COX, in a similar manner as it acts to activate guanylyl cyclase.[17] We went on to show that NO and PGE_2 play an important role in controlling the release of not only corticotropin-releasing hormone (CRH), but also luteinizing hormone-releasing hormone from the hypothalamus, and that stress acts to release CRH by activating NOS followed by COX.[19,20] We hypothesized that this pathway may be active not only in the hypothalamus, but also in the target gland of adrenocorticotropin (ACTH), the adrenal cortex. Consequently, we evaluated the effect of chronic neurogenic stress and/or ethyl alcohol (ETOH) on the activity of NOS and COX in the adrenal gland. The possible interactions between ETOH, NO, and PGE in the adrenal gland and their effects on corticosterone release *in vitro* were evaluated as well.

METHODS

Adult male Sprague-Dawley rats (250–300 g) purchased from FUCAL Buenos Aires, Argentina, were used. The animals were fed laboratory chow and water ad libitum and were maintained under controlled conditions of light (lights on at 6:00 AM, lights off at 8:00 PM) and temperature (22–24°C). Animals were kept in our animal room for 10 days before the experiment. They were divided into several experimental groups of 6–8 each and then transferred to a separate room during the experiments. The experimental procedures reported here were approved by the Animal Care Committee of the Center of Experimental Pharmacology and Botanical

Studies of the National Council for Research of Argentina (CEFYBO-CONICET) and carried out in accord with the Declaration of Helsinki.

In Vivo *Studies*

All rats were implanted with an intragastric cannula using the procedure of Dees *et al.*[21] The gastric cannula was implanted surgically 1 week before the experiment. Rats were divided into four groups:

Control Group. Rats received 5 ml of tap water intragastrically twice a day at 10:00 AM and 6:00 PM for 5 days and were killed between 11:00 and 12:00 AM, 1 hour after the last water administration on the fifth day.

ETOH Group. Rats received ETOH intragastrically (3 g/kg in 5 ml of water) twice a day at 10:00 AM and 6:00 PM for 5 days and were killed 1 hour after the last ETOH administration between 11:00 and 12:00 in the morning.

Repetitive Restraint Stress (RRS) Group. Rats were exposed to 120 minutes of restraint once a day for 5 days using plastic cylinders (diameter = 18 cm; length = 52 cm) provided with several holes along the length of the tubes. The RRS was alternatively applied 1 day in the morning and the subsequent day in the afternoon. On the fifth day, rats were sacrificed immediately after the end of the 2-hour restraint period at about noon on that day.

ETOH and RRS Group. Rats in this group received ETOH intragastrically (3 g/kg in 5 ml of water) twice a day at 10:00 AM and 6:00 PM for 5 days and were exposed to 120 minutes of restraint once a day, as just described. The ETOH was administered 1 hour after the beginning of RRS each day, and the rats were sacrificed immediately after the end of the restraint period on the fifth day, after 2 hours of restraint, and 1 hour after ETOH administration around noon of the fifth day.

Immediately after decapitation and collection of trunk blood into tubes containing sodium and potassium EDTA salts, the samples were centrifuged and the plasma was frozen for corticosterone measurements. The adrenal glands were removed, weighed, and frozen individually, first in dry ice and stored at –70°C until used for individual determinations of constitutive NOS (cNOS) and iNOS activities or eicoisanoid determination.

Measurement of NOS Activity. NOS activity was measured by a modification[22] of the [^{14}C]-citrulline method of Bredt and Snyder.[23] Calcium-dependent and calcium-independent NOS activity was determined as previously described.[22,25] Because NOS converts arginine into equimolar quantities of NO and citrulline, the data were expressed as NO produced per adrenal gland per minute.

Measurements of Eicoisanoids. The eicoisanoid production by adrenals was determined by radioconversion assay of [^{14}C] AA to eicoisanoids. This was performed by chromatography of ethylacetate extracts of adrenals and counting of the labeled eicoisanoids, as previously reported.[26] The area of each of the radioactive peaks corresponding to authentic eicoisanoids was calculated and expressed as a percentage of the total radioactivity of the plates.

In Vitro *Studies*

The adrenal glands dissected immediately after decapitation of untreated normal male rats were cut in half, and both halves were put in the same tube and preincubated in Krebs-Ringer bicarbonate-buffered medium (pH 7.4) containing 0.1% glucose for 15 minutes prior to replacement with fresh medium or medium containing the compounds to be tested. Incubation was continued for 15 minutes, and then the medium and tissues were removed and stored at −70°C. Corticosterone and prostaglandin E_2 (PGE_2) released into the incubation medium were determined by radioimmunoassay (RIA) and NOS activity in the tissue by the [^{14}C]-citrulline method. Incubations were carried out in a Dubnoff metabolic shaker (50 cycles per min, 95% O_2/5% CO_2).

The adrenals were incubated in the following conditions: (**A**) (1) Krebs-Ringer buffer (control group), (2) NP (600 μM) as NO donor, (3) NP plus hemoglobin (2 μg/ml) as scavenger of NO, (4) ETOH (100 mM), (5) ETOH plus NP, and (6) ETOH plus NP plus hemoglobin. In these groups, we measured corticosterone and PGE_2 released into the medium by RIA. (B) Another set of adrenals was incubated with PGE_2 (10^{-5}M, 10^{-7}M, and 10^{-9}M) for 15 minutes. Corticosterone in the media was measured by RIA and NOS activity in the tissue by the [^{14}C]-citrulline method as just described (*in vivo* studies). Corticosterone and PGE were determined by RIA using rabbit antiserum from the Sigma Chemical Co.

Statistics. Data are presented as the means + SEM. Comparisons between groups were performed using Student's *t* test or one-way analysis of variance (ANOVA) followed by Student-Newman-Keuls' multiple comparison test for unequal replicates, using Graph-Pad Prism 3.0 software. Differences were considered significant when P values were <0.05.

RESULTS

In Vivo *Studies*

Adrenal weight was significantly increased after treatment for 5 days with ETOH and/or RRS (FIG. 1A). These effects were not additive, which suggests that both acted as stressors probably through the same pathway. Ingestion of alcohol failed to decrease adrenal weight of the RRS rats.

RRS caused a significant increase in plasma corticosterone as compared to that of the control group (FIG. 1B). Although ETOH slightly, but not significantly, increased plasma corticosterone levels, when administered with RRS, it prevented the increase in plasma corticosterone levels, suggesting that alcohol diminished the release of ACTH induced by immobilization.

The total NOS in adrenal glands after all treatments was decreased compared to that of the control group (FIG. 2A). This decrease paralleled the decrease in constitutive NOS (cNOS) (FIG. 2B), which represents almost 98% of the total NOS. Although the percentage of iNOS activity is very small, it was not affected by RRS, but it presented an important decrease after ETOH treatment, and this decrease was even more pronounced when both treatments (ETOH + RRS) were applied together (FIG. 2C). The presence of iNOS in control adrenals was confirmed by the expression of iNOS measured by Western blot (data not shown).

The radioconversion assay measuring the products of COX and 5-LOX showed a significant inhibitory effect of alcohol on PGE_2 and $PGF_{2\alpha}$ synthesis (FIG. 3A and B) and a slight but not significant decrease in 5-HETE (FIG. 3C). On the other hand,

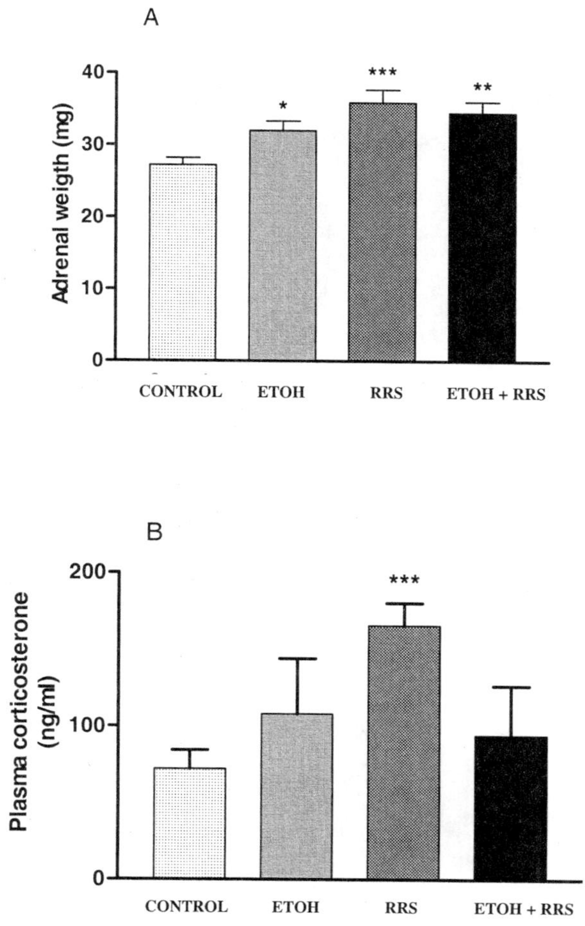

FIGURE 1. Effect of 5 days of ethanol (ETOH), repeated restraint stress (RRS), or both on adrenal weight (**A**) and plasma corticosterone levels (**B**). Values are means ± SEM (n = 6–8 animals/group); *P <0.05; **P <0.01; ***P <0.001 vs control group.

RRS produced a significant increase in PGE_2 and $PGF_{2\alpha}$ production (FIG. 3A and B) and a slight decrease in 5-HETE (FIG. 3C), but when ETOH and RRS were combined, the inhibiting effect of ETOH on PGE_2 and $PGF_{2\alpha}$ production was not counteracted by RRS. The combined treatment significantly inhibited the production of 5-HETE (FIG. 3A, B, and C). The inhibiting effect of ETOH on PG and HETE synthesis is probably caused by inhibition of COX and LOX; however, we cannot rule out an inhibitory effect of alcohol on PLA_2 that would also suppress PG and HETE synthesis, as reported by Basavarajappa.[27]

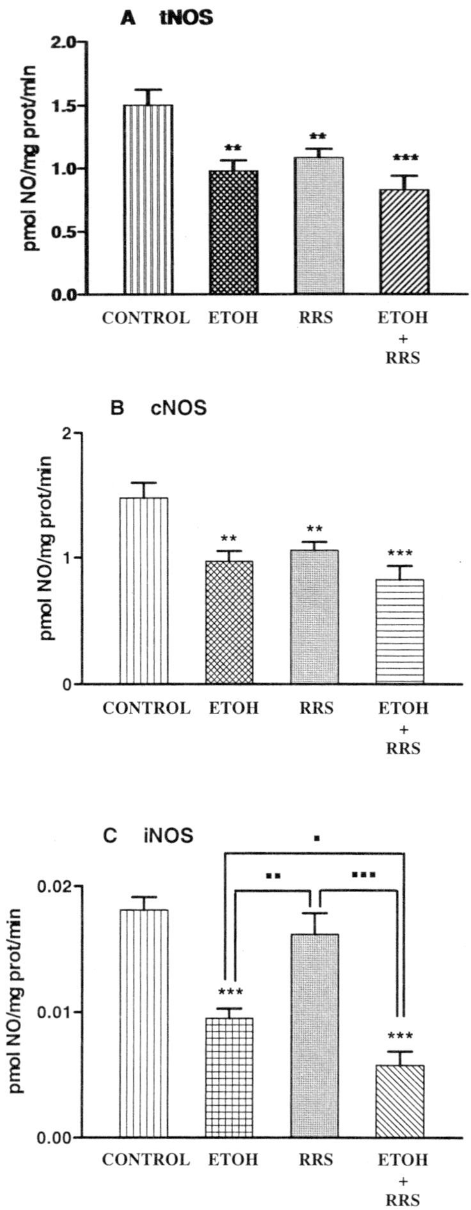

FIGURE 2. Effect of 5 days of ethanol (ETOH), repeated restraint stress (RRS), or both on nitric oxide synthase (NOS) activity in adrenal glands at the end of the fifth day. (**A**) Total NOS activity; (**B**) cNOS activity; and (**C**) iNOS activity. Values are means ± SEM (n = 6–8 adrenals/group); $^{**}P$ <0.01; $^{***}P$ <0.001 vs control and ■ P <0.05, ■■ P <0.01, ■■■ P <0.001 between groups.

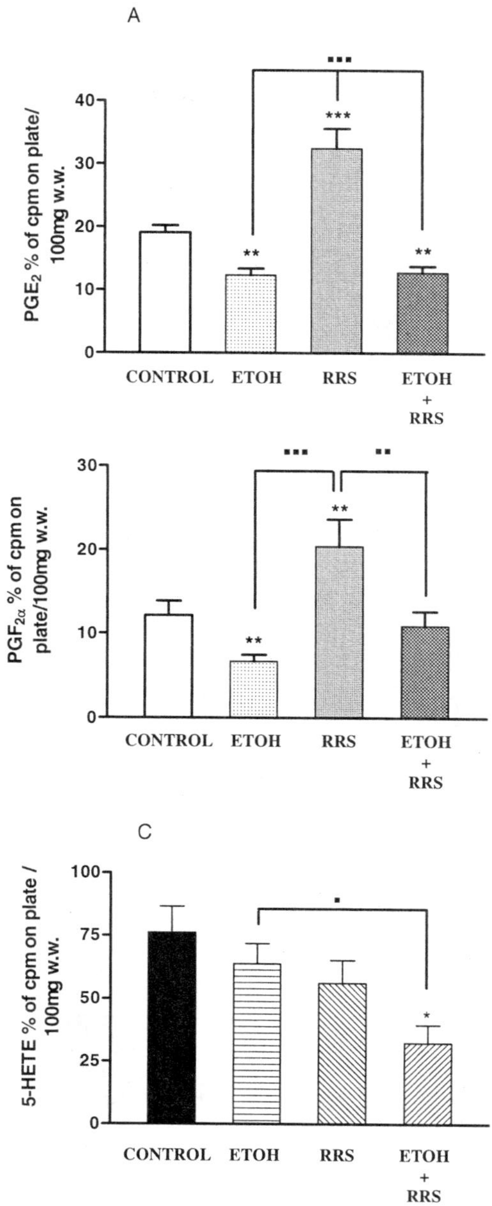

FIGURE 3. Effect of 5 days of ethanol (ETOH), repeated restraint stress (RRS), or both on prostaglandins in adrenal glands. Values are means ± SEM (n = 6–8 adrenals/group); *P <0.05, **P <0.01, ***P <0.001 vs respective control group in **A**, **B**, and **C**. (**A**) Production of PGE_2, ■■■ P <0.001 RRS vs ETOH group and ETOH+RRS group. (**B**) Production of $PGF_{2\alpha}$ ■■ P <0.01 RRS vs ETOH+RRS group, ■■■ P <0.001, RRS vs ETOH group. (**C**) Production of 5-HETE metabolite of 5-LOX in adrenal glands. ■ P <0.05 ETOH vs ETOH+RRS.

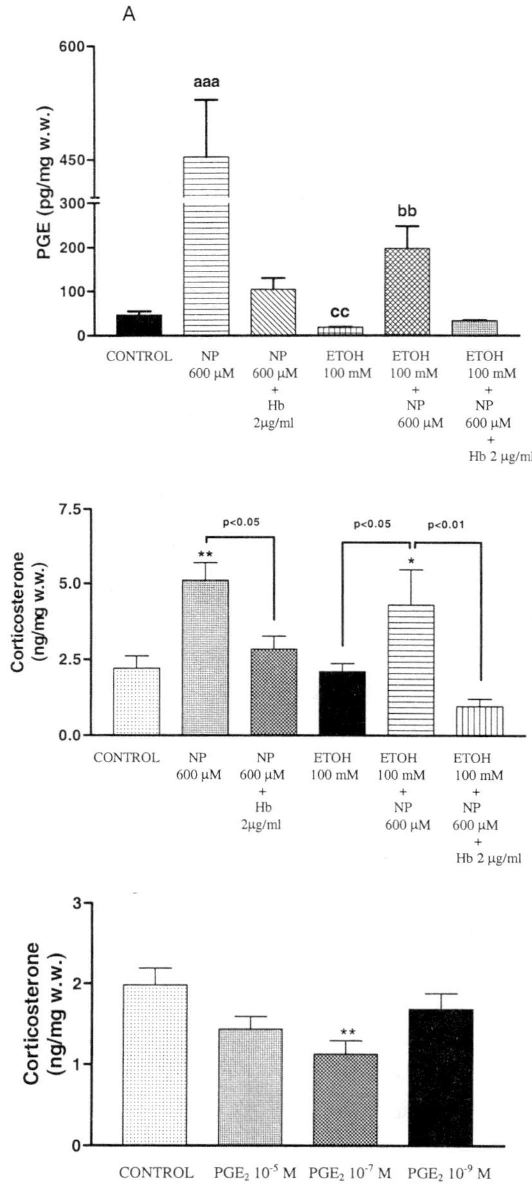

FIGURE 4. (**A**) Effect of sodium nitroprusside (NP), NP+hemoglobin(Hb), ETOH, ETOH+NP, and ETOH+NP+Hb on PGE release from adrenal glands *in vitro*. The effect of NP was aaa $P<0.001$ vs all groups; bb $P<0.01$ vs control; ETOH and ETOH+NP group (ANOVA-Newman-Keuls); cc $P<0.01$ vs control group by Student's *t* test. (**B**) Effect of NP, NP+Hb, ETOH, ETOH+NP, and ETOH+NP+Hb on corticosterone release from adrenals *in vitro*. $^*P<0.05$, $^{**}P<0.01$ vs control group. (**C**) Effect of PGE_2 on corticosterone release from adrenals *in vitro*. $^{**}P<0.01$ vs control group. All values are means ± SEM (n = 8–10 adrenals/group).

In Vitro *Studies*

Incubation of adrenal glands in the presence of NP, a donor of NO, produced a dramatic increase in PGE release that was abolished by the NO scavenger hemoglobin (FIG. 4A). ETOH inhibited basal release of PGs. These effects were similar to those seen previously in a preparation of hypothalamic explants incubated *in vitro* with NP and alcohol.[21] Furthermore, the coincubation of adrenal glands with NP in the presence of alcohol produced an augmentation of PGE release, but of much lesser magnitude than that of NP alone (FIG. 4A). Again, hemoglobin effectively abolished the effect of NO released by NP. As reported in other tissues, such as the hypothalamus[18] and uterus,[26] NO interacts with the iron-heme-center of COX, increasing PGE_2 synthesis followed by a prompt release, because it has been shown that PGs are not stored for further release.[28]

The stimulatory effect of NO on corticosterone release from adrenals *in vitro* followed a similar pattern as for PGE_2 (FIG. 5B), but alcohol present in the incubation medium was without effect on corticosterone release. The incubation of adrenal glands with PGE_2 (10^{-7}M) did not modify NOS activity (data not shown), and when the adrenal glands were incubated with PGE_2 (10^{-5} M–10^{-9} M), only the 10^{-7} M concentration had a significant inhibitory effect on corticosterone release (FIG. 5C).

DISCUSSION

Our experiments confirmed our hypothesis that interactions between NO and PGs would occur in the adrenal cortex as had previously been shown to occur in the hypothalamus, where stress-induced release of ACTH occurs by afferent input into the hypothalamus, activating nNOS. The NO released then activates CRH release by activating COX with subsequent release of PGE_2 coupled with activation of guanylyl cyclase followed by increased cGMP release, which causes the release of CRH into the portal vessels.[20] In the chronic stress experiment, as expected, there was an increase in adrenal weight and plasma corticosterone that surprisingly was coupled with a decrease in cNOS, but interestingly no change in iNOS. Administration of ETOH, although not increasing plasma corticosterone significantly, did increase adrenal weight, suggesting that ETOH was also causing release of ACTH, which acted on the adrenal and produced a similar reduction in cNOS as that seen with RRS. However, ETOH produced a marked reduction in iNOS in contrast to RRS that did not change iNOS from that of controls. When ETOH was administered together with RRS, adrenal weight was increased slightly less than that in the RRS rats, but there was no significant difference in adrenal weight among these three groups. However, ETOH together with RRS resulted in a decrease in plasma corticosterone, such that it was no longer significantly greater than that of the control animals. At the same time, ETOH combined with RRS, although not significantly altering the decrease in cNOS observed with RRS or ETOH alone, decreased iNOS below the control level observed in rats subjected to RRS alone and even below the level of the animals given only ETOH. Thus, ETOH is definitely having an inhibitory effect on the adrenal response to restraint stress. The explanation for the lowered levels of cNOS by all of the treatments may be related to the chronic stimulation of the adrenal, which decreases synthesis of cNOS. ETOH actually lowered iNOS values below control, suggesting that it was blocking the stimulatory effect of stress on iNOS.

PGE_2 and $PGF_{2\alpha}$, both products of COX, were increased by RRS even though cNOS was decreased. Thus, the increases must be mediated by the maintained level of iNOS. Ethanol alone decreased both of these PGs. The control levels of PGs and the effect of RRS to increase them were suppressed by ETOH, presumably because it decreased iNOS by itself and even more when combined with RRS. These results suggest that ETOH is decreasing ACTH release, at least at the time of sacrifice of the rats, and that the decreased ACTH release decreased iNOS activity, suppressing production and release of PGs. The fact that RRS increased PG production in the presence of a decrease in cNOS and no change in iNOS is puzzling. We hypothesize that the iNOS associated with the release of corticosterone is increased, but levels elsewhere in the cortical cells are lowered, so that the total iNOS measured here was unchanged.

The incubation of hemiadrenals proved a convenient way to study direct effects of various substances on the adrenal. NP, a releaser of NO, produced dramatic stimulation of not only PGE release, but also corticosterone release into the media. That this was a specific effect of NO was indicated by the fact that it was quenched by adding hemoglobin to the medium. ETOH had an effect by itself at a relatively high dose of 100 mM to reduce PGE, but not corticosterone release, and it effectively counteracted partially the effect of NP to stimulate prostaglandin release. In contrast to these effects, ETOH had no significant effect to reduce the increase in corticosterone induced by NP. Therefore, although the results clearly show that NO stimulates the release of corticosterone, they also show that there was no effect of ETOH on the adrenals *in vitro*, except to reduce PGE release.

Interestingly enough, although NO stimulated corticosterone release, PGE_2 reduced corticosterone release at concentrations from 10^{-6} to 10^{-8} M. The maximal inhibitory effect at 10^{-7} M was highly significant. Therefore, we conclude from the *in vitro* experiments that NO stimulates PGE release by activation of COX and that this effect is antagonized by ETOH presumably by direct inhibition of COX activity. On the other hand, corticosterone secretion induced by NO is not due to activation of COX, because PGE_2 had only an inhibitory action on corticosterone release, but instead the release of corticosterone induced by NO is most probably related to activation of guanylyl cyclase and production of cGMP that, in turn, acts on protein kinase G to evoke corticosterone secretion.

The inhibitory effect of PGE_2 on corticosterone release suggests that it acts by negative feedback in the adrenal to suppress corticosterone release, either by an inhibitory effect on NOS, or alternatively on guanylyl cyclase or by both methods. Since PGE_2 had no effect in NOS activity, we hypothesize that it inhibits the activation of guanylyl cyclase by NO. Our results from incubation of adrenals indicate that the effects in the *in vivo* experiments are probably related to increased ACTH release induced by RRS that is partially blocked by action within the brain of ethanol to decrease ACTH release. Importantly, we have shown a dramatic action of NO within the adrenal not only to activate COX, but also to induce corticosterone secretion that may be inhibited by a short-loop negative feedback of the PGE_2 released.

ACKNOWLEDGMENTS

This work was supported by grants from Ministerio de Salud: Beca Ramón Carrillo-Arturo Oñativia, Agencia Nacional de Promoción Científica y Tecnológica, Argentina (PICT 99#5-6117) and the National Institute of Mental Health (NIMH) (S.M.M.). We also thank Ana Inés Casella for her administrative help and Judy Scott and Nicole Mestayer for their excellent secretarial assistance.

REFERENCES

1. SELYE, H. 1936. Thymus and adrenals in the response of the organism to injuries and intoxication. Br. J. Exp. Pathol. **17:** 234-248.
2. Csermely, P. (Ed.) 1998. Stress of Life. From Molecules to Man. Ann. N.Y. Acad. Sci. vol. 851.
3. MCCANN, S.M., J.M. LIPTON, E.M. STERNBERG, *et al.* (Eds.) 1998. *In* Neuroimmunomodulation. Molecular Aspects, Integrative Systems, and Clinical Advances. Ann. N.Y. Acad. Sci. vol. 840.
4. POHORECKY, L.A. 1991. Stress and alcohol interaction: an update of human research. Alcohol Clin. Exp. Res. **15:** 438-459.
5. HILAKIVI, C.L. & R. LISTER. 1992. Social status and voluntary alcohol consumption in mice: interaction with stress. Psychopharmacology **108:** 276–282.
6. SPENCER, R. & B. MC EWEN. 1990. Adaptation of the hypothalamic pituitary axis to chronic ethanol stress. Neuroendocrinology **52:** 481-489.
7. KALANT, H. 1990. Stress-related effect of ethanol in mammals. Crit. Rev. Biotechnol. **9:** 265-272.
8. MC DONALD, L.J. & F. MURAD. 1996. Nitric oxide and cyclic GMP signaling. Proc. Soc. Exp. Biol. Med. **211:** 1–6.
9. DAWSON, V.L. & T.M. DAWSON. 1996. Nitric oxide in neuronal degeneration. Proc. Soc. Exp. Biol. Med. **211:** 333–340.
10. BREDT, D.S., P.M. HWANG & S.H. SNYDER. 1990. Localization of nitric oxide synthase indicating a neural role of nitric oxide. Nature (Lond.) **347:** 768–770.
11. BATES, T., A. LOESCH, G. BURSTOK & J. CLARK. 1995. Immunocytochemical evidence for a mitochondrially located nitric oxide synthase in brain and liver. Biochem. Biophys. Res. Commun. **213:** 896–900.
12. GIUVILI, C., J. PODEROSO & A. BOVERIS. 1998. Production of nitric oxide by mitochondria. J. Biol. Chem. **273:** 11038–11043.
13. NELSON, N.A., R.C. KELLY & R.A. JOHNSON. 1982. Prostaglandins and the arachidonic acid cascade. Chem. Engineering News **60:** 30–37.
14. ROBERTSON, R.P. 1994. Eicosanoids and human diseases. *In* Principles of Internal Medicine. K. Iselbacher *et al.,* Eds. :431-435. McGraw-Hill Press.
15. WU, K.K. 1995. Inducible cyclooxygenase and nitric oxide synthase. Adv. Pharmacol. **33:** 179–207.
16. KALEY, G. & A. KOLLER. 1995. Prostaglandin-nitric oxide interactions in the microcirculation. Adv. Prostaglandin Thromboxane Leukot. Res. **23:** 485–490.
17. RETTORI, V., M. GIMENO, K. LYSON & S.M. MCCANN. 1992. Nitric oxide mediates norepinephrine-induced prostaglandin E_2 release from the hypothalamus. Proc. Natl. Acad. Sci. USA **89:** 11543–11546.
18. SALVEMINI, D., T.P. MISKO, J.L. MASFERRER, *et al.* 1993. Nitric oxide activates cyclooxygenase enzymes. Proc. Natl. Acad. Sci. USA **90:** 7240–7244.
19. RETTORI, V., N. BELOVA, W.L. DEES, *et al.* 1993. Role of nitric oxide in the control of luteinizing hormone-releasing hormone release *in vivo* and *in vitro*. Proc. Natl. Acad. Sci. USA **90:** 10130–10134.
20. KARANTH, S., K. LYSON & S.M. MCCANN. 1993. Role of nitric oxide in interleukin 2-induced corticotropin-releasing factor release from incubated hypothalami. Proc. Natl. Acad. Sci.USA **90:** 3383–3387.

21. DEES, W.L., C.W. SKELLEY & G.P. KOZLOWSKI. 1984. Intragastric cannulation as a method of ethanol administration for neuroendocrine studies. Alcohol **1:** 177–180.
22. CANTEROS, G., V. RETTORI, A. FRANCHI, *et al.* 1995. Ethanol inhibits luteinizing hormone releasing hormone (LHRH) secretion by blocking the response of LHRH neuronal terminals to nitric oxide. Proc. Natl. Acad. Sci. USA **92:** 3416–3420.
23. BREDT, D. & H. SNYDER. 1990. Isolation of nitric oxide synthase, a calmodulin requiring enzyme. Proc Natl. Acad. Sci. USA **87:** 682–685.
24. WEINER, C.P., Y. LIZASOAIN, S.A. BALIS, *et al.* 1994. Induction of calcium-dependent nitric oxide synthases by sex hormones. Proc. Natl. Acad. Sci. USA **91:** 5212–5216.
25. LOMNICZI, A., S. CEBRAL, G. CANTEROS, *et al.* 2000. Methylene blue inhibits the increase of inducible nitric oxide synthase activity induced by stress and lipopolysaccharide in the medial basal hypothalamus of rats. Neuroimmunomodulation **8:** 122–127.
26. FRANCHI, A.M., M. CHAUD, V. RETTORI, *et al.* 1994. Role of nitric oxide in eicosanoid synthesis and uterine motility in estrogen-treated rat uteri. Proc. Natl. Acad. Sci. USA **91:** 539–543.
27. BASAVARAJAPPA, B.S., T.B. COOPER & B.L. HUNGUND. 1998. Effect of chronic ethanol exposure in mouse brain arachidonic acid specific phospholipase A2. Biochem. Pharmacol. **15:** 515–521
28. SAMUELSSON, B. 1987. An elucidation of the arachidonic acid cascade. Discovery of prostaglandins, thromboxane and leukotrienes. Drugs **3:** 2–9.

Hypothalamo-Pituitary-Adrenal Axis and Chronic Immune Activation

MICHAEL S. HARBUZ, ANJO J. CHOVER-GONZALEZ,[a] AND DAVID S. JESSOP

URC Neuroendocrinology, University of Bristol, Bristol, BS2 8HW, UK

ABSTRACT: Corticosteroids have potent immunosuppressive and anti-inflammatory effects. Although corticosteroids are an important weapon in the clinical arsenal for treating inflammatory episodes, the mechanisms underlying the actions and regulation of endogenous corticosteroids remain obscure. In the late 1980s and early 1990s, a hypothesis was proposed that suggested that susceptibility to autoimmune disease was linked to a hypoactive hypothalamo-pituitary-adrenal (HPA) axis. It was further suggested that this defect in regulation of the HPA axis was situated at the level of the hypothalamus. This compelling hypothesis directly linked control of the HPA axis with susceptibility to disease rather than just severity of inflammation. The initial findings acted as a stimulus to further research, and over the next decade the hypothesis was tested. Recent studies suggest that the original hypothesis is in need of modification and that susceptibility is more complex and requires the involvement of more than a single parameter. These data are discussed together with recent developments concerning regulation of the HPA in disease in preclinical models and patients with rheumatoid arthritis. The latter studies in patients with rheumatoid arthritis provide evidence for the existence of a subpopulation of these patients with altered negative feedback regulation of the HPA axis.

KEYWORDS: hypothalamo-pituitary-adrenal (HPA) axis; corticosteroids; inflammation; arthritis

THE HYPOTHALAMO-PITUITARY-ADRENAL AXIS

Regulation of the hypothalamo-pituitary-adrenal (HPA) axis is coordinated at the level of the paraventricular nucleus (PVN) located in the hypothalamus. It is in the parvocellular cells of the PVN that the major corticotrophin-releasing factors, corticotrophin-releasing factor$_{1\text{-}41}$ (CRF) and arginine vasopressin (AVP), are synthesized and released into the hypophysial portal blood from terminals in the external zone of the median eminence. CRF and AVP exert a synergistic action on the release of ACTH from the anterior pituitary. ACTH stimulates the synthesis and release of corticosteroids (cortisol in man and corticosterone in rodents) from the adrenal cortex. Following exposure to an acute stressor there is activation of the HPA axis at

[a]Present address: Department of Neuroscience, University of Cadiz, Cadiz, Spain.

Address for correspondence: Dr. Michael S. Harbuz, URC Neuroendocrinology, University of Bristol, BRI Marlborough Street, Bristol, BS2 8HW, UK. Voice: 0117 928 3400; fax: 0117 928 3315.

m.s.harbuz@bristol.ac.uk

Ann. N.Y. Acad. Sci. 992: 99–106 (2003). © 2003 New York Academy of Sciences.

all levels, resulting in release of CRF and AVP into the hypophysial portal blood and elevated circulating levels of ACTH and corticosteroids.[1]

DYNAMICS OF CORTICOSTERONE RELEASE

The diurnal rhythm of corticosteroid release is firmly established. In man, cortisol levels increase to peak after waking and fall towards the evening. In rodents, levels of corticosterone are at a nadir during the morning, when these nocturnal animals are resting, to peak at around the onset of their activity period in the evening. Recent studies using an automated blood sampling system capable of sampling at 10-minute intervals have allowed much more detailed analysis of the dynamics underlying corticosterone release. These studies have revealed that in female rats regular pulses of approximately 1-hour duration occur throughout 24 hours with thepulses following one after another.[2] Comparison of individual pulses with the half- life of corticosterone (less than 10 minutes in the rat) suggests that the rising phase reflects a period of hormone release and that the falling phase of the pulse reflects a period when hormone release has ceased. Individual pulses can reach high corticosterone concentrations followed by a rapid decrease to undetectable levels. Therefore, the body is seeing not only varying concentrations throughout 24 hours but also markedly different levels each hour. A clear circadian rhythm was observed in these studies with smaller pulses seen in the morning than in the evening. However, pulse frequency did not alter over 24 hours, suggesting that the pulse-initiating mechanism has a constant periodicity throughout the day.

HPA AXIS AND DISEASE

Endogenous corticosteroids are essential for regulating inflammatory disease activity. Blocking cortisol release in patients with rheumatoid arthritis (RA) results in an immediate flare in disease activity.[3] Adrenalectomy will also facilitate an earlier onset and increase in severity of disease in adjuvant-induced arthritis (AA) and experimental allergic encephalomyelitis (EAE).[4,5] These effects can be prevented by corticosteroid replacement. Corticosterone replacement can also reduce inflammation in the streptococcal cell-wall model of arthritis in the susceptible Lewis strain. In addition, the resistant Fischer strain of rat will develop arthritis if the corticosteroid receptor is blocked.[6]

ADJUVANT-INDUCED ARTHRITIS

Injection of a suspension of heat-killed, ground *Mycobacterium butyricum* in paraffin oil results in the development of hind paw inflammation 12–13 days after injection. There is an associated chronic elevation in circulating ACTH and corticosterone and a loss in the normal diurnal rhythm. Despite the increase in activity of the pituitary-adrenal system, at the level of the PVN there is a paradoxical decrease in CRF mRNA and a decrease in the release of the mature peptide into the hypophysial portal blood. This decrease in CRF expression is apparent at the time of onset of inflammation and reaches a nadir at the time of maximum severity.[7] Decreased CRF

TABLE 1. CRF in chronic inflammatory disease models

Disease	Species	CRF	References
AA	Rat	Decreased	7–9
EAE	Rat	Decreased	10
Eosinophilia myalgia syndrome	Rat	Decreased	8
Systemic lupus erythematosus	Mouse	Decreased	11
Leishmania donovani infection	Mouse	Decreased	12
MS	Human	Suggested[a]	13, 14
MS	Human	Suggested[b]	15

[a]Increased activity in CRF+/AVP+ neurons.
[b]Increased response to AVP.

expression has been reported in the Piebald-Viral-Glaxo (PVG) strain of rat,[7] the Lewis rat,[8] and the Wistar rat.[9] These data suggest that this is a common mechanism associated with inflammation in AA. Decreased CRF has been noted in a number of chronic inflammatory disease models (TABLE 1).

Arginine vasopressin may take over as the major drive to the HPA axis under conditions of chronic inflammatory stress. An increase in AVP mRNA in the parvocellular cells of the PVN and an increased release of AVP into the hypophysial portal blood have been noted in AA.[7,16] These data suggest a switch in hypothalamic regulation in response to chronic inflammation with a shift from CRF to AVP as the major driving factor regulating the HPA axis. Similar findings have been reported in repeated and chronic stress models. The role of AVP in RA, multiple sclerosis, and other autoimmune diseases was recently reviewed.[17] From the available evidence it appears that AVP takes over as the major stimulator of the HPA axis, whereas CRF provides a secondary permissive role in chronic inflammatory stress. This alteration in the hypothalamic control of the HPA axis in these disease models and in autoimmune disease suggests that this change may be part of the adaptive response to chronic immune-mediated disease/inflammatory stressors across species.

HYPOTHALAMIC SWITCH AND RESPONSE TO STRESS

The hypothalamic switch from a predominantly CRF to a vasopressinergic drive has profound implications for the ability of animals with AA to respond to acute stress. Neither predominantly psychological stressors nor physical stress can increase circulating levels of corticosterone or CRF mRNA in the PVN.[5,18,19] Analysis of the pulsatile release patterns of corticosterone in rats with AA has revealed alterations in pulse frequency associated with the development of inflammation.[19] These changes are not apparent 7 days after injection of the adjuvant, when inflammation is not yet apparent, suggesting that the changes are a response to the development of hind-paw inflammation rather than injection of the adjuvant. Non-AA control animals show 13 ± 1 pulse in 24 hours. When hind-paw inflammation is apparent, this rises to 22 ± 1 pulse in 24 hours. The elevation in plasma corticosterone in AA is due not to an increase in pulse amplitude, but to the increased frequency of pulses. Further analysis of individual pulse profiles revealed that the rising phase was relatively shorter and the falling phase longer in AA rats than in controls. The ability to respond to stress appears to depend on whether the onset of stress occurs in conjunction with a rising or falling phase of corticosterone. These studies revealed that the AA rat can, in fact, respond to stress. However, the combination of the increased number of pulses, the diminished interpulse interval, and the reduced time spent in the rising stimulatory phase means that it is statistically less likely that stress will coincide with a rising phase and generate a response. In these studies the stress only coincided with a rising phase in 4 of 19 AA rats. Overall, the response was significantly less than that seen in the control animals.[19]

A similar inability to respond to stress has been noted in patients with RA undergoing surgery to replace hip or knee joints. In contrast, patients with osteoarthritis (OA) undergoing the same surgery did mount a cortisol response. A normal response to a CRF stimulation test in RA patients suggested intact pituitary and adrenal responses, supporting the case for a hypothalamic defect in RA.[20] By contrast, however, a normal response to surgical stress in RA patients was reported,[21] indicating the need for further study into stress responses in RA patients.

IS SUSCEPTIBILITY TO AUTOIMMUNE DISEASE RELATED TO AN IMPAIRED STRESS RESPONSE?

In the late 1980s and early 1990s it was hypothesized that susceptibility to autoimmune disease was a consequence of a hypoactive response to stress, resulting in an inability to prevent immune activation attacking self.[6,22,23] This hypothesis developed from comparison of the susceptible Lewis rat, which is considered to have a poor stress response, with resistant strains that exhibit a robust response to stress. Although a compelling hypothesis, evidence has accumulated to question its usefulness. First, although the PVG strain of rat has a robust response to stress, protecting it from experimental allergic encephalomyelitis , it is susceptible to AA.[5] Second, some laboratories have failed to observe differences in stress responses between the Lewis (hypoactive HPA axis and susceptible) and Fischer (hyperactive and resistant) strains.[24–26] Third, relative HPA axis responsiveness in a number of strains was not correlated with disease susceptibility.[27] Fourth, these studies have compared different strains of rat. The difference in HPA axis responsivity is likely to be only one of many differences between them. It is likely that other genetic variations between strains, resulting in altered neuroendocrine and immune parameters, will impact on their susceptibility to disease. To resolve this question we recently investigated single populations of the same strain of rat divided into subpopulations on the basis of their responses in behavioral tests. The Open Field test is a measure of anxiety, and a population can readily be divided into low and high anxiety animals. A significant difference in plasma corticosterone was determined between these groups; however, this did not relate to a difference in either susceptibility or severity of AA.[28]

Learned Helplessness (LH) has been used as a model of depression. In this model, animals are exposed to an inescapable footshock. They are subsequently placed into a shuttle-box where following a light an electric current is applied to the floor of the cage. The learned helpless (LH+) animals do not move and are considered to exhibit symptoms of depression. By contrast, the LH– animals very quickly learn to avoid the footshock by moving into the other compartment of the shuttle-box. A significant difference in plasma corticosterone was revealed, comparing the learned helpless (LH+), depressive-like animals, with the LH– animals in response to the shock; with the LH– animals having the greater response. The hypothesis would predict that the LH– rats should be relatively protected by the larger increase in plasma corticosterone. However, the LH– rats developed inflammation sooner and the severity was increased compared with that of the LH+ rats.[9] These data suggest that HPA axis responsivity alone is not a good predictor of susceptibility to AA.

Establishing whether a hypoactive HPA axis is contributory to disease in man is somewhat problematic. However, it has been demonstrated that individuals with sleeping sickness (infection with the potentially lethal parasite *Trypanosoma brucei)* are unable to generate a cortisol response to either CRF or ACTH.[29] Following successful treatment and elimination of the parasite, responses to CRF and ACTH are normal, suggesting that as in the animal models the defective HPA axis appears to be an adaptation to the disease and not an inherent quality in these individuals. On the basis of our current knowledge, it seems unlikely that HPA axis responsivity is a good predictor of susceptibility to immune-mediated disease.

DO PATIENTS WITH AUTOIMMUNE DISEASE HAVE AN ALTERED HPA AXIS?

Despite the obvious importance of the endogenous corticosteroids in regulating the immune response in autoimmune disease, the precise role of the HPA axis has yet to be resolved. In RA, published evidence suggests that the HPA axis is not significantly different from that in normal subjects.[30] This raises the possibility that any impairment lies in the inability of the HPA axis in RA to be activated in response to elevated stimulatory cytokines. Challenging the system has helped to reveal some differences between individuals with autoimmune disease and normal subjects. Injection of CRF and AVP has suggested that AVP may be more important than CRF in regulating HPA axis activity in patients with MS.[31] Responses to such challenges may differ depending on whether the disease is newly diagnosed or established.[32,33]

The dexamethasone-CRF test has been used extensively to assess HPA axis function in psychiatric disorders.[34,35] Depressed individuals exhibit an altered feedback regulation, so that the dose of dexamethasone is unable to fully suppress the cortisol response to CRF challenge. As a consequence, cortisol levels are elevated in depressed individuals, but remain suppressed in normal subjects, reflecting lower glucocorticoid receptor sensitivity in depressed patients.[36] Approximately 50% of MS patients did not suppress cortisol after dexamethasone administration,[37] a figure similar to that in patients with major depression and much greater than that in a normal population. Subsequent studies have confirmed that MS patients can escape from dexamethasone suppression following challenge with CRF, suggesting hyperactivity of the HPA axis that is significantly correlated with disease activity.[38–40] In patients with RA, three of seven patients escaped dexamethasone suppression, whereas four remained suppressed. No correlation between disease activity or severity and nonsuppression was noted, suggesting the existence of subpopulations of RA with differential HPA axis responses. The impact of these differences in HPA axis responsivity on disease progression in RA remains to be elucidated.[41]

SUMMARY

The underlying causes of autoimmune disease remain obscure. The HPA axis is essential in regulating severity of disease, as blocking or removing corticosteroids results in increased disease activity. It is clear that the development of disease can alter HPA axis responses, although increasing evidence suggests that a hypo-responsive axis is not necessarily an indicator of susceptibility. This may depend on many factors including behavioral responses, and these are likely to impact on neuroendocrine and immune parameters. The use of challenges such as the dexamethasone suppression test and the dexamethasone-CRF test suggest subpopulations of patients with RA and MS. These subpopulations may have confounded earlier conflicting studies. Wider use of HPA axis challenges in the clinic may reveal further subpopulations of patients with autoimmune disease and permit the development of therapies specific for subtypes of the disease.

REFERENCES

1. Buckingham, J.C. *et al.* 1997. The neuroendocrine system: anatomy, physiology and responses to stress. *In* Stress, Stress Hormones & the Immune System. J.C. Buckingham, A.-M. Cowell & G. Gillies, Eds. :9–47. John Wiley & Sons. Chichester, UK.
2. Windle, R.J. *et al.* 1998. Ultradian rhythm of basal corticosterone release in the female rat: dynamic interaction with the response to acute stress. Endocrinology **139:** 443–450.
3. Panayi, G.S. 1992. Neuroendocrine modulation of disease expression in rheumatoid arthritis. EULAR Congress Reports **2:** 2–12.
4. Mason, D. *et al.* 1990. The role of the neuroendocrine system in determining genetic susceptibility to experimental encephalomyelitis in the rat. Immunology **70:** 1–5.
5. Harbuz, M.S. *et al.* 1993. Hypothalamo-pituitary responses to acute stress and changes in circulating glucocorticoids during chronic adjuvant-induced arthritis in the rat. Am. J. Physiol. **264:** R179–R185.
6. Sternberg, E.M. *et al.* 1989. A central nervous system defect in biosynthesis of corticotropin-releasing hormone is associated with the susceptibility to streptococcal cell wall-induced arthritis in Lewis rats. Proc. Natl Acad. Sci. USA **86:** 4771–4775.
7. Harbuz, M.S. *et al.* 1992. Paradoxical responses of hypothalamic CRF mRNA and CRF-41 peptide and adenohypophyseal POMC mRNA during chronic inflammatory stress. Endocrinology **130:** 1394–1400.
8. Brady, L.S. *et al.* 1994. 1′1-Ethylidenebis[L-Tryptophan], a contaminant implicated in L-tryptophan eosinophilia myalgia syndrome, suppresses mRNA expression of hypothalamic corticotropin-releasing hormone in Lewis (LEW/N) rat brain. Neuroimmunomodulation **1:** 59–65.
9. Chover-Gonzalez, A.J. *et al.* 2000. Onset and severity of inflammation in rats exposed to the learned helplessness paradigm. Rheumatology **39:** 764–771.
10. Harbuz, M.S. *et al.* 1993. Changes in hypothalamic corticotrophin-releasing factor and anterior pituitary pro-opiomelanocortin mRNA during the course of experimental allergic encephalomyelitis. J. Neuroimmunol. **45:** 127–132.
11. Shanks, N. *et al.* 1999. Alterations in hypothalamic-pituitary-adrenal function correlated with the onset of murine SLE in MRL +/+ and lpr/lpr mice. Brain Behav. Immunol. **13:** 348–360.

12. Harbuz, M.S. *et al.* 1995. Evidence for altered control of hypothalamic CRF in immune-mediated diseases. Ann. N.Y. Acad. Sci. **771:** 449–458.
13. Erkut, Z.A. *et al.* 1995. Increased activity of hypothalamic corticotropin-releasing hormone neurons in multiple sclerosis. J. Neuroimmunol. **62:** 27–33.
14. Purba, J.S. *et al.* 1995. Increased number of corticotropin-releasing hormone expressing neurons in the hypothalamic paraventricular nucleus of patients with multiple sclerosis. Neuroendocrinology **62:** 62–70.
15. Michelson, D. *et al.* 1994. Multiple sclerosis is associated with alterations in hypothalamic-pituitary-adrenal axis function. J. Clin. Endocrinol. Metab. **79:** 848–853.
16. Chowdrey, H.S. *et al.* 1995. Evidence for arginine vasopressin as the primary activator of the HPA axis during adjuvant-induced arthritis. Br. J. Pharmacol. **116:** 2417–2424.
17. Chikanza, I.C. *et al.* 2000. Perturbations of arginine vasopressin secretion during inflammatory stress. Pathophysiologic implications. Ann. N.Y. Acad. Sci. **917:** 825–834.
18. Aguilera, G. *et al.* 1997. Biphasic regulation of hypothalamic-pituitary corticotropin releasing hormone receptors during development of adjuvant-induced arthritis in the rat. J. Endocrinol. **153:** 185–191.
19. Windle, R.J. *et al.* 2001. Increased corticosterone pulse frequency during adjuvant-induced arthritis and its relationship to alterations in stress responsiveness. J. Neuroendocrinol. **13:** 905–911.
20. Chikanza, I.C. *et al.* 1992. Defective hypothalamic response to immune and inflammatory stimuli in patients with rheumatoid arthritis. Arth. Rheum. **35:** 1281–1288.
21. Eijsbouts, A. *et al.* 1998. Similar response of adrenocorticotrophic hormone, cortisol and prolactin to surgery in rheumatoid arthritis and osteoarthritis. Br. J. Rheumatol. **37:** 1138–1139.
22. Sternberg, E.M. *et al.* 1989. Inflammatory mediator-induced hypothalamic-pituitary-adrenal axis activation is defective in streptococcal cell wall arthritis susceptible Lewis rats. Proc. Natl. Acad. Sci. USA **86:** 2374–2378.
23. Mason, D. 1991. Genetic variation in the stress response; susceptibility to experimental allergic encephalomyelitis and implications for human inflammatory disease. Immunol. Today **12:** 57–60.
24. Rivest, S. & C. Rivier. 1994. Stress and interleukin-1 beta-induced activation of c-fos, NGFI-B and CRF gene expression in the hypothalamic PVN: comparison between Sprague-Dawley, Fisher-344 and Lewis rats. J. Neuroendocrinol. **6:** 101–117.
25. Dhabhar, F.S. *et al.* 1993. Stress response, adrenal steroid receptor levels and corticosteroid-binding globulin levels: a comparison between Sprague-Dawley, Fischer 344 and Lewis rats. Brain Res. **16:** 89-98.
26. Grota, L.J. *et al.* 1997. Corticosterone responses of adult Lewis and Fischer rats. J. Neuroimmunol. **74:** 95–101.
27. Stefferl, A. *et al.* 1999. Susceptibility and resistance to experimental allergic encephalomyelitis: relationship with hypothalamic-pituitary-adrenocortical axis responsiveness in the rat. Endocrinology **140:** 4932–4938.
28. Chover-Gonzalez, A.J. 1998. A differential response to stress is not a prediction of susceptibility or severity in adjuvant-induced arthritis. Stress **2:** 221–226.
29. Reincke, M. *et al.* 1994. Impairment of adrenocortical function associated with increased plasma tumour necrosis factor-alpha and interleukin-6 concentrations in african trypanosomiasis. Neuroimmunology **1:** 14–22.
30. Harbuz, M.S. & D.S. Jessop. 1999. Is there a defect in cortisol production in rheumatoid arthritis? Rheumatology **38:** 298–302.
31. Wei, T. & S.L. Lightman. 1997. The neuroendocrine axis in patients with multiple sclerosis. Brain **120:** 1067–1076.
32. Gudbjornsson, B. *et al.* 1996. Intact adrenocorticotropic hormone-secretion but impaired cortisol response in patients with active rheumatoid arthritis-effect of glucocorticoids. J. Rheumatol. **23:** 596–602.
33. Templ, E. *et al.* 1996. Anterior pituitary function in patients with newly-diagnosed rheumatoid arthritis. Br. J. Rheumatol. **35:** 350–356
34. Holsboer, F. *et al.* 1985. ACTH, cortisol, and corticosterone output after ovine corticotropin-releasing factor challenge during depression and after recovery. Biol. Psych. **20:** 276–286.

35. ZOBEL, A.W. *et al.* 2001. Cortisol response in the combined dexamethasone/CRH test as predictor of relapse in patients with remitted depression. A prospective study. J. Psych. Res. **35:** 83–94.
36. MODELL, S. *et al.* 1997. Corticosteroid receptor function is decreased in depressed patients. Neuroendocrinology **65:** 216–222.
37. REDER, A.T. *et al.* 1994. Adrenal size is increased in mulitple sclerosis. Arch. Neurol. **51:** 151–154.
38. FASSBENDER, K. *et al.* 1998. Mood disorders and dysfunction of the hypothalamic-pituitary-adrenal axis in multiple sclerosis: association with cerebral inflammation. Arch. Neurol. **55:** 66–72.
39. THEN BERGH, F. *et al.* 2001. Combined treatment with corticosteroids and moclobemide favors normalization of hypothalamo-pituitary-adrenal axis dysregulation in relapsing-remitting multiple sclerosis: a randomized, double blind trial. J. Clin. Endocrinol. Metab. **86:** 1610–1615.
40. KUMPFEL, T. *et al.* 1999. Dehydroepiandrosterone response to the adrenocorticotropin test and the combined dexamethasone and corticotropin-releasing hormone test in patients with multiple sclerosis. Neuroendocrinology **70:** 431–438.
41. HARBUZ, M.S. *et al.* 2003. HPA axis dysregulation in patients with rheumatoid arthritis following the dexamethasone-CRF test. J. Endocrinol. In press.

Hypothalamic-Pituitary-Adrenocortical and Gonadal Functions in Rheumatoid Arthritis

M. CUTOLO, A. SULLI, C. PIZZORNI, C. CRAVIOTTO, AND R.H. STRAUB[a]

Research Laboratory and Division of Rheumatology, Department of Internal Medicine, University of Genoa, 16136, Genoa, Italy

[a]Laboratory of Neuroendocrinoimmunology, Department of Internal Medicine I, University Hospital of Regensburg, 93042 Regensburg, Germany

ABSTRACT: Rheumatoid arthritis (RA) as well as most autoimmune disorders results from a combination of several predisposing factors including the relations between epitopes of the trigger agent (i.e., virus, self-antigens) and histocompatibility epitopes (i.e., HLA), the status of the stress response system including the hypothalamic-pituitary-adrenocortical axis (HPA) and the sympathetic nervous system (SNS), as well as the gonadal hormones (hypothalamic-pituitary-gonadal axis, HPG), with estrogens implicated as enhancers of the immune response and androgens and progesterone as natural suppressors. The regular observation of reduced cortisol and adrenal androgen secretion during testing in RA patients not treated with glucocoticoids should clearly be regarded as "relative adrenal insufficiency" in the setting of a sustained inflammatory process, as shown by high interleukin (IL)-6 levels. In polymyalgia rheumatica, several pathogenetic and clinical aspects of the disease might well overlap RA, at least with elderly onset RA (EORA). Therefore, reduced production of adrenal hormones (i.e., cortisol, DHEAS) at baseline in active and untreated patients with polymyalgia rheumatica was detected. The defect was mainly related to altered adrenal responsiveness to ACTH stimulation (i.e., increased 17-OHP), at least in untreated patients with polymyalgia rheumatica. Finally, normal serum estrogen and low androgen levels, but high synovial fluid estrogen and much lower androgen levels, have been found in RA patients, supporting the fundamental role of the peripheral sex hormone metabolism in the manifestations of the disease.

KEYWORDS: hypothalamic-pituitary-adrenocortical axis (HPA); gonadal axis; rheumatoid arthritis

INTRODUCTION

Autoimmune disorders result from a combination of several predisposing factors including the relations between epitopes of the trigger agent (i.e., virus, self-antigens) and histocompatibility epitopes (i.e., HLA), the status of the stress response system including the hypothalamic-pituitary-adrenocortical axis (HPA) and the sympathetic

Address for correspondence: Dr. M. Cutolo, Research Laboratory and Division of Rheumatology, Department of Internal Medicine, University of Genoa, Viale Benedetto XV, 6, 16136, Genoa, Italy. Voice: 0039 010 353 7994; fax: 0039 010 353 8885.
mcutolo@unige.it

Ann. N.Y. Acad. Sci. 992: 107–117 (2003).

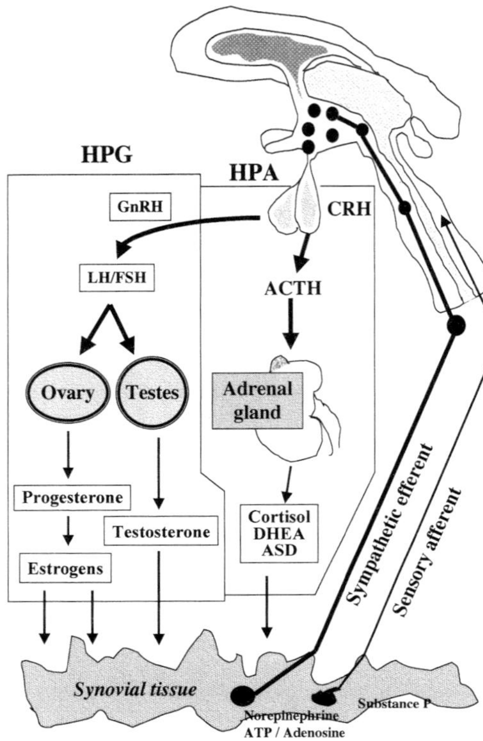

FIGURE 1. The hypothalamic-pituitary-adrenocortical axis (HPA) and the hypothalamic-pituitary-gonadal axis (HPG) together with the sympathetic nervous system (SNS) are represented with the target tisssue (synovial tissue) of their end products (adrenal hormones, gonadal hormones, and neurotransmitters) in rheumatoid arthritis.

nervous system (SNS), as well as the gonadal hormones (hypothalamic-pituitary-gonadal axis, HPG), with estrogens implicated as enhancers of the immune response and androgens and progesterone as natural suppressors[1–4] (FIG. 1).

Autoimmune disorders such as rheumatoid arthritis (RA), systemic lupus erythematosus (SLE), systemic sclerosis (SSc), and Sjögren's syndrome (SS) are inflammatory chronic diseases with very similar neuroendocrine pathogenetic mechanisms.[1] However, how these variables interact with one another and how they ultimately influence the disease process in these conditions is only partially known. Nonetheless, research clearly demonstrates links between the stress system and alterations in disease activity and the associated outcomes (i.e., pain, disability) in autoimmune disorders.[5]

In particular, the stress response system (HPA+SNS), which is pivotal in these conditions, is made up of psychological and neuroendocrine components that can be activated by a range of physical and psychological stressors. Stressors are all events that activate the stress response system which, in turn, attempts to return the organism to homeostatic balance.[6,7]

Research clearly demonstrates that the HPA axis and HPG axis functioning are altered in RA patients, and both are major components of the stress response system.[8] For example, cortisol levels are often inappropriately low for the inflammatory status of RA, and low levels of gonadal and adrenal androgens have been found in premenopausal RA patients.[9]

As stated, the immune system seems directly linked to the stress system and is profoundly influenced by the effectors of the stress response. Therefore, the stress response is associated with activation of several neuroendocrine systems including the HPA and HPG axes and the SNS[10] (FIG. 1). Activation of the HPA axis may occur when confronted by a psychosocial stressor that, if appraised as threatening, can result in associated affective and behavioral (i.e., coping) responses as well as elevated serum levels of cortisol. Therefore, the HPA axis provides an essential interface between the internal and external environments and enables the individual to adapt to different noxious stimuli, whether they be psychological or physical.[11]

The role of increased cortisol release is adaptational and attempts to modulate the effects of stressors in order to reestablish homeostasis. However, failure to mount an appropriate HPA axis response to a stress trigger, as following chronic exposure to the stressors, may be detrimental and may represent a significant contributory factor in the etiology of a variety of disease processes, including autoimmune and inflammatory autoimmune diseases.[12]

As a matter of fact, evidence from *in vitro* animal and human studies demonstrates that activation of the immune system may constitute *per se* a stressor to which the HPA axis responds.[13] On the other hand, interpersonal stressors may have the greatest effect on the physiological and psychological functioning of individuals with autoimmune diseases, at least in RA.[13]

As just noted, major versus minor stressors appear to have differential effects, and these differences may be mediated by disparate physiologic mechanisms involving the HPA and the SNS, which influence the immune system. The length and intensity of exposure to the stressors may also play a critical role. Short-term acute stressors tend to elicit immediate, but relatively transient changes in physiologic parameters, whereas chronic stressors may lead to relatively stable changes in baseline physiologic levels.[14,15]

Prior stress history also plays an important role in determining how individuals respond to subsequent stressors. For example, in animal models, chronic intermittent exposure to a stressor of low intensity may lead to decreased sympathetic activity, whereas frequent exposure to a stressor of high intensity increases sympathetic activity.[16] Therefore, a number of physiologic stress systems (i.e., HPA and SNS) are associated with autoimmune diseases and appear to mediate the relation between environmental stressors and disease pathophysiology.[18] In particular, chronic exposure to stressors seems to reduce the efficacy of the stress system response and increases the risk of an altered immune response to antigenic stimuli.[19]

HYPOTHALAMIC-PITUITARY-ADRENOCORTICAL FUNCTION IN RHEUMATOID ARTHRITIS

The inflammatory cytokines (i.e., interleukin [IL]-6, IL-1, and tumor necrosis factor-alpha [TNF-α]) as soluble products of the activated immune system stimulate the production of corticotropin-releasing hormone (CRH) in the hypothalamus. CRH release leads to pituitary production of adrenocorticotropic hormone (ACTH), followed by glucocorticoid secretion by the adrenal cortex and indirect perturbations of gonadal function.[20,21]

It is now recognized that young females affected by recent intensive stressful conditions (interpersonal stressors, surgical or infectious events) activating the HPA, with associated low plasma adrenal androgens (i.e., dehydroepiandrosterone sulfate [DHEAS]) and recent use of contraceptive pills, are the best candidates for the onset of autoimmune disorders, including RA.[22–24]

The stress system has multiple levels and is comprised of neuroendocrinological (i.e., HPA axis), psychological, and environmental components.[25] The physiologic balance between the stress and the immune system may be disrupted as a consequence of various pathological insults, including sustained exposure to stress, abnormal immune reactions to infections, or both.[26]

Recently, intact ACTH secretion, but impaired cortisol response, in patients with active RA was described, and this observation was consistent with relative adrenal glucocorticoid insufficiency, the latter already suggested 40 years earlier.[27,28] Increased HPA axis function is a normal response to the stress of inflammation and might be mediated by central and peripheral actions of circulating cytokines.

Besides IL-1 and TNF-α, IL-6 appears to be a major factor mediating interactions between the activated immune system and both anterior pituitary cells and adrenal steroidogenesis[29] (FIG. 2). However, recent studies in RA patients have shown that overall activity of the HPA axis remains inappropriately normal and is apparently insufficient to inhibit ongoing inflammation at least in early untreated arthritic patients.[30]

More recently, another study showed a significantly altered secretion of adrenal androgens in non-glucocorticoid–treated premenopausal RA patients.[24]

Baseline concentrations of dehydroepiandrosterone (DHEA) and its sulfate metabolite DHEAS were significantly lower in patients with chronic RA than in normal subjects. In addition, during low-dose ACTH testing, DHEA production was significantly lower in patients with chronic RA than in controls.[24] Low levels of plasma DHEA and DHEAS in the same study were found to be significantly correlated with early morning low cortisol concentrations and high basal levels of IL-6 in RA patients.[24] Early morning IL-6 peak values were recently found to be higher in patients with RA than in controls and were significantly correlated to morning CRP levels and Ritchie's index.[31]

The observation of reduced DHEA production combined with normal cortisol production during oCRH and ACTH testing further support the concept of the presence of adrenal hypofunction in active RA patients.[32]

IL-6 had a strong effect on steroid release and may be one of the factors controlling the long-term adrenal response to stress, because this cytokine can act synergistically with ACTH on the adrenal cells to stimulate the release of corticosterone.[33,34] Therefore, the reduced cortisol and adrenal androgen secretion observed during testing in RA patients not treated with glucocoticoids should clearly be regarded as "relative adrenal insufficiency" in the setting of a sustained inflammatory process, as shown by high IL-6 levels.[35]

In a very recent investigation on salivary cortisol levels in patients with recent-onset RA, afternoon concentrations in patients with high disease activity did not

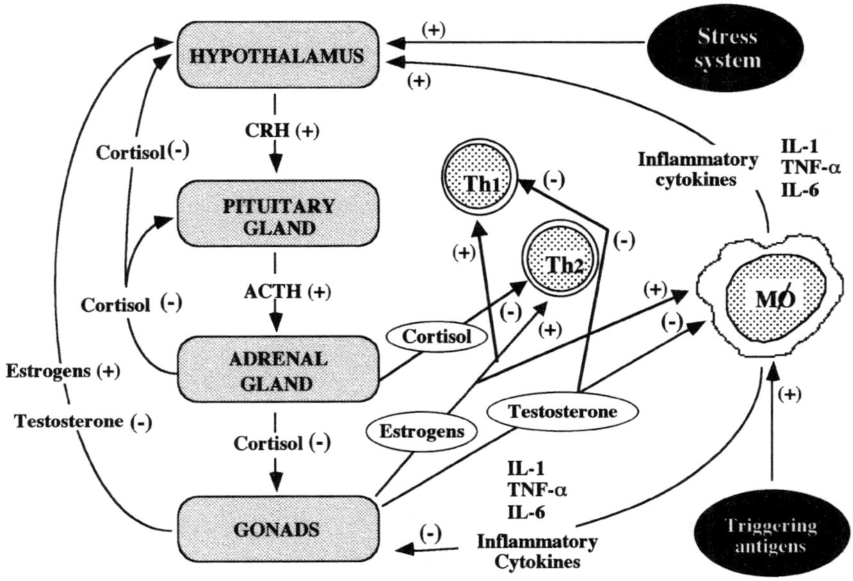

FIGURE 2. Effects of the adrenal and gonadal hormones on the cells involved in the immune response. On the other hand, the inflammatory cytokines (interleukin [IL]-1, tumor necrosis factor [TNF]-alpha, and IL-6) modulate the function of the hypothalamic-pituitary-adrenal axis (HPA) and of the hypothalamic-pituitary-gonadal axis (HPG) through direct effects on the hypothalamus and gonads, respectively.

decrease, as did cortisol levels in healthy controls and RA patients with low disease activity.[36] This indicates that activation of the HPA axis is possible but insufficient.

HYPOTHALAMIC-PITUITARY ADRENOCORTICAL FUNCTION IN POLYMYALGIA RHEUMATICA

Although currently polymyalgia rheumatica (PMR) is not properly considered an autoimmune disorder, several pathogenetic and clinical aspects of the disease might well overlap RA, at least with elderly onset RA (EORA).[37]

These aspects include female sex prevalence, joint synovitis, involvement of cytokines expressed in Th1-dependent processes, the presence of activated monocytes/macrophages in pathological lesions, a common association with the HLA-DRB1 phenotype, a role for infectious factors, the favorable effects of combination and immunosuppressive therapies such as steroids and methotrexate, or antimalarials or azathioprine as well as elderly onset.

PMR is a common disorder in the elderly characterized by aching and morning stiffness in the neck, shoulders, and pelvic girdle, along with constitutional symptoms (malaise, weight loss, and fever) and marked serologic acute phase response.[37]

Although PMR occurs in patients older than 50 years of age and PMR incidence increases with age, age-associated pathogenic factors are not yet known.[38] The natural decline of several hormones, including DHEA/DHEAS and androstenedione (ASD) during aging may well represent one such factor.[39] The decrease of adrenal/gonadal hormones is different in both sexes (healthy subjects), for example cortisol and 17-hydroxyprogesterone (17-OHP) decrease in female subjects but not in male subjects.[40]

However, in both sexes, cortisol serum levels are relatively low in relation to plasma adrenocorticotropic hormone (ACTH), which indicates that despite increased ACTH, the production of cortisol decreases during aging.[41] Nevertheless, cortisol serum levels remain relatively high in relation to serum levels of other adrenal and gonadal hormones during aging.[41]

In addition, aging is characterized by altered innate immune system function with a loss of phagocytic capacity and an increase of "early" cytokines such as IL-6 and TNF.[41] Recently, it was demonstrated that DHEA and ASD have a direct inhibitory effect on IL-6 secretion in monocytes and macrophages.[42] All of these findings might well support a possible link between endocrinosenescence and immunosenescence in the pathogenesis of PMR.[37]

The abrupt onset of PMR, with clinical features similar to the steroid withdrawal syndrome (i.e., musculoskeletal pain, malaise, fever) or adrenal insufficiency, as well as the dramatic and rapid disappearance of these symptoms following glucocorticoid administration, may be a strong clinical argument for an altered function of the hypothalamic-pituitary-adrenal axis (HPA) in these patients.[37]

A recent study has partially clarified this point, by analyzing the interrelation between basal inflammatory cytokines (IL-6, TNF) and adrenal hormones (cortisol, DHEAS, ASD) levels in more than one hundred PMR patients with both beginning and chronic disease.[43] As expected, basal serum IL-6 levels were found to be significantly higher in untreated PMR patients as compared to age-matched normal subjects and were positively correlated with basal serum cortisol, DHEAS and ASD levels, irrespective of glucocorticoid treatment. However, basal serum levels of cortisol in PMR patients with or without glucocorticoid, were found lower than expected by considering the inflammatory status (increased IL-6).[57] Furthermore, IL-6 plasma concentrations and clinical symptoms during 14 months of glucocorticoid therapy are correlated in PMR patients.[44]

In a recent study, the HPA axis function and possible correlations between adrenal hormone levels, IL-6 and other acute-phase reactants were evaluated in patients with recent-onset PMR not previously treated with glucocorticoids.[45] Forty-one PMR patients of both sexes, with recent-onset disease were included into a longitudinal study. Female and male PMR patients were monitored for serum cortisol, DHEAS, ASD, clinical and laboratory parameters of disease activity such as C-reactive protein (CRP) and IL-6 concentrations at baseline and 1, 3, 6, 9, and 12 months of glucocorticoid treatment. Furthermore, in order to assess dynamic HPA axis function, serum cortisol and plasma ACTH levels, were evaluated in another eight glucocorticoid-untreated recent-onset PMR patients, in comparison to healthy age-matched controls using the ovine corticotropin releasing hormone (oCRH) test. In addition, serum cortisol and 17-OHP levels were evaluated after stimulation with low dose intravenous ACTH.[44]

Serum cortisol levels of all PMR patients at baseline, did not differ from the cortisol levels of control subjects. During the follow-up, cortisol levels dipped at 1 and 3 months. Serum DHEAS levels in all PMR patients, were found to be significantly lower than in control subjects at baseline. Serum ASD levels of all PMR patients at basal time, did not differ from the ASD levels of control subjects. In female PMR patients a significant correlation was found at baseline between cortisol levels and duration of the disease. Serum concentrations of IL-6 at baseline were found to be significantly higher in PMR patients than in sex- and age-matched healthy controls. During the follow-up, IL-6 levels after a significant decrease, remained stable in all PMR patients and did not increase again despite tapering of the glucocorticoid dose. After oCRH stimulation, a similar cortisol response was found in PMR patients and control subjects. After ACTH administration, a significant cortisol peak was detected in PMR patients and in controls, whereas, no significant difference in cortisol AUC was found between the groups. In contrast, ACTH induced a significant peak of 17-OHP at +30 minutes only in PMR patients and the 17-OHP AUC was found to be significantly higher in PMR patients as compared to healthy controls.

In conclusion, the study showed reduced production of adrenal hormones (i.e., cortisol, DHEAS) at baseline in active and untreated PMR patients. The defect was found mainly related to altered adrenal responsiveness to the ACTH stimulation (i.e., increased 17-OHP) at least in untreated PMR patients. The 12-month glucocorticoid treatment of PMR patients, reduced in a stable manner the production of inflammatory mediator levels (i.e., IL-6) that showed to persist even after the tapering phase of the glucocorticoids.[45]

HYPOTHALAMIC-PITUITARY GONADAL FUNCTION IN RHEUMATOID ARTHRITIS

Generally, androgens exert suppressive effects on both humoral and cellular immune responses and seem to represent natural anti-inflammatory hormones; on the contrary, estrogens exert immunoenhancing activities.[46]

Physiological low doses of estrogens, in particular, seem to enhance the Th1 cytokine network (cellular immunity, i.e., RA), whereas pharmacological high doses of estrogens seem to enhance the Th2 cytokine network (humoral response, i.e., SLE) (FIG. 3).

Low gonadal (testosterone [T]/dihydrotestosterone [DHT]) and adrenal androgen (dehydroepiandrosterone [DHEA] and its sulfate [DHEAS]) levels as well as reduced androgen/estrogen ratios have been detected in body fluids (i.e., blood, synovial fluid, smears, saliva) of both male and female RA patients, supporting the possible pathogenic role for decreased levels of the immunosuppressive androgens.

Interestingly, serum estrogen levels were found to be normal in RA patients. Several physiological, pathological, and therapeutic conditions may change the sex hormone milieu and/or peripheral conversion, including the menstrual cycle, pregnancy, postpartum period, menopause, chronic stress, inflammatory cytokines, and the use of corticosteroids, oral contraceptives, and steroid hormonal replacements, inducing altered androgen/estrogen ratios and related effects.[47] Therefore, sex hormone balance, still a crucial factor in the regulation of immune and inflammatory responses,

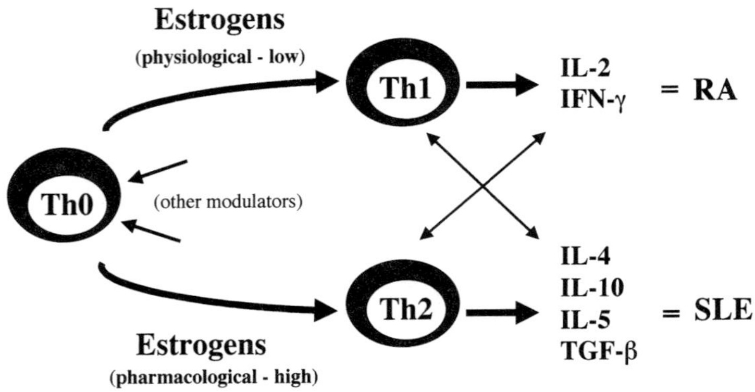

FIGURE 3. Effects of low physiological estrogens levels and high pharmacological estrogen levels on Th0 differentiation into Th1 and Th2 cytokine networks (including the paradigmatic diseases rheumatoid arthritis [RA] and systemic lupus erythematosus [SLE]).

and its therapeutic modulation should represent part of the advanced biological treatment for RA and other autoimmune rheumatic diseases.

Recently, considerable interest has been devoted to endocrine disruption, a new area of endocrinology concerned with chemicals that mimic hormones, particularly sex steroids.[48] Chemicals that mimic estrogens (so-called estrogenic xenobiotics) have been the main focus of the research. By blocking androgen action, exposure to these antiandrogens may cause changes similar to those associated with estrogen exposure.[49] Furthermore, genetic polymorphism affecting levels or function of androgens and estrogens may lead to an imbalance in the complex hormonal-immune system interaction and might contribute to RA etiology.

One of the most promising fields is the study of the localized metabolism of the sex hormones at the site of the inflammatory reaction in RA, but also in other conditions. Recently, we detected lower androgen and higher estrogen levels in both female and male RA synovial fluids. The appropriate explanation might originate from recent studies showing that the inflammatory cytokines (i.e., IL-6, IL-1, TNF-α) can markedly stimulate the aromatase activity in peripheral tissues.[50–52] As a matter of fact, the aromatase enzyme complex is involved in the peripheral conversion of androgens (testosterone and androstenedione) to estrogens (estrone and estradiol, respectively).

In tissues rich in macrophages a significant correlation was found between aromatase activity and IL-6 production.[52] Therefore, increased aromatase activity induced by locally produced inflammatory cytokines (i.e., TNF-α, IL-1, and IL-6) might explain the altered balance resulting in lower androgen and higher estrogen levels in synovial RA fluids as well as their mitogenic and proliferative effects on synovial cells.[53]

In addition, IL-6 has been found to mediate an increase in reductive 17β-hydroxysteroid dehydrogenase (17β-HSD) activity which converts estrone to the biologically more active 17β-estradiol.[54]

The role of local sex hormone concentrations at the level of inflammatory foci is of great value in better explaining the modulatory effects exerted by the hormones on the immune-inflammatory reaction.[55,56]

In practice, high estrogen levels in the synovial milieu, as here reported, might locally induce a Th2 cytokine network and explain the synovial production of rheumatoid factors and the high number of activated B cells.

REFERENCES

1. STRAUB, R. & M. CUTOLO. 2001. Impact of the hypothalamic-pituitary-adrenal/gonadal axes and the peripheral nervous system in rheumatoid arthritis: a systemic pathogenic view point. Arthritis Rheum. **44:** 493–507.
2. WILDER, R.L. 1995. Neuroendocrine-immune system interactions and autoimmunity. Annu. Rev. Immunol. **13:** 307–338.
3. CUTOLO, M., A. SULLI, B. SERIOLO, ***et al.*** 1995. Estrogens, the immune response and autoimmunity. Clin. Exp. Rheumatol. **13:** 217–226.
4. CUTOLO, M. & L. CASTAGNETTA. 1996. Immunomodulatory mechanisms mediated by sex hormones in rheumatoid arthritis. Ann. N.Y. Acad. Sci. **784:** 534–541.
5. HERRMANN, M., J. SCHÖLMERICH & R.H. STRAUB. 2000. Stress and rheumatic diseases. Rheum. Dis. Clin. North Am. **26:** 737–761.
6. CHROUSOS, G.P. & P.W. GOLD. 1992. The concepts of stress and stress system disorders: overview of physical and behavioral homeostasis. JAMA **267:** 1244–1252.
7. STERNBERG, E. 1997. Neuroendocrine immune interactions: principles and relevance to systemic lupus erythematosus. *In* Dubois' Lupus Erythematosus. D.J. Wallace & B.H. Hahn, Eds. :232–233. Williams & Wilkins. Baltimore.
8. MASI, A.T. & M. CUTOLO. 1996. Perturbations of the hypothalamic pituitary gonadal axis in rheumatoid arthritis. *In* Neuroendocrine Immune Mechanisms of Rheumatic Diseases. I.C. Chikanza, Ed. Ballière's Clin. Rheumatol. **10:** 295–331.
9. BIJLSMA, J.W.J., M. CUTOLO, A.T. MASI & I. CHIKANZA. 1999. Neuroendocrine immune basis of the rheumatic diseases. Immunol. Today **20:** 298–301.
10. BIJLSMA, J.W.J., R.H. STRAUB, A.T. MASI, *et al.* 2002. Neuroendocrine immune mechanisms in rheumatic diseases. Trends Immunol. **23:** 59–61.
11. O'LEARY A. 1990. Stress, emotion, and human immune function. Psychol. Bull. **108:** 363–382.
12. CUTOLO, M., C. PRETE & J. WALKER. 1999. Is stress a factor in the pathogenesis in autoimmune rheumatic diseases? Clin. Exp. Rheum. **17:** 515–518.
13. ZAUTRA, A.J., M.H. BURLESON, K.S. MATT, *et al.* 1994. Interpersonal stress, depression, and disease activity in rheumatoid arthritis and osteoarthritis patients. Health Psychol. **13:** 139–148.
14. HERBERT, T.B. & S. COHEN. 1993. Stress and immunity in humans: a meta-analytic review. Psychosom. Med. **55:** 364–379.
15. BASEDOVSKY, H.O., A.E. DEL REY & E. SORKIN. 1985. Immune-neuroendocrine interactions. J. Immunol. **135:** 750–753.
16. MCCARTY, R. & P.E. GOLD. 1996. Catecholamines, stress and disease: a psychobiological perspective. Psychosom. Med. **58:** 590–597.
17. DA SILVA, J.A.P., A. PINTO, M. CUTOLO & A. PORTO. 1999. Gender differences in adrenal and gonadal responses in inflammatory aggression. Ann. N.Y. Acad. Sci. **876:** 148–151.
18. STRAUB, R.H., C. GUNZLER, L.E. MILLER, *et al.* 2002. Antiinflammatory cooperativity of corticosteroids and norepinephrine in rheumatoid arthritis synovial tissue *in vivo* and *in vitro*. Cortisol FASEB J. **16:** 993–1000.
19. MASI, A.T., J.W.J. BIJLSMA, I.C. CHIKANZA, *et al.* 1999. Neuroendocrine, immunological, and microvascular systems interactions in rheumatoid arthritis; physiopathogenetic and therapeutic perspectives. Sem. Arthritis Rheum. **29:** 65–81.

20. MASI, A.T., S.L. FEIGENBAUM, R.T. CHATTERON & M. CUTOLO. 1995. Integrated hormonal-immunological-vascular ("H-I-V" triad) system interactions in rheumatic diseases. Clin. Exp. Rheumatol. **13:** 203–216.
21. CHROUSOS, G.P. 1995. The hypothalamic-pituitary-adrenal axis and immune-mediated inflammation. N. Engl. J. Med. **332:** 1351–1362.
22. MAN, K.S., M. BURLESON, Z. CASTRO, *et al.* 1992. Effects of stress on the neuroendocrine axis in rheumatoid arthritis and osteoarthritis. Arthritis Rheum. **35:** 24–27.
23. HALLER, C., B. HOLZNER, E. MUR & G. GUNTHER. 1997. The impact of live events on patients with rheumatoid arthritis: a psychological myth? Clin. Exp. Rheumatol. **15:** 175–179.
24. CUTOLO, M., L. FOPPIANI, C. PRETE, *et al.* 1999. Hypothalamic-pituitary-adrenocortical axis in premenopausal rheumatoid arthritis patients not treated with glucocorticoids. J. Rheumatol. **26:** 282–388.
25. WALKER, J.G., G. LITTLEJOHN, N.E. MCMURRAY & M. CUTOLO. 1999. Stress system activation in rheumatoid arthritis: a multilevel approach. Rheumatology **38:** 1050–1057.
26. Pietrini, P. & M. Guazzelli. 1997. Life events in the course of chronic diseases: a psychological or a psycho-neuro-biochemical loop? Clin. Exp. Rheumatol. **15:** 125–138.
27. GUDBJÖRNSSON, B., B. SKOGSEID, B. ÖBERG, *et al.* 1996. Intact adrenocorticotropic hormone secretion but impaired cortisol response in patients with active rheumatoid arthritis. Effect of glucocorticoids. J. Rheumatol. **23:** 596–602.
28. WEST, H.F. 1993. Corticosteroid metabolism and rheumatoid arthritis. Ann. Rheum. Dis. **16:** 173–181.
29. CROFFORD, L.J., K.T. KALOGERAS, G. MASTORAKOS, *et al.* 1997. Circadian relationship between interleukin (IL)-6 and hypothalamus-pituitary-adrenocortical axis hormones: failure of IL-6 to cause hypercortisolism in patients with early untreated rheumatoid arthritis. J. Clin. Endocr. Metab. **82:** 1279–1283.
30. MASI, A.T. & G.P. CHROUSOS. 1996. Hypothalamic-pituitary-adrenal-glucocorticoid axis function in rheumatoid arthritis. J. Rheumatol. **23:** 577–581.
31. ARVIDSON, G.N., G. GUDBJØRSSON, L. ELFMAN, *et al.* 2000. Circadian rhythm of serum interleukin-6 in rheumatoid arthritis. Ann. Rheum. Dis. **53:** 521–524.
32. TEMPL, E., M. KOELLER, M. RIEDL, *et al.* 1996. Anterior pituitary function in patients with newly diagnosed rheumatoid arthritis. Br. J. Rheumatol. **35:** 350–356.
33. MASTORAKOS, G., G.P. CHROUSOS & J.S. WEBER. 1993. Recombinant interleukin-6 activates the hypothalamic-pituitary-adrenal axis in human. J. Clin. Endocr. Metab. **77:** 1690–1694.
34. EHRHART-BORNSTEIN, M., J.P. HINSON, S.R. BORNSTEIN. *et al.* 1998. Intraadrenal interactions in the regulation of adrenocortical steroidogenesis. Endocr. Rev. **19:** 101–143.
35. DEKKERS, J.K., R. GREENEN, G.L.R. GODAERT, *et al.* 2000. Diurnal rhythm of salivary cortisol levels in patients with recent-onset rheumatoid arthritis. Arthritis Rheum. **43:** 465–467.
36. STRAUB, R.H., L. PAIMELA, R. PELTOMAA, *et al.* 2002. Inadequately low serum levels of steroid hormones in relation to IL-6 and TNF in untreated patients with early rheumatoid arthritis and reactive arthritis. Arthritis Rheum. **46:** 654–662.
37. CUTOLO, M. & R.H. STRAUB. 2000. Polymyalgia rheumatica: evidence for a hypothalamic-pituitary-adrenal axis-driven disease. Clin. Exp. Rheumatol. **18:** 655–658.
38. SALVARANI, C., S.E. GABRIEL, W.M. O'FALLON & G.G. HUNDER. 1995. Epidemiology of polymyalgia rheumatica in Olmsted Country, Minnesota, 1970–1991. Arthritis Rheum. **38:** 369–373.
39. ORENTREICH, N., J.L. BRIND, R.L. RIZER & J.H. VOGELMAN. 1984. Age changes and sex differences in serum dehydroepiandrosterone sulfate concentrations throughout the adulthood. J. Clin. Endocrinol. Metab. **59:** 551–555.
40. STRAUB, R.H., L.E. MILLER, J. SCHÖLMERICH & B. ZIETZ. 2000. Cytokines and hormones as possible links between endocrinosenescence and immunosenescence. J. Neuroimmunol. **109:** 10–15.
41. PAWALEC, G. & R. SOLANA. 1997. Immunosenescence. Immunol. Today **18:** 514–516.
42. STRAUB, R.H., L. KONECNA, S. HRACH, *et al.* 1998 Serum dehydroepiandrosterone (DHEA) and DHEA sulfate are negatively correlated with serum interleukin-6 (IL-

6), and DHEA inhibits IL-6 secretion from mononuclear cells in man *in vitro*: possible link between endocrinosenescence and immunosenescence. J. Clin. Endocrinol. Metab. **83:** 2012–2017.
43. STRAUB, R.H., T. GLÜCK, M. CUTOLO, *et al.* 2000. The adrenal steroid status in relation to inflammatory cytokines (interleukin-6 and tumor necrosis factor) in polymyalgia rheumatica. Rheumatology **39:** 624–631.
44. ROCHE, N.E., J.W. FULBRIGHT, A.D. WAGNER, *et al.* 1993. Correlation of interleukin-6 and disease activity in polymyalgia rheumatica and giant cell arteritis. Arthritis Rheum. **9:** 1286–1294.
45. CUTOLO, M., C. SALVARANI, A. SULLI, *et al.* 2002. Adrenal gland hypofunction in early-onset polymyalgia rheumatica. Effects of 12 months of corticosteroid treatment on adrenal hormones and IL-6 levels. J. Rheumatol. **29:** 748–756.
46. CUTOLO, M., B. SERIOLO, B. VILLAGGIO, *et al.* 2002. Androgens and estrogens modulate the immune and inflammatory responses in rheumatoid arthritis. Ann. N.Y. Acad. Sci. **966:** 131–142.
47. CUTOLO, M. 1998. The roles of steroid hormones in arthritis. Br. J. Rheumatol. **37:** 597–601.
48. SOHONI, P. & J.P. SUMPTER. 1998. Several environmental estrogens are also anti-androgens. J. Endocrinol. **158:** 327–333.
49. KELCE, W.R., C.R. STONE, S.C. LAWS, *et al.* 1995. Persistent DDT metabolite p,p′-DDE is a potent androgen receptor antagonist. Nature **375:** 581–588.
50. NESTLER, J.E. 1993. Interleukin-1 stimulates aromatase activity of human placental cytotrophoblasts. Endocrinology **132:** 566–570.
51. MACDIARMID, F., D. WANG & L.G. DUNCAN. 1994. Stimulation of aromatase activity in breast fibroblasts by tumor necrosis factor a. Mol. Cell. Endocrinol. **106:** 17–21.
52. PUROHIT, A., M.W. GHILCHIC & L. DUNCAN. 1995. Aromatase activity and interleukin-6 production by normal and malignant breast tissues. J. Clin. Endocrinol. Metab. **80:** 3052–3058.
53. CUTOLO, M. & L. CASTAGNETTA. 1996. Immunomodulatory mechanisms mediated by sex hormones in rheumatoid arthritis. Ann. N.Y. Acad. Sci. **784:** 534–541.
54. SPEIRS, V., E.F. ADAMS & M.C. WHITE. 1993. The anti-estrogen tamoxifen blocks the stimulatory effects of interleukin-6 on 17?-hydroxysteroid dehydrogenase activity in MCF-7 cells. J. Steroid. Biochem. Molec. Biol. **46:** 605–611.
55. CID, M.C. 2002. Estrogens and the vascular endothelium. Ann. N.Y. Acad. Sci. **966:** 143–157.
56. ELENKOV, I. & G.P. CHROUSOS. 2002. Sex hormones, proinflammatory and antiinflammatory cytokines, and autoimmunity. Ann. N.Y. Acad. Sci. **966:** 290–304.

The Hypothalamo-Pituitary-Adrenal Axis in Multiple Sclerosis

INGE HUITINGA, ZEYNEL A. ERKUT, DENIS VAN BEURDEN, AND DICK F. SWAAB

Netherlands Institute for Brain Research, Amsterdam, the Netherlands

ABSTRACT: During multiple sclerosis (MS), an inflammatory demyelinating disease of the central nervous system (CNS), activation of the hypothalamo-pituitary-adrenal (HPA) axis is considered to modulate the immune system in such a way that the probability of recovery from a relapse is increased. In a series of postmortem studies we observed a significant activation of corticotropin releasing hormone (CRH) neurons and increased cortisol in the cerebrospinal fluid (CSF) of MS patients, indicating activation of the HPA axis in this disease. On the other hand, sepsis, while elevating cortisol in control subjects, did not associate with a further increase of cortisol in MS patients. Thus, the activated HPA-system in MS does not respond to an acute inflammatory stimulus. In order to investigate the role of chronic inflammation in the CNS in the activation of the HPA axis in MS, MS lesions in the hypothalamus were quantified and interleukin (IL)-6 levels in the CSF were determined. There was no difference in IL-6 levels between MS and control patients. A positive correlation was found between cortisol and IL-6 in control subjects with sepsis, but not in MS patients with sepsis or MS and control groups without sepsis. Thus, IL-6 in the CSF of MS patients is not the cause of the activation of the HPA system in MS. We found a remarkably high incidence (95% of the patients) of MS lesions in the hypothalamus, of which the majority (60%) were active. The more active lesions were present in the hypothalamus, the shorter the disease duration to the moment of death, indicative of a worse disease course. Preliminary data show suppression of the activation of CRH neurons by active hypothalamic MS lesions. We propose that this suppression of CRH neurons by active hypothalamic MS lesions causes the concomitant unfavorable disease course via an inadequate cortisol response during relapses of MS.

KEYWORDS: multiple sclerosis; hypothalamus; cortisol; interleukin-6

INTRODUCTION

Multiple sclerosis (MS) is a demyelinating inflammatory condition of the central nervous system (CNS). Several studies indicate that the hypothalamo-pituitary-adrenal (HPA) axis (the "stress axis") plays a crucial role in the control of the disease process in MS. Stress influences the course of the disease.[1,2] Cortisol, the end prod-

Address for correspondence: Inge Huitinga, Netherlands Institute for Brain Research, Meibergdreef 33, 1105 AZ Amsterdam, the Netherlands. Voice: +31-20-5665503; fax: +31-20-6961006.

i.huitinga@nih.knaw.nl

Ann. N.Y. Acad. Sci. 992: 118–128 (2003). © 2003 New York Academy of Sciences.

uct of the HPA axis, has immune modulatory effects and synthetic glucocorticoids are used to treat relapses of MS.[3,4] Pioneer studies using experimental allergic encephalomyelitis (EAE) as a model for MS showed that low reactivity of the HPA system increases the susceptibility to the disease and decreases the recovery rate from a relapse.[5–8] All these findings lead to the assumption that MS patients may, like the EAE-susceptible Lewis rat, also have a hyporesponsive HPA system that would make these subjects more susceptible to the disease. However, subsequent studies generally revealed the opposite—that MS patients had a hyperresponsive HPA axis. They appeared to have enlarged adrenal glands and increased numbers of corticotropin releasing hormone (CRH)–expressing neurons, which show colocalization of vasopressin as a sign of hyperactivity.[9,11] In addition, these patients have elevated resting cortisol levels in plasma and an enhanced response in the dexamethasone suppression test,[12–15] which are all indications of an activated HPA axis.

The mechanism underlying the chronic activation of the HPA system in MS is not clear. For obvious reasons the HPA system has been investigated only after the onset of the disease, when the CNS contains multiple MS lesions. Since proinflammatory cytokines that are produced in MS lesions such as interleukin (IL)-1, IL-6, and TNF-α, are powerful activators of CRH neurons,[16,17] these lesions can be responsible for the activation of the HPA axis in MS. Therefore, cortisol and IL-6 levels were measured in postmortem CSF and related to each other. In addition, numbers of CRH neurons were counted as a measure for activation of the HPA axis and related to the MS lesion load in the hypothalamus.

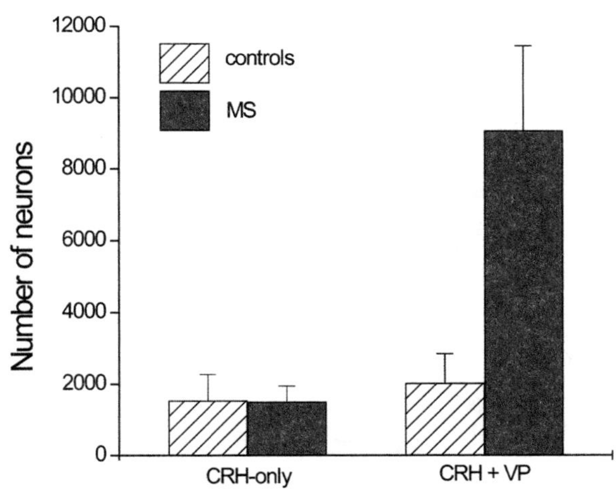

FIGURE 1. Numbers of CRH neurons that do not localize VP (CRH-only) or that localize VP (CRH + VP) in the PVN of 8 MS patients and 8 controls.[9] Tissue was obtained from the Netherlands Brain Bank (Amsterdam). Clinicopathological data (mean ± SEM):age, 51.0 ± 3.8 years (MS), 52.6 ± 5.0 years (controls); postmortem delay, 12.9 ± 5.6 h (MS), 13.9 + 3.9 h (controls); fixation time, 49 ± 14.0 h (MS), 36.7 ± 4.3 h (controls); duration of MS, 23 years; primary progressive MS, 2/8 and secondary progressive MS, 6/8. Neurons are counted in the PVN after immunohistochemical double staining of VP and CRH as described.[9] The difference in numbers of CRH/VP neurons between the MS and the control group is significant ($P = 0.046$).

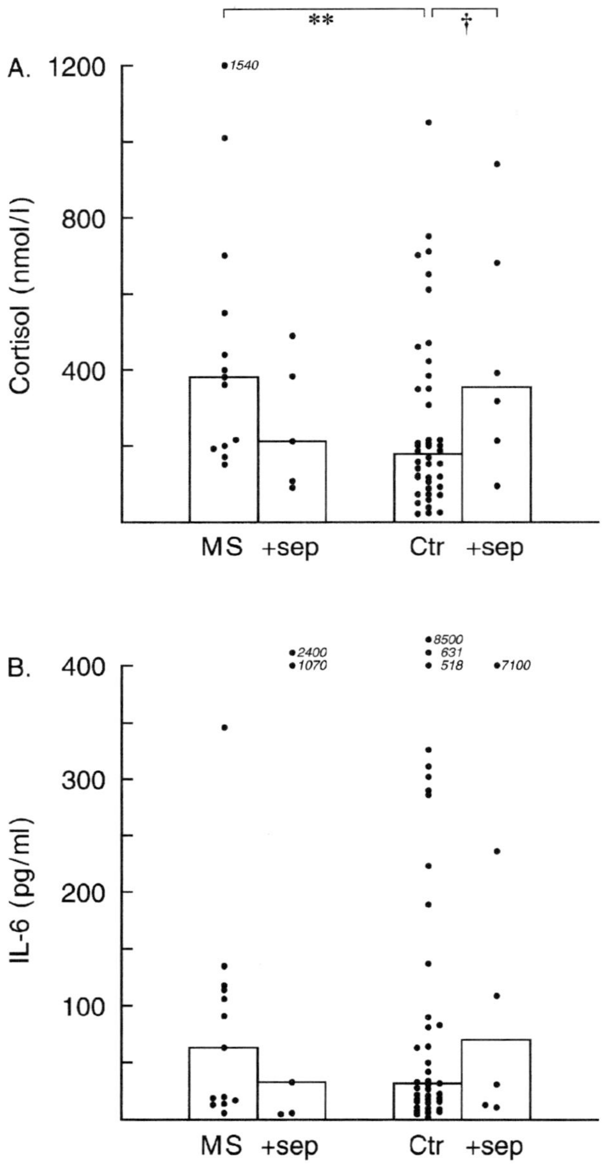

FIGURE 2. Individual values and medians of cortisol **(A)** and IL-6 **(B)** in postmortem CSF of MS patients without sepsis ($n = 13$) and with sepsis ($n = 5$), controls without sepsis ($n = 44$) and with sepsis ($n = 6$).[10] $^{**}P < 0.01$, †$0.05 < P < 0.1$. CSF was taken from the lateral ventricles during brain autopsy performed in the framework of the Netherlands Brain Bank (Amsterdam), cells were spinned down, and supernatant was kept at −80 °C. Clinicopathological data are given in TABLE 1. Cortisol was analyzed by RIA (DPC, LA), and IL-6 was determined by ELISA (CLB, the Netherlands). (Reproduced from Erkut *et al.* with permission.[10])

THE HPA AXIS IS ACTIVATED BUT UNRESPONSIVE TO SEPSIS IN MS

In postmortem tissue of 8 MS patients and 8 control subjects CRH neurons were counted in the paraventricular nucleus (PVN) of the hypothalamus that coexpressed vasopressin (CRH/VP neurons) or did not coexpress VP (CRH-only neurons). VP cosecretion potentiates adrenocorticotropin hormone (ACTH) release up to 20-fold and is thus an important measure of hyperactivation of the HPA system.[18] We found a significant 4.5-fold increase in the CRH/VP neurons in the MS patients ($P < 0.05$; FIG. 1).[9] There was no difference in the numbers of CRH-only neurons between the groups. Multiple regression analysis performed with sex, age, disease state, age at onset of disease, and duration of disease showed that none of these factors made a significant contribution to the total number of CRH and CRH/VP cells in both groups. We conclude that the increased numbers of CRH/VP neurons in MS is a sign of activation of the HPA system in MS.

In addition we measured cortisol levels in postmortem CSF of 18 MS patients and 50 control subjects from which 5 MS patients and 6 control patients died of sepsis.[10] The median CSF levels were 381 nmol/L for the MS group without sepsis and 178 nmol/L for the control subjects without sepsis, which differed significantly from each other ($P = 0.008$; FIG. 2a). Control subjects with sepsis had twofold higher cortisol levels as compared to the control group without sepsis (median 345 nmol/L, $P = 0.08$; FIG. 2a), while sepsis was associated with a nonsignificant 40% decrease in MS patients (median 212 nmol/L, $P = 0.2$; FIG. 2a). The cortisol levels in postmortem serum and CSF of 33 subjects were highly correlated ($r = 0.76$, $P < 0.001$); therefore, CSF cortisol levels reflect plasma cortisol levels. Thus, in line with the activated state of the CRH neurons, cortisol also is elevated in the group of MS patients. However, the cortisol response is impaired in sepsis.

IL-6 LEVEL IN CSF IS NOT RESPONSIBLE FOR ACTIVATION OF THE HPA AXIS IN MS

The CSF IL-6 levels of the MS patients and control subjects were not significantly different from each other (medians 63 and 32 pg/mL, respectively, $P > 0.7$; FIG. 2b).[10] Also, sepsis was not associated with significant changes in IL-6 levels of either control or MS patients ($P > 0.3$). There was no significant correlation between the cortisol and IL-6 levels within the MS or control group ($r = 0.43$, $P = 0.14$ and $r = 0.26$, $P = 0.08$, respectively; FIG. 3a and 3b). Control subjects with sepsis, on the other hand, showed a strong positive correlation between cortisol and IL-6 ($r = 0.89$, $P = 0.019$; FIG. 3c), whereas such a correlation was not present in MS patients with sepsis ($r = -0.29$, $P = 0.49$). Thus, IL-6 does not seem to be the cause of the elevated levels of cortisol CSF in MS. In control subjects IL-6 is related to increased cortisol

---

FIGURE 3. Scatter graphs showing postmortem CSF cortisol and IL-6 relationships in subgroups of MS patients **(A)**, controls **(B)**, and MS patients and controls with sepsis **(C)** (clinicopathological data are given in TABLE 1). There are no significant correlations between cortisol and IL-6 levels in any group except for the control subjects with sepsis (MS: $r = 0.43$, $P = 0.14$; controls: $r = 0.26$, $P = 0.08$; MS with sepsis: $r = -0.29$, $P = 0.49$ and controls with sepsis: $r = 0.89$, $P = 0.019$). (Reproduced from Erkut *et al.* with permission.[10])

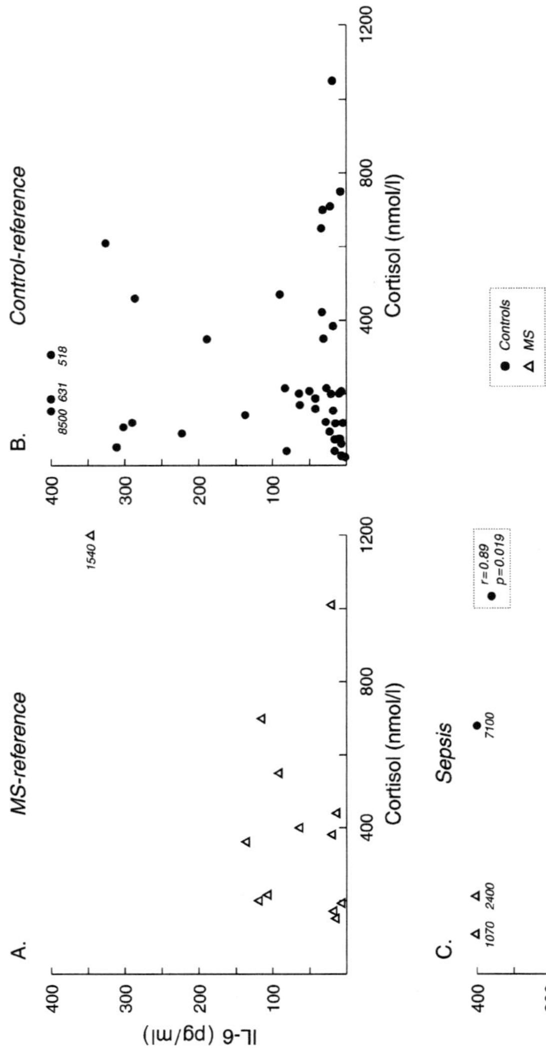

FIGURE 3. *See previous page for legend.*

levels, suggesting that IL-6 may be involved in the activation of the HPA axis during sepsis.

HIGH INCIDENCE OF ACTIVE MS LESIONS IN THE HYPOTHALAMUS

In order to assess the lesion load in myelinated bundles in or adjacent to the hypothalamus (FX: fornix; IC: internal capsule; AC: anterior commissure; OS: optic system),[19] the hypothalami of 17 MS patients were examined. The presence of (p)reactive (activated microglial cells and perivascular cuffing of leukocytes but no demyelination), active lesions (active demyelination and foamy macrophages), or chronic inactive MS lesions (gliotic demyelinated hypocellular lesions) was assessed according to the classification system of MS lesions in postmortem CNS tissue.[20] The incidence of active + (p)reactive lesions (the "active lesion score") and chronic inactive lesions (the "chronic inactive lesion score") were scored on a scale of 1–4.

MS lesions were found in the hypothalamus of 16 out of 17 MS patients (95%). The lesion load varied from a single small lesion in one of the myelinated bundles to complete demyelination of the bundles analyzed. In most of the cases, active and chronic inactive lesions were found within one hypothalamus. However, in one patient only chronic inactive lesions were found, and 3 out of 16 MS patients had only (p)reactive lesions. The total incidence of active MS lesions was high (60%), and the active lesion score was significantly higher in the IC (P = 0.005); whereas both scores were not significantly different in the AC (P = 0.44), the FX (P = 0.29) and the optic system (P = 0.20; FIG. 4A).

ACTIVE HYPOTHALAMIC LESION LOAD SHOWED A STRONG NEGATIVE RELATIONSHIP WITH DISEASE DURATION

The active lesion score showed a strong negative correlation with the duration of MS ($r = -0.72$, $P = 0.001$; FIG. 4B), whereas there was no significant relationship between the chronic inactive lesion score and the disease duration ($r = -0.41$, $P = 0.10$). A short disease duration until the moment of death in MS reflects an unfavorable course of the disease, as these patients die sooner as a result of MS.

TABLE 1. Clinicopathological data of MS patients and control subjects used for the CSF studies

Patient	*n*	M/F	Age	PMD	Onset of MS	Duration of MS
MS	13	1/12	55 ± 4	361 ± 20	34 ± 3	22 ± 4
MS sepsis	5	2/3	62 ± 6	344 ± 69	31 ± 3	30 ± 7
Controls	44	30/14	72 ± 1	413 ± 27		
Controls sepsis	6	4/2	72 ± 5	563 ± 135		

ABBREVIATIONS: M/F = male/female; PMD = postmortem delay (hours).

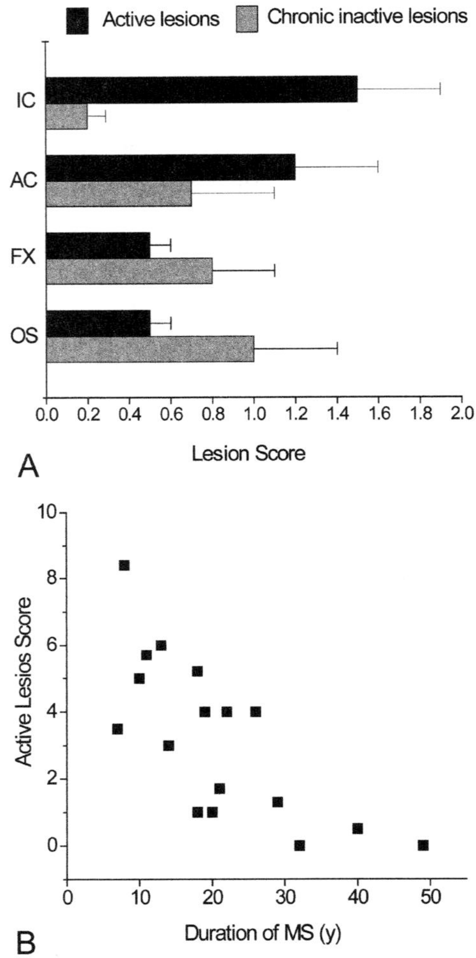

FIGURE 4. Active and chronic inactive MS lesion score in the hypothalamus of 17 MS patients in different myelin bundles in the hypothalamus **(A)** (IC = internal capsule, AC = anterior commissure, FX = fornix, OS = optic system); and relationship between the active MS lesion score in the hypothalamus and the duration of MS **(B)**. Clinicopathological data (mean ± SEM): age, MS 54.3 ± 3.6 years, controls 53.3 ± 3.6 years; postmortem delay, MS 838 ± 197 hours, controls 575 ± 164 hours; fixation, MS 34.6 ± 2.9 days, controls 33.9 ± 4.1 days; duration of MS 20.9 ± 2.7 years. The active lesion score comprises both (p)reactive (containing activated microglial cells but no demyelination) and active demyelinating MS lesions (containing lipid-laden demyelinating macrophages), whereas the chronic inactive lesion score concerns hypocellular inactive gliotic demyelinated lesions. Note the high incidence of active MS lesions in a group with a mean duration of 21 years and the highly significant negative relationship between the active lesion score and the disease duration ($r = -0.72$, $P = 0.001$); whereas there is no relationship between the chronic inactive lesion score and the duration of MS ($r = -0.41$, $P = 0.10$). Short disease duration until death points to an unfavorable disease course, as these patients died sooner as a result of MS. (Reproduced from Huitinga *et al.* with permission.[19])

DISCUSSION AND CONCLUSIONS

Increased numbers of CRH neurons colocalizing VP in the hypothalamus of MS patients and increased levels of cortisol in the CSF show that the HPA axis of MS patients is activated. These postmortem data confirm the results of endocrine studies in living MS patients that show that they have elevated resting cortisol levels in plasma and an enhanced response to the dexamethasone suppression test,[12–15] all indications of an activated HPA axis. The fact that only the numbers of CRH neurons that colocalize VP are elevated is a sign of hyperactivity, and upregulation of VP expression in CRH neurons is also seen in animal models of chronic inflammation.[21,22] However, in these models CRH mRNA expression is reduced in the presence of upregulation of VP.[22,23] It is thought that sustained activation of the hippocampal-hypothalamus feedback loop during the chronic inflammatory stress in these models leads to enhancement of the inhibitory signal from the hippocampus to the paraventricular nucleus and thereby to reduced mRNA expression.[22,23] VP upregulation in this situation may act as a compensatory mechanism that sustains HPA axis activity when CRH neurons become less efficient.[22] Thus, the increased coexpression of VP in CRH neurons in MS may be an additional support of the activation of the CRH neurons by the chronic inflammation in the CNS during MS.

Interestingly, in a model of MS, chronic experimental allergic encephalomyelitis (EAE), CRH neurons show a decreased sensitivity to IL-1 during the course of the disease, but not to noninflammatory stress stimuli.[8] Decreased sensitivity of the HPA axis to acute inflammatory stimuli during MS was also found in our study, illustrated by the absence of a cortisol response during systemic infection. In our group of MS patients that died with sepsis, cortisol levels were not increased as they were in control subjects with sepsis. Failure to elevate endogenous cortisol levels under severe disease conditions like sepsis can have a serious negative impact on the prognosis of the MS patients. Indeed, patients with adrenal insufficiency have a worse disease prognosis and benefit from a high-dose gluocorticoid treatment in severe septic conditions.[24]

IL-6 levels were not different between MS patients and control subjects, which is in agreement with the CSF results of others,[25,26] but not with the report of Maimone *et al.*[27] Differences in IL-6 levels between the studies could be caused by differences in clinical subtypes and activity level of the disease, since the MS patients in the latter study had active MS. We did not find a correlation between IL-6 and cortisol in MS patients. Therefore, we do not have any evidence to imply IL-6 as a major cause of cortisol release during MS. However, we did find a strong positive correlation between IL-6 and cortisol in control patients who died with sepsis, indicating that an interaction between the two is present in acute inflammatory situations. It was indeed shown that IL-6 can activate the HPA axis in humans.[28]

The postmortem IL-6 CSF levels in our study are two- to threefold higher than the findings of some studies[25,26] and almost 20 times higher than the findings of others in lumbar CSF.[13] A possible explanation for this difference can be an increase in IL-6 CSF levels during the process of dying. Importantly, the cortisol levels are also 10–20 times higher than the *in vivo* levels measured in lumbar CSF. This is in accordance with our earlier study on postmortem CSF.[29] The high cortisol levels in postmortem CSF in both controls and MS patients is likely due to the fatal condition during the process of dying (Erkut *et al.*, submitted).

Unexpected was the high lesion load found in myelin bundles in and adjacent to the hypothalamus.[19] All but one of the MS patients had hypthalamic lesions, varying from a small focal lesion in one of the bundles to completely demyelinated hypothalami. Moreover, more than 50% of these lesions were immunologically active—that is, contained lipid-laden foamy macrophages and activated microglial cells. The mean duration of disease was 21 ± 3 years in the group of MS patients studied; thus, active demyelination is an ongoing process even during an extremely long disease course. Demyelination of fiber bundles in and adjacent to the hypothalamus has likely implications for the conduction of action potentials in the axons and thereby affects their functions. Demyelination in the optic nerve may lead to visual problems; in the anterior commissure it may lead to impaired temporal functions such as memory and olfactory deficits; lesions in the fornix may lead to disturbed memory functions, and lesions in the internal capsule to disturbed motor functions. Clearly the presence of many active lesions in the hypothalamus leads to an unfavorable disease course since the disease duration leading to death shows highly significant negative correlations with the active lesion score. Since the presence of many lesions in the hypothalamus is accompanied by a similarly high lesion load elsewhere in the CNS,[19] this relationship reflects a positive correlation between disease duration and high lesion load anywhere in the CNS, rather than MS lesions in the hypothalamus alone.

Since the majority of the MS lesions in the hypothalamus contain activated macrophages and microglial cells, inflammatory mediators produced in these lesions may diffuse towards the CRH neurons and modulate their activity.[30] Consequently, active MS lesions may have a strong impact on the activity of the HPA axis.[16] Preliminary data indeed show a strong negative relationship between the presence of active hypothalamic MS lesions and the state of activation of the neurons. Interestingly, the nearer these active MS lesions are situated to the CRH neurons, the stronger the effect, suggesting that the MS lesions actively suppress the activity of the CRH neurons. Thus, active MS lesions in the hypothalamus suppress the HPA axis, and active hypothalamic lesions also relate to a worse disease course given their negative relationship with the duration of MS. Given the beneficial effects of glucocorticoids on EAE and MS, we postulate that the suppression of CRH neurons by active hypothalamic MS lesions causes an unfavorable disease course of MS via an inadequate cortisol response during relapses of MS.

REFERENCES

1. Martinelli, V. 2000. Trauma, stress and multiple sclerosis. Neurol. Sci. **21:** S849–852.
2. Goodin D.S., G. Ebers, K.P. Johnson, *et al.* 1999. The relationship of MS of physical trauma and psychological stress. Report of the Therapeutics and Technology Assessment Subcommittee of the American Academy of Neurology. Neurology **52:** 1737–1745.
3. Polman, C.H & B.M.J. Uitdehaag. 2000. Drug treament in multiple sclerosis. Brit. Med. J. **321:** 490–494.
4. Gold, R., F. Burgereit & K.V. Toyka. 2001. Mechanism of glucocorticoid hormones: possible implications for therapy of neuroimmunological disorders. J. Neuroimmunol. **117:** 1–8.
5. MacPhee, I.A., F. Antoni & D.W. Mason. 1989. Spontaneous recovery of rats from experimental allergic encephalomyelitis is dependent on regulation of the immune system by endogenous adrenal corticosteroids. J. Exp. Med. **169:** 431–445.

6. MASON, D. 1991. Genetic variation in the stress response: susceptibility to experimental allergic encephalomyelitis and implications for human inflammatory diseases. Immunol. Today **12:** 57–61.
7. STERNBERG, E.M. 2001. Neuroendocrine regulation of autoimmune/inflammatory disease. J. Endocrinol. **169:** 429–435.
8. STEFFERL, A., M.K. STORCH, C. LININGTON, *et al.* 2001. Disease progression in chronic relapsing experimental allergic encephalomyelitis is associated with reduced inflammation driven production of corticosterone. Endocrinology **142:** 3616–3624.
9. ERKUT, Z.A., M.A. HOFMAN, R. RAVID & D.F. SWAAB. 1995. Increased activity of hypothalamic corticotropin-releasing hormone neurons in multiple sclerosis. J. Neuroimmunol. **62:** 27–33.
10. ERKUT, Z.A., E. ENDERT, I. HUITINGA & D. SWAAB. 2002. Cortisol is increased in post mortem cerebrospinal fluid of multiple sclerosis patients: relationship with cytokines. Multiple Sclerosis **8:** 229–236.
11. REDER, A.T., R.L. MACKOWIEC & M.T. LOWY. 1994. Adrenal size is increased in multiple sclerosis. Arch. Neurol. **51:** 151–154.
12. MICHELSON, D., L. STONE, E. GALLIVEN, *et al.* 1994. Multiple sclerosis is associated with alterations in hypothalamic-pituitary-adrenal axis function. J. Clin. Endocrinol. Metabol. **79:** 848–853.
13. FASSBENDER, K., R. SCHMIDT, R. MÖßNER, *et al.* 1998. Mood disorders and dysfunction of the hypothalamus-pituitary-adrenal axis in multiple sclerosis. Arch. Neurol. **55:** 66–72.
14. GRASSER, A., A. MÖLLER, H. BACKMUND, *et al.* 1996. Heterogeneity of the hypothalamic-pituitary-adrenal system response to a combined dexamethasone-CRH test in multiple sclerosis. Exp. Clin. Endocrinol. **104:** 31–37.
15. THEN BERGH, F., T. KÜMPFEL, C. TRENKWALDER, *et al.* 1999. Dysregulation of the hypothalamo-pituitary-adrenal axis is related to the clinical course of MS. Neurology **53:** 772–777.
16. TURNBULL, A.V. & C.L. RIVIER. 1999. Regulation of the hypothalamic-pituitary-adrenal axis by cytokines: actions and mechanisms of action. Physiol. Rev. **79:** 1–71.
17. BROSNAN, C.F., B. CANELLA, L. BATTISTINI & C.S. RAINE. 1995. Cytokine localization in multiple sclerosis lesions: correlation with adhesion molecule expression and reactive oxygen species. Neurology **45:** S16–S21.
18. WHITNALL, M.H. 1993. Regulation of the hypothalamic corticotropin-releasing hormone secretory system. Progr. Neurobiol. **40:** 573–629.
19. HUITINGA, I., C.J.A. DE GROOT, P. VAN DER VALK, *et al.* 2001. Hypothalamic lesions in multiple sclerosis. J. Neuropathol. Exp. Neurol. **60:**1208–1218.
20. DEGROOT, C.J.A., L. BERGERS, W. KAMPHORTS, *et al.* 2001. Postmortem MRI-guided sampling of multiple sclerosis brain lesions: increased yield of active demyelinating and (p)reactive lesions. Brain **124:** 1635–1645.
21. CHOWDREY, H.S., P.J. LARSEN, M.S. HARBUZ, *et al.* 1995. Evidence for arginine vasopressin as the primary activator of the HPA axis during adjuvant arthritis. Br. J. Pharmacol. **116:** 2417–2424.
22. SAKIC, B., N. LAFLAMME, L.S. CRNIC, *et al.* 1999. Reduced corticotropin-releasing factor and enhanced vasopressin gene expression in brains of mice with autoimmunity-induced behavioural dysfunction. J. Neuroimmunol. **96:** 80–91.
23. GRINEVICH, V., X.M. MA, J.P. HERMAN, *et al.* 2001. Effect of repeated polysaccharide administration on tissue cytokine expression and hypothalamus pituitary axis activity in rats. J. Neuroendocrinol. **13:** 711–723.
24. MEDURI, G.U. & G.P. CHROUSOS. 1998. Duration of glucocorticoid treatment and the outcome in sepsis: is the right drug used in the wrong way? Chest **114:** 355–360.
25. HAUSER, S.L., T.H. DOOLITTLE, R. LINCOLN, *et al.* 1990. Cytokine accumulations in CSF of multiple sclerosis patients. Neurology **40:** 1735–1739.
26. SEKIZAWA, T., H. OPENSHAW, K. OHBO, *et al.* 1998. CSF IL-6 in amyotropic lateral sclerosis: immunological parameter for comparison with inflammatory and non-inflammatory central nervous system diseases. J. Neurol. Sci. **154:** 194–199.
27. MAIMONE, D., S. GREGORY, B.G. ARNASON & A.T. REDER. 1991. Cytokine levels in cerebrospinal fluid and serum of patients with multiple sclerosis. J. Neuroimmunol. **32:** 67–74.

28. MASTORAKIS, G., G. CHROUSOS & J.S. WEBER. 1993. Recombinant IL-6 activates the HPA-axis in humans. J. Clin. Endocrinol. Metabol. **77:** 1690–1694.
29. SWAAB, D.F., F.C. RAADSHEER, E. ENDERT, *et al.* 1994. Increased cortisol levels in aging and Alzheimer's disease in post mortem CSF. J. Neuroendocrinol. **6:** 681–687.
30. KONSMAN, J.P., V. TRIDON & R. DANTZER. 2000. Diffusion and action of intracerebroventricularly injected interleukin-1 in the CNS. Neuroscience **101:** 957–967.

Effects of *in Vitro* and *in Vivo* Opioids on the Production of IL-12 and IL-10 by Murine Macrophages

PAOLA SACERDOTE

Department of Pharmacology, University of Milan, Milan, Italy

ABSTRACT: We evaluated the ability of the specific μ opioid receptor agonist DAMGO, the κ-specific agonist U-50488 *in vitro,* and exogenous opioid morphine administered *in vivo* both acutely and chronically to modulate IL-12 and IL-10 production by murine peritoneal macrophages. DAMGO and U-50488 at the concentrations of 10^{-6} and 10^{-8} M decreased the production of IL-12 without affecting IL-10. One hour after the acute administration of 5, 10, and 20 mg/kg of morphine a dose-related decrease of both IL-10 and IL-12 levels was present. The pretreatment with naltrexone at doses up to 20 mg/kg did not prevent the decrease of IL-10 and IL-12 induced by morphine. When the drug was administered chronically, a differential development of tolerance to the immune effects was observed. After 3 days of treatment the effect of the acute challenge with 20 mg/kg of morphine on IL-12 was lost. In contrast, morphine-induced inhibition of IL-10 disappeared between 10 and 12 days of treatment, in parallel with tolerance to the antinociceptive effect. These results suggest that opioids modulate macrophage cytokine production. However, the effects exerted by the *in vivo* administration of morphine are not superimposable onto those induced by the *in vitro* administration of specific opioid agonists.

KEYWORDS: morphine; opioids; cytokines; macrophages; interleukin-10; interleukin-12; tolerance

INTRODUCTION

It is well known that endogenous opioid peptides and exogenous opioid compounds, such as morphine, affect both natural and adaptive immunity in the experimental animal as well as in the human.[1–3] Surprisingly, however, the modulation exerted by the endogenous opioids does not always coincide with the effects obtained with morphine, and different results have also been obtained in *in vitro* vs. *in vivo* experiments.[4] Macrophages play a central role in both innate and adaptive immunity. Interleukin (IL)-1, IL-6 and tumor necrosis factor (TNF)-α produced by macrophages are prominent inflammatory cytokines.[5,6] Moreover, monocytes/macrophages and professional antigen presenting cells are the main producers of IL-12,[7] the critical factor driving the development of T helper (Th)-1 cells,[8] linked to cellular

Address for correspondence: Paola Sacerdote, Department of Pharmacology, University of Milan, via Vanvitelli 32, 20129 Milan, Italy. Voice: +39-02-503-16929; fax:+39-02-503-16933.
paola.sacerdote@unimi.it

Ann. N.Y. Acad. Sci. 992: 129–140 (2003).

immune responses and tissue injury. Conversely, Th-2 cells, responsible for humoral responses and allergy,[8] are stimulated by the T lymphocyte cytokine IL-4 and by IL-10,[8] produced by T lymphocytes as well as by monocytes/macrophages.

Therefore, on considering the importance of macrophage cytokines in orchestrating the immune response, we studied the effect of the *in vitro* administration of the specific opioid agonists for the μ receptor DAMGO and for the κ receptor U-50488 on IL-12 and IL-10 production by murine peritoneal macrophages. Moreover, considering that morphine is still the drug of first choice for the treatment of severe acute and chronic pain conditions, we analyzed the effects exerted by the *in vivo* administration of morphine on macrophage cytokine production. Although it is well known that tolerance develops to many of the effects of morphine, the timing of the development of tolerance to the immune effects of morphine has been scarcely taken into consideration. Therefore we paid particular attention to the development of tolerance to the effect of morphine on IL-10 and IL-12 cytokines and its relation with the antinociceptive effect of the drug.

MATERIALS AND METHODS

Preparation of Macrophages

BALB/CJ male mice, 18 to 20 g body weight (Charles River, Calco, Italy), were inoculated intraperitoneally (i.p.) with 2 mL of 3% Brewer's thioglycollate medium (Difco, Detroit, MI) for macrophage elicitation. Four days later, peritoneal exudate cells (PECs) were harvested in cold RPMI-1640 medium (Sigma, St Louis, MO) plus 10% of fetal calf serum (FCS) (GIBCO BRL, Life Technology, Italy). Isolation and purification of macrophages were carried out by adherence to culture plates. After a period of 2 h, nonadherent cells were removed with the medium and adherent cells washed twice with warm RPMI plus 10% FCS. Elicited macrophages were primed with 1 μg/mL of LPS (Sigma) for IL-10 production or with 1 μg/mL LPS and 50 U/mL IFN-γ (Pharmingen, San Diego, CA) for IL-12 stimulation.

In Vitro *Treatments*

PECs obtained from 6 animals were pooled and macrophages isolated as described. The specific μ agonist DAMGO and the κ agonist U-50488 (Tocris Cookson, UK) were added to the macrophage cultures at the concentrations of 10^{-6}, 10^{8},10^{-10}, and 10^{-12} M. After 24 h of incubation medium was collected for cytokine evaluation.

In Vivo *Treatments*

In the acute experiments, morphine hydrochloride (S.A.L.A.R.S., Como, Italy) was injected subcutaneously (s.c.) 4 days after the macrophage elicitation at doses of 5, 10, or 20 mg/kg. Control animals were treated with the same volume of saline. Naltrexone (S.A.L.A.R.S., Como, Italy) was injected s.c. at doses of 10 mg/kg and 20 mg/kg, alone or 15 minutes before 20 mg/kg of morphine. Starting from the thioglycollate injection day, 24 animals were treated s.c. with morphine twice daily at the doses of 10 mg/kg for 2 days and 20 mg/kg for the following days. Control groups (24 animals) received the same volume of saline. At the 3rd, 7th, and 12th days of treatment, 16 animals (8 morphine + 8 saline) were sacrificed for evaluation of cytokine production. In all experiments animals received the last morphine injection 1 h before sacrifice for macrophage collection. PECs were harvested and stimulated as described above.

Cytokine Evaluation

The levels of IL-12 (p70 protein) and of IL-10 were determined by enzyme-linked immunosorbent assay (ELISA) protocol as standardized by Pharmingen (San Diego, CA) and previously described in detail.[9]

Evaluation of Tolerance to Antinociception

The hot-plate test was used to assess nociceptive thresholds.[3] In order to evaluate the development of tolerance to the analgesic effect of morphine, the antinociceptive response was recorded 60 minutes after challenge with 5 mg/kg morphine every other day of chronic treatment. The results are expressed as percentage of the maximal possible effect (%MPE); MPE = [(TL–BL)/(ML–BL)] × 100, where BL is the mean basal latency, TL is the test latency measured after treatments, and ML is the maximal latency accepted (30 seconds).

Statistical Analysis

Significant differences between groups were assessed by one-way ANOVA, followed by Bonferroni's *t* test for multiple comparisons. %MPE was evaluated by the Kruskall Wallis analysis of variance for nonparametric data.

RESULTS

In Vitro *Experiments*

FIGURE 1 reports the effect of the addition of the specific μ agonist DAMGO and of the κ agonist U-50488 to macrophage cultures on the production of IL-10 and IL-12 stimulated with LPS or LPS + IFN-γ, respectively. Both DAMGO and U-50488 decreased the production of IL-12 when added to cultures at the concentrations of $10^{-6}$and 10^{-8} (upper panel). In contrast the opioid agonists did not exert any significant effect on IL-10 production (lower panel).

In Vivo *Experiments*

Acute Experiments

One hour after the acute administration of 5, 10, and 20 mg/kg of morphine to mice, peritoneal macrophages were incubated for 24 h in the presence of stimuli for the production of cytokines. As reported in FIGURE 2, acute morphine administration decreased the production of both IL-12 (upper panel) and IL-10 (lower panel) by thioglycollate-elicited macrophages. The effect on IL-12 started to be present at 10 mg/kg of morphine, but reached statistical significance only with 20 mg/kg of the

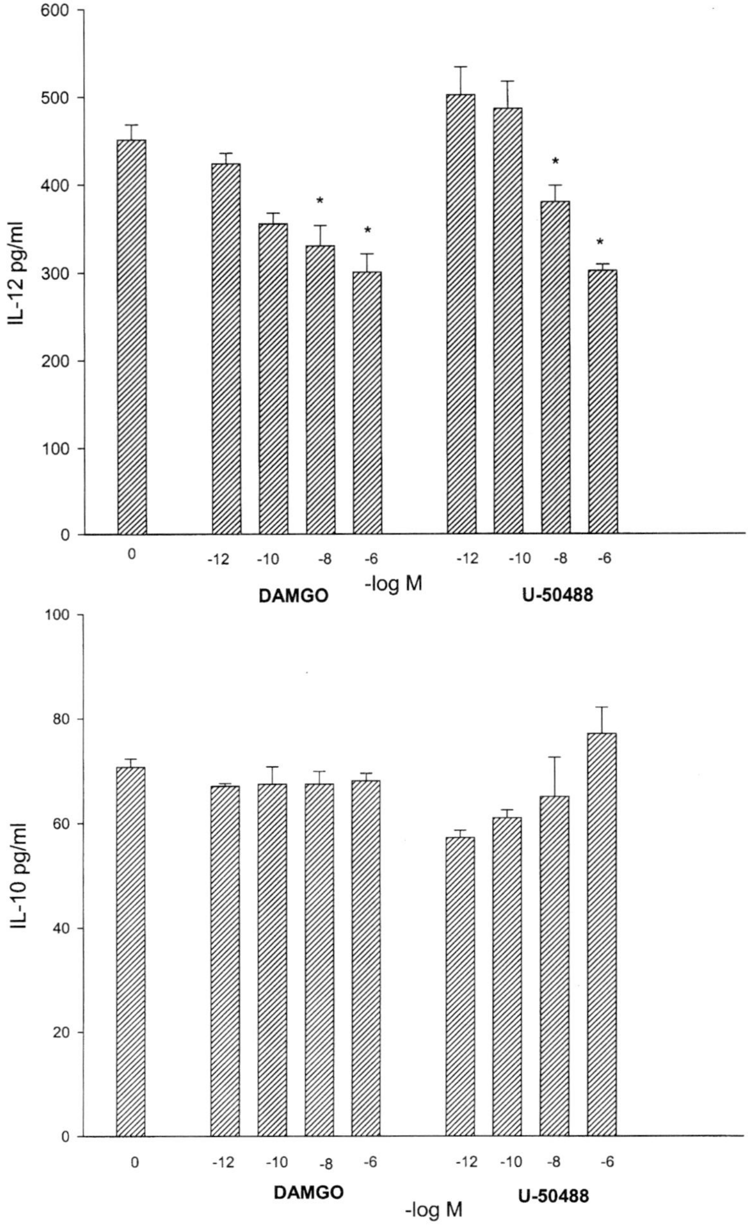

FIGURE 1. Effect of DAMGO and U-50488 on the production of IL-12 **(upper panel)** and IL-10 **(lower panel)** by macrophages *in vitro*. The opioid agonists were added at the reported concentrations to macrophages at the moment of stimulation with LPS (IL-10) or LPS + IFN-γ (IL-12). Cytokines were evaluated in the medium 24 h later. Values are means ± SD of 3 experiments. $^*P < 0.05$ vs. control (medium only).

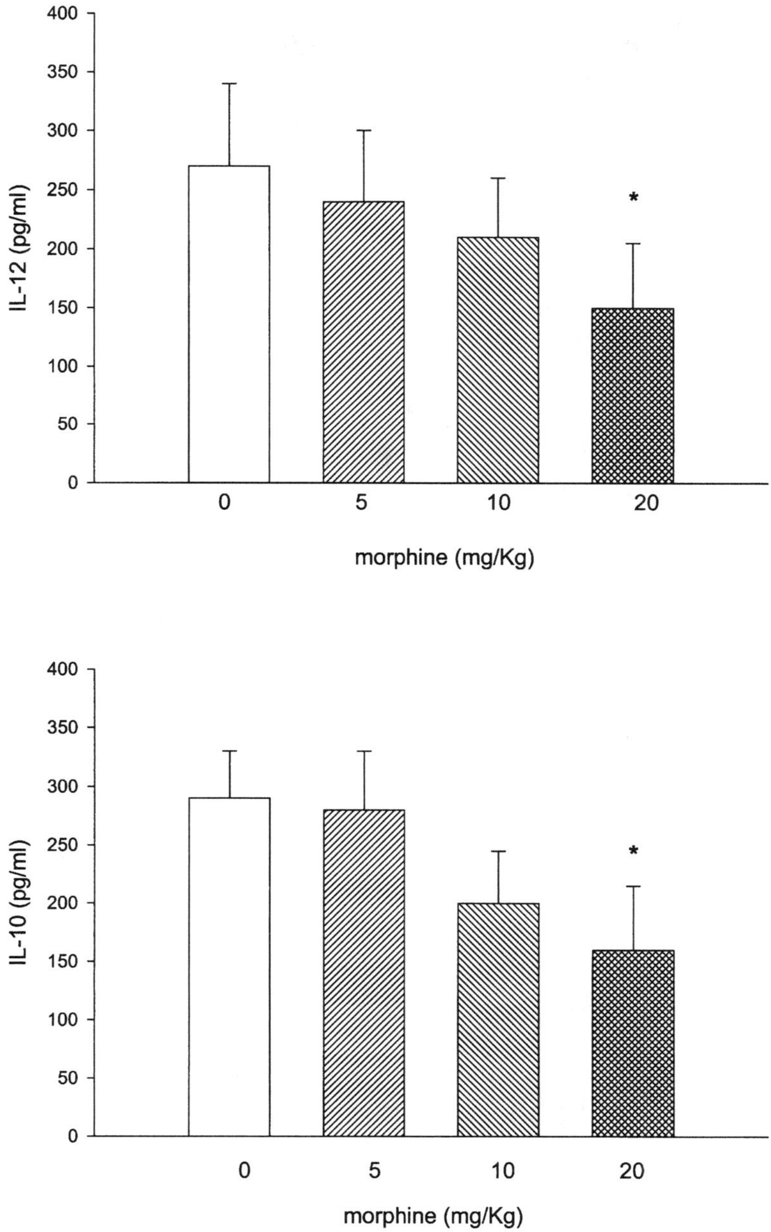

FIGURE 2. Effect of the acute administration of three doses of morphine on IL-12 **(upper panel)** and IL-10 **(lower panel)** production by thioglycollate-elicited murine peritoneal macrophages. Values are means ± SD of 8 animals (1 experimental session). The experiments were repeated three times with similar results. * $P < 0.01$ vs. saline-treated animals (0).

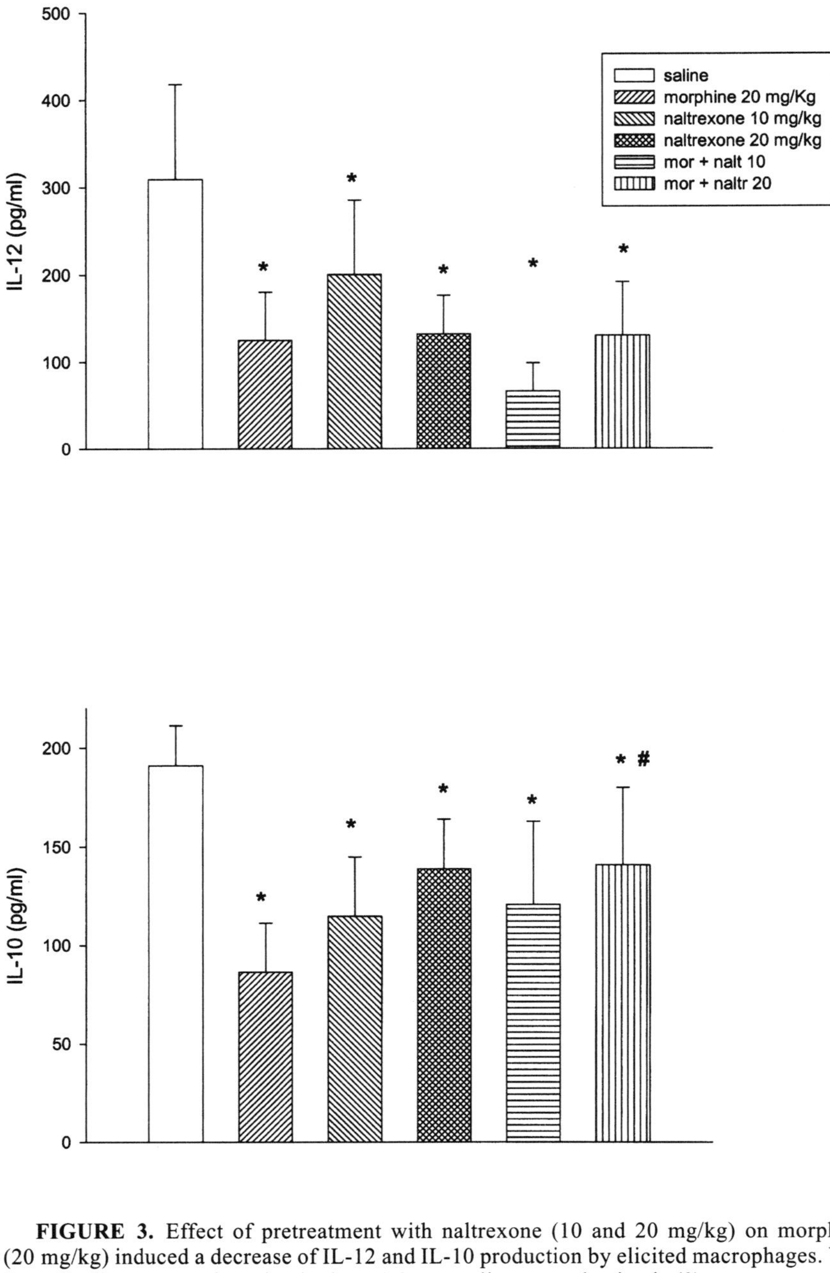

FIGURE 3. Effect of pretreatment with naltrexone (10 and 20 mg/kg) on morphine (20 mg/kg) induced a decrease of IL-12 and IL-10 production by elicited macrophages. Values are means ± SD of 8 animals. *$P < 0.01$ vs. saline-treated animals (0).

opiate drug. Also IL-10 was significantly reduced only by the highest dose of morphine.

Effect of Naltrexone Pretreatment

FIGURE 3 reports the effects of the acute administration of 10 and 20 mg/kg of naltrexone alone or in combination with 20 mg/kg of morphine on IL-12 (upper panel) and IL-10 (lower panel) production. Both doses of the opiate antagonist were able to induce a slight, but significant, decrease of IL-12 and IL-10 production by elicited peritoneal macrophages. When the antagonist doses were administered 15 minutes before 20 mg/kg of morphine, IL-12 remained significantly lower than that in saline-treated animals. As far as IL-10 is concerned, at the high dose of 20 mg/kg naltrexone seems to partially prevent the morphine-induced IL-10 reduction.

Chronic Experiments

In order to study the development of tolerance to the antinociceptive and immunosuppressive effects of morphine, animals were treated for 12 days with morphine. FIGURE 4 reports the development of tolerance to the antinociceptive effect of morphine. Each point represents the mean response of 8 mice that were going to be killed the following day for immune evaluation. Tolerance started by the 6th day of treatment and was complete at the 11th day of chronic morphine administration. In fact,

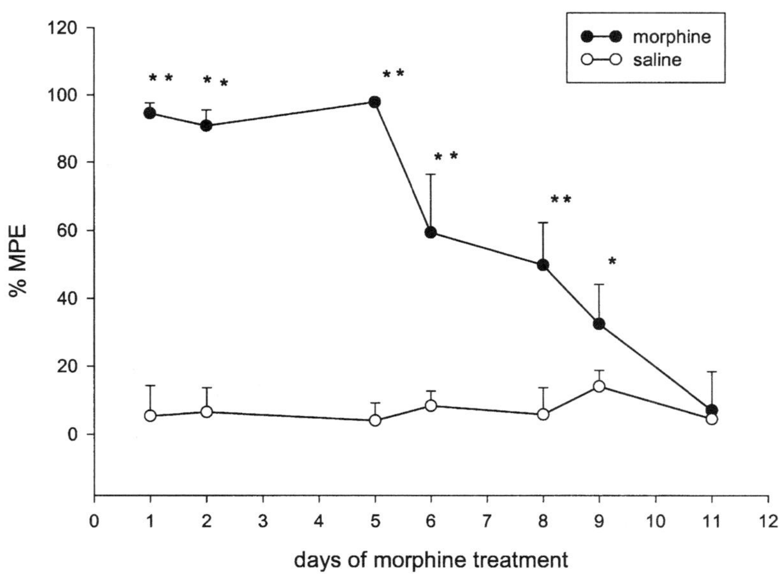

FIGURE 4. Analgesic responses to acute administration of morphine (5 mg/kg) in mice chronically treated with morphine. Nociceptive thresholds were measured using the hot-plate test immediately before and 60 min after acute morphine treatment. As controls, animals chronically treated with saline were used. Values are means ± SD of 8 animals. $*P < 0.05$ vs. saline-treated animals $**P < 0.001$ vs. saline-treated animals.

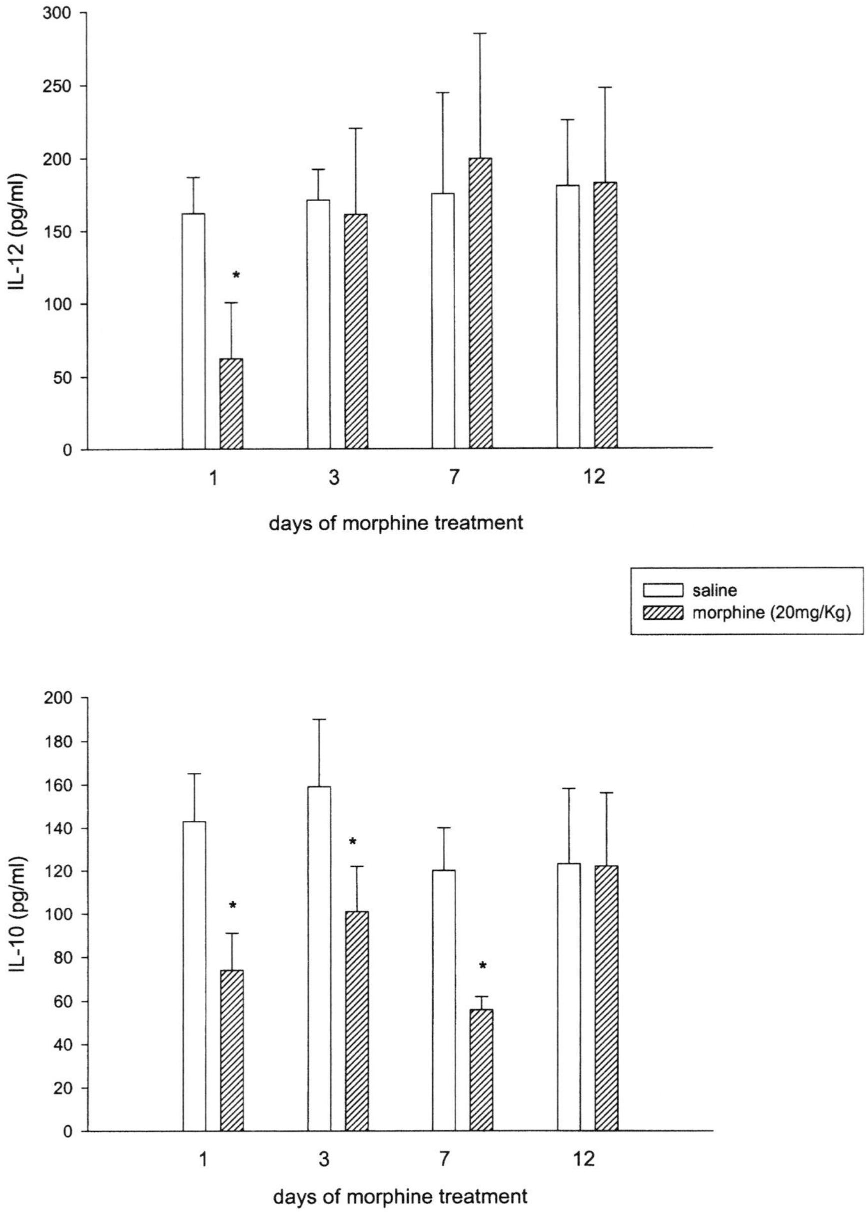

FIGURE 5. Development of tolerance to morphine-induced decrease of IL-10 and IL-12 production by peritoneal macrophages. Mice chronically treated with morphine for the time indicated were challenged with 20 mg/kg of morphine. One hour after morphine administration macrophages were stimulated *in vitro* for 24 h in the presence of LPS (IL-10) or LPS + IFN-γ (IL-12). Values are means ± SD of 8 animals (1 experimental session). Eexperiments were repeated three times with similar results. *$P < 0.01$ vs. saline-treated animals.

at this time the acute challenge with 5 mg/kg of morphine did not elicit any significant antinociceptive effect in comparison to saline-treated animals. The effects of chronic morphine on cytokine production are reported in FIGURE 5. As shown in the upper panel, tolerance developed very rapidly to the suppressive effect of morphine on IL-12 since it appeared between the 1st and 3rd day of treatment; after 3 days of treatment, indeed, no reduction of this cytokine was present after 20 mg/kg of morphine. In contrast, the effect of the opiate on IL-10 decrease persisted longer, since it disappeared between the 7th and the 12th day, in parallel with the development of tolerance to the antinociceptive effect.

DISCUSSION

This study shows that opioids affect the production of the macrophage cytokines IL-12 and IL-10. *In vitro* addition of opioid receptor–specific agonists significantly decreases IL-12 production, without affecting IL-10 production; μ and κ opioid receptor agonists are equally able to modulate IL-12 production *in vitro*. IL-12, a heterodimeric cytokine produced mainly by monocytes/macrophages, is a central inducer of cell-mediated immunity that promotes the development, proliferation, and function of Th1 cells.[7,8] Th1 cells promote the activation and function of natural killer cells and of T cell cytotoxicity and produce IL-2 and IFN-γ.[8] In contrast IL-10, produced as a result of activation of Th2 cells, B lymphocytes, and macrophages, is an endogenous inhibitor of IL-12 and Th1 responses, while stimulating the Th2 cell population and humoral immunity.[8,9] In previous work we showed that endogenous opioid peptides have a role in regulating the Th1/Th2 pattern, as they skew the balance towards Th2, by decreasing Th1 and increasing Th2 cytokines.[10] Considering the effect of the opioid agonists on macrophages *in vitro*, it can be suggested that the effects exerted by endogenous opioids on the Th1/Th2 pattern are mediated by their action on IL-12 production by macrophages. The diminished production of IL-12 can, in fact, be at the basis of a Th2 shift. This hypothesis is further supported by the observation that when DAMGO and U-50488 are added *in vitro* to purified T cells, they do not directly affect the production of IL-2, IFN-γ, or IL-4 (Sacerdote *et al.*, unpublished results). However, when the exogenous opioid morphine is given *in vivo* to mice, different results were obtained. Indeed, the acute administration of morphine significantly decreased both IL-12 and IL-10 production by LPS and IFN-γ–stimulated murine peritoneal macrophages.

The question of the development of tolerance to the immunological effects of morphine is still an open one. A certain degree of tolerance has been shown to develop to some, although not all, immune effects of morphine. West *et al.*,[11,12] employing a model with morphine delivered in drinking water, reported that tolerance developed to the suppression of natural killer (NK) activity in parallel to tolerance to antinociception, while the lymphoproliferation suppression did not seem to go into tolerance. In contrast, other authors,[13,14] with a twice-daily injection protocol, showed that the suppression of Con-A lymphoproliferation induced by morphine underwent tolerance in 4–8 days in parallel to antinociceptive tolerance. Also, in a recent paper[15] development of tolerance to morphine inhibition of lymphoproliferation was reported; while, in this case, no tolerance to suppression of NK activity was observed up to the 8th day of chronic morphine treatment. On the whole, it seems clear that the development of tolerance to morphine effects can depend upon many factors, such as the immune parameter evaluated and the way of drug administration. Our data on the effects of chronic morphine on macrophage cytokines seem to confirm this observation. When, in fact, the effects of morphine and the production of IL-12 completely disappeared after 3 days of morphine treatment, the reduction of IL-10 was still present. It has, therefore, to be considered that the final status of the immune responses can vary with different morphine regimens.

It is difficult to hypothesize how the modifications of macrophage cytokine production induced by acute or chronic morphine can impact on Th1/Th2 balance, especially considering that a complex regulatory loop exists between Th1 and Th2 cytokines.[7–9] The results of the present study indicate that *in vivo* morphine seems to be a potent inhibitor of macrophage activity, suppressing both IL-12 and IL-10 secretion. In theory, these modifications should diminish both Th1 and Th2 responses, or, in any case, should not particularly affect one of the T subsets. Consistently, the data present in the literature report that morphine affects both cellular and humoral immune responses,[4,16,17] as well as the production of Th1 cytokines (IL-2 and IFN-γ)[3,4] and Th2 cytokines such as IL-4.[18]

The differential development of tolerance to immune effects of morphine can be relevant when considering the chronic morphine treatment of patients. The final effect of morphine on immune function can, in fact, vary over time, depending on the balance of the effects still present at different moments. The effects induced by the administration of the opioid antagonist naltrexone on IL-12 and IL-10 production are surprising. The antagonist, in fact, seems to possess some agonistic activity, since it slightly decreases the cytokine levels, similarly to the effects exerted by morphine. Moreover, the pretreatment with the antagonist does not block the morphine-induced decrease of IL-12, and only at the high dose of 20 mg/kg seems to slightly block IL-10 reduction. However, we are aware that this dose is very high and that any specificity at the μ opioid receptor should be lost. Two possible scenarios can be envisaged in order to explain these results.

The most obvious explanation can be that the effects induced by morphine are not mediated by a classical opioid receptor. In the literature most, but not all, of the immune effects of morphine have been shown to be blocked by the antagonists and therefore to be mediated by the μ opioid receptors.[4,19] However, several papers have reported on the existence of nonclassical opioid binding sites on a different cell population that can mediate the non-naloxone reversible effects of morphine.[19,20]

Another explanation could be that under our experimental conditions, naltrexone could behave as an agonist. Conditions where the opioid antagonists naloxone and naltrexone behave as agonists have already been described for the main opioid effect—centrally and peripherally mediated analgesia.[21–24] Further studies are in any case needed in order to better understand the effects of naltrexone.

In conclusion, although it is evident that opioids can regulate several aspects of macrophage functions, much remains to be elucidated. In future studies, we must be aware that morphine has particular immunomodulating properties that are not always superimposable onto those exerted by either endogenous opioids or specific receptor agonists. Moreover, the experimental protocols, such as *in vitro* vs. *in vivo* experiments or acute vs. chronic administration, can deeply condition the final results.

REFERENCES

1. Lysle, D.T., M.E. Coussons, V.J. Watts, *et al.* 1993. Morphine-induced alterations of immune status: dose dependency, compartment specificity and antagonism by naltrexone. J. Pharmacol. Exp. Ther. **265:** 1071–1078.
2. Panerai, A.E. & P. Sacerdote. 1997. Beta-endorphin in the immune system: a role at last. Immunol. Today **18:** 317–319.
3. Sacerdote, P., B. Manfredi, P. Mantegazza & A.E. Panerai. 1997. Antinociceptive and immunosuppressive effects of opiate drugs: a structure-related activity study. Br. J. Pharmacol. **121:** 834–840.
4. Eisenstein, T.K. & M.E. Hillburger. 1998. Opioid modulation of immune responses: effects on phagocyte and lymphoyd cell populations. J. Neuroimmunol. **83:** 36–44.
5. Miller, J.A., S.J. Hopkins & G.N. Luheshi. 1997. Sites of action of IL-1 in the development of fever and cytokine responses to tissue inflammation in the rat. Br. J. Pharmacol. **120:** 1274–1279.
6. Beutler, B. & A. Cerami. 1989. The biology of cachectin/TNF—a primary mediator of the host response. Annu. Rev. Immunol. **7:** 625–655.
7. Trincheri, G. 1995. Interleukin-12: a proinflammatory cytokine with immunoregulatory functions that bridge innate resistance and antigen specific adaptive immunity. Annu. Rev. Immunol. **13:** 251–276.
8. Mosman, T.R. & S. Sad. 1996. The expanding universe of T-cell subsets; Th1,Th2 and more. Immunol. Today **17:** 138–146.
9. Limiroli, E., L. Gaspani, A.E. Panerai & P. Sacerdote. 2002. Differential tolerance development in the modulation of macrophage cytokine production in mice. J. Leukocyte Biol. **72:** 43–48.
10. Sacerdote, P., B. Manfredi, L. Gaspani & A.E. Panerai. 2000. The opioid antagonist naloxone induces a shift from type 1 cytokine pattern to type 2 cytokine pattern in balb/cJ mice. Blood **95:** 2031–2036.
11. West, J.P., L.A. Dykstra & D.T. Lysle. 1997. Tolerance development to morphine-induced alterations of immune status administration. Drug Alcohol Depend. **46:** 147–157.
12. West, J.P., L.A. Dykstra & D.T. Lysle. 1998. Differential tolerance to morphine's immunomodulatory effects following continuous administration. Drug Alcohol Depend. **53:** 31–38.
13. Bayer, B.M., M.C. Hernandez & X.Z. Ding. 1994. Tolerance and crosstolerance to the suppressive effects of cocaine and morphine on lymphocyte proliferation. Pharmacol. Biochem. Behav. **53:** 227–234.
14. Bayer, B.M., R.M. Brechio, X.Z. Ding & M.C. Hernandez. 1994. Enhanced susceptibility of the immune system to stress in morphine-tolerant rats. Brain Behav. Immun. **8:** 173–184.
15. Massi, P., A. Vaccani, S. Romorini & D. Parolaro. 2001. Comparative characterization in the rat of the interaction between cannabinoids and opiates for their immunosuppressive and analgesic effects. J. Neuroimmunol. **117:** 116–124.
16. Bryant, H.U., E.W. Bernton & J.W. Holaday. 1988. Morphine pellet-induced immunomodulation in mice: temporal relationships. J. Pharmacol. Exp. Ther. **246:** 913–920.
17. Bussiere, L.J., M.W. Adler, T.J. Rogers & T.K. Eisenstein. 1993. Cytokine reversal of morphine-induced suppression of the antibody response. J. Pharmacol. Exp. Ther. **264:** 591–597.
18. Bhargava, H.N., P.T. Thomas, S. Thorat & R.V. House. 1994. Effect of morphine tolerance and abstinence on cellular immune responses. Brain Res. **642:** 1–10.
19. McCarthy, L., M. Wetzel, J.K. Sliker & T.K. Eisenstein, *et al.* 2001. Opioids, opioid receptors and the immune response. Drug Alcohol Depend. **62:** 111–123.
20. Madden, J.J., W.L. Whaley, D. Ketelsen & R.M. Donahoe. 2001. The morphine-binding site on human activated T-cells is not related to the mu opioid receptor. Drug Alcohol Depend. **62:** 131–139.
21. Sacerdote P., P. Mantegazza & A.E. Panerai. 1985. Analgesic effects of mu antagonists after naloxone non-reversible stress induced analgesia. Brain Res. **359:** 34–38.

22. BIANCHI, M., P. SACERDOTE, L. LOCATELLI, P. MANTEGAZZA, *et al.* 1991. Corticotropin releasing hormone, interleukin 1-alpha, and tumor necrosis factor alpha share characteristics of stress mediators. Brain Res. **546:** 139–142.
23. BIANCHI, M. & A.E. PANERAI. 1993. Naloxone-induced analgesia; involvement of k-opiate receptors. Pharmacol. Biochem. Behav. **46:** 145–148.
24. FERREIRA, S.H. 1980. Peripheral analgesia: mechanism of the analgesic action of aspirin-like drugs and opiate antagonists. Br. J. Clin. Pharmacol. **2:** 237–245.

PACAP in Immunity and Inflammation

MARIO DELGADO, CATALINA ABAD, CARMEN MARTINEZ, M. GUILLERMA JUARRANZ, JAVIER LECETA, DOINA GANEA,[a] AND ROSA P. GOMARIZ

Department of Cell Biology, School of Biology, Complutense University, Madrid 28040, Spain

[a]*Rutgers University, Department of Biological Sciences, Newark, New Jersey 07102, USA*

ABSTRACT: The pituitary adenylate cyclase-activating polypeptide (PACAP) is a neuropeptide belonging to the VIP/secretin/glucagon family of peptides, produced by the lymphoid cells, which exerts a wide spectrum of immunological functions controlling the homeostasis of immune system through different receptors expressed in various immunocompetent cells. In the last decade, PACAP has been clearly identified as a potent anti-inflammatory factor that exerts its function by regulating the production of both anti- and proinflammatory mediators. In this sense, PACAP prevents death by septic shock, an acute inflammatory disease with a high mortality. In addition, PACAP regulates the expression of costimulatory molecules, inasmuch as this related to the modulation in the shift from Th1 towards Th2 differentiation. We recently reported that PACAP prevents the deleterious effects of arthritis by downregulating both inflammatory and autoimmune components of the disease. Therefore, PACAP and analogs have been proposed as very promising candidates, alternative to other existing treatments, for treating acute and chronic inflammatory and autoimmune diseases, such as septic shock, arthritis, multiple sclerosis, Crohn's disease, or autoimmune diabetes.

KEYWORDS: neuroimmunology; inflammation; autoimmune diseases; rheumatoid arthritis; activation-induced cell death; neuropeptides; endotoxic shock; cytokines; chemokines; endotoxin; apoptosis; costimulatory response; differentiation; Th1 and Th2 cells; anti-inflammatory agents; therapeutic application; TNF-α; transcription factors; macrophages; vasoactive intestinal peptide (VIP)

INTRODUCTION

The inflammatory process is vital to the survival of all complex organisms, and its functions play a profound role in health and disease. Although it is a localized protective response that serves to destroy the injurious agent, the sustained production of inflammatory mediators can lead to serious pathological conditions. The accumulation and subsequent activation of leukocytes are central events in the

Address for correspondence: M. Delgado, Instituto de Parasitologia y Biomedicina Lopez Neyra, CSIC, Granada 18001, Spain. Voice: 34-958-805056; fax: 34-958-203323.
mdelgado@ipb.csic.es

Ann. N.Y. Acad. Sci. 992: 141–157 (2003). © 2003 New York Academy of Sciences.

pathogenesis of virtually all forms of inflammation. The elimination of the foreign material proceeds by a series of integrated steps, the first one being recognition of the agent.

Inflammatory responses are self-controlled by anti-inflammatory mediators secreted during the ongoing process. The ability to control an inflammatory state depends on the local balance between pro- and anti-inflammatory factors. An insufficient response could compromise the viability of the organismm but an excessive response could lead to pathological conditions such as the systemic inflammatory response syndrome or inflammatory bowel disease.[1–3] Inflammation is also a key aspect of autoimmunity. Diseases such as multiple sclerosis, rheumatoid arthritis, and insulin-dependent diabetes mellitus are initiated by a small number of antigen-specific T cells that recognize a tissue antigen. Additional cells, namely, T cells, B cells, macrophages, and other antigen-presenting cells (APCs) that can also activate resident cells, are recruited to the site.[4–6] The role of inflammation in autoimmune diseases has generally been thought of as a tissue destructive one.

Current strategies in the treatment of inflammatory and autoimmune diseases have focused on individually blocking the main mediators of the inflammatory processes. Anti-inflammatory cytokines such as interleukin (IL)-10, antibodies that neutralize proinflammatory cytokines such as anti-tumor necrosis factor (TNF), and agents targeted to prevent gene activation of inflammatory mediators such as corticosteroids and nonsteroidal anti-inflammatory drugs have been used to block cytokines and chemokine actions, cell adhesion molecule expression, and recruitment of inflammatory cells.[7–10] However, the tissue specificity of each inflammatory process, its multistep nature, and the cellular and molecular heterogeneity of the different pathological conditions have yielded some controversial results. In the last decade, neuropeptides, hormones, and other components of the neuroendocrine system, which are also produced by cells of the immune system, have been included in the list of potential candidates to treat inflammatory and autoimmune disorders.[11–13]

The circuit between the three main systems involved in homeostasis, nervous, endocrine, and immune, is well established. An important fact in the behavior of this circuit is that their cells synthesize and secrete common substances and share the same receptors for them. This represents the suppression of traditional differences between neurotransmitters, hormones, and immune mediators. To date, at least 27 different neuroendocrine mediators could be produced by cells of central and peripheral lymphoid organs, and the most recent members added are: glucocorticoids,[14] calcitonin gene-related peptide,[15] and pituitary adenylate cyclase-activating polypeptide (PACAP).[16,17]

PACAP was first isolated from ovine hypothalamic tissue by Arimura and coworkers in 1989.[18] The peptide belongs to the vasoactive intestinal peptide (VIP)/secretin/glucagon family of peptides. The N-terminal sequence of PACAP shows a 68% homology with VIP. PACAP is present in two amidated forms, PACAP27 and PACAP38, PACAP38 being the predominant form, and the PACAP38/PACAP27 ratio varies among tissues, especially in the central nervous system, adrenal, and testis, suggesting different processing in different tissues. From a functional point of view, PACAP was first identified as a novel hypothalamic hormone that stimulates adenylate cyclase in pituitary cells;[18] we now know that the peptide has a wider spectrum of biological actions.[19,20] Moreover, PACAP sequence has been markedly well conserved during evolution, suggesting that PACAP could exert significant physiological functions. Although the central nervous system contains the highest tissue concentration of PACAP, the peptide has been located in numerous tissues, such as pituitary, adrenal medulla, testis, gastrointestinal tract, and pancreas.[19,20]

PACAP IS PRODUCED BY LYMPHOCYTES

PACAP is considered an important signal molecule of the neuroendocrine network that is present in lymphoid tissues. Indeed, PACAP immunoreactivity has been shown in cells with lymphocyte morphology in rat bone marrow, thymus, spleen, lymph nodes, and duodenal mucosa.[16] In addition, we have recently supported and extended these previous studies, providing evidence of the presence of PACAP immunoreactivity and mRNA expression in isolated murine lymphocytes.[17] Similarly, as in other peripheral tissues in which both VIP and PACAP appear to be co-expressed in the same cells, PACAP storage and gene expression in central (thymus) and peripheral (spleen and lymph nodes) lymphoid organs appear in exactly the same lymphocyte subpopulations as does VIP. Thus, VIP and PACAP are co-expressed in single- and double-positive ($CD4^{+}CD8^{+}$) thymocytes and in T and B lymphocytes from spleen and lymph nodes. Moreover, there are few differential functions between VIP and PACAP in the immune system, because most of the actions exerted by VIP are also shared by PACAP.

PACAP RECEPTORS IN IMMUNE CELLS

PACAP exerts its biological actions through three different receptors of the family 2 of G protein-coupled receptors that are shared with VIP. To date, three types of VIP/PACAP receptors have been cloned that, according to International Union of Pharmacology (IUPHAR) nomenclature,[21] have been classified as follows: the VPAC1 receptor (also known as VIP1, VIP/PACAP type II, or PVR2) and the VPAC2 receptor (also termed VIP2, VIP/PACAP type III, or PVR3), both of which bind VIP and PACAP with equal affinity and activate primarily the adenylate cyclase pathway; and the PAC1 receptor (also known as VIP/PACAP type I receptor, or PVR1); the PACAP preferring receptor, which binds PACAP with a 300- to 1,000-fold higher affinity than does VIP and it activates both adenylate cyclase and phospholypase C.[20]

Our group recently studied the expression and distribution of the different VIP/PACAP receptors in various immune cell populations. VPAC1 is expressed in rat thymocytes, peripheral T and B lymphocytes, murine thymocytes, and peripheral CD4 and CD8 T lymphocytes, murine macrophages, and human monocytes.[22–35] By contrast to VPAC1, which seems to be constitutively expressed in both unstimulated and stimulated lymphocytes and macrophages, VPAC2 is expressed only following stimulation through the TCR-associated CD3 molecule in lymphocytes[33] or endotoxin in macrophages[34] and represents the only VIP receptor expressed in T cell lines such as EL4.IL-2, D10-G4.1, 2B4.11, and A1.1.[33,36,37] The physiological significance of the distinct anatomical distribution and regulation of VPAC1 and

VPAC2 is unresolved at the present time, but it seems to be a general characteristic because in most organs VPAC1 and VPAC2 do not overlap anatomically, and in some cases, particularly in the brain, the distribution is complementary.[38] Also, the expression of VPAC2 appears to be developmentally regulated in several systems.[38] The expression of VPAC1 and VPAC2 in T lymphocytes and macrophages seems to follow a similar pattern, with VPAC2 mRNA being induced during lymphocyte and macrophage activation. Involvement of different transduction signals could explain the differential distribution and regulation of both receptors. The best characterized effect of PACAP and VIP in various tissues, including immune cells, is the accumulation of intracellular cAMP and the subsequent activation of protein kinase A.[21] Although both VPAC1 and VPAC2 induce intracellular cAMP accumulation, more subtle differences may exist between transduction pathways affected specifically by both receptors.

Regarding PAC1, macrophages and monocytes are the only immunocompetent cells that have been shown to constitutively express PAC1.[39,40] Although a high preference of this receptor for PACAP versus VIP, mainly in the central nervous system, has been extensively reported, we have shown that PAC1 expressed in peritoneal macrophages binds PACAP and VIP with similar affinity;[39] moreover, both neuropeptides activate in a similar way the protein kinase C/phospholypase C system coupled to PAC1,[39] suggesting that PAC1 expressed in macrophages is essentially different from that expressed in the nervous system, because at least five different subtypes of this receptor have been described .[41]

ROLE OF PACAP ON IMMUNITY

Host defense mechanisms implicate several cell types responsible for different functions, whose goal is the elimination of pathogens, as well as transformed or altered self-cells. Inflammation is a vital process that involves both non-antigen–specific and antigen-specific mechanisms. The two main cellular types of players of these mechanisms are macrophages and lymphocytes.

Macrophages play a crucial role in the fight against pathogens by contributing to integratopm of both non-antigen–specific and antigen-specific defense mechanisms. Phagocytosis of pathogens is the main characteristic of macrophages, leading to their activation in terms of cytokine production and antigen presentation and to the reduction of the pathogen load. Macrophages initiate the inflammatory response through the secretion of inflammatory cytokines and production of reactive oxygen and nitrogen intermediates.

Antigen-specific–mechanisms are based on clonal activation of T and B lymphocytes that is triggered in cooperation with both antigen-specific and non-antigen–specific cell populations. Signals from accessory populations include antigen presentation and mediators, such as cytokines, that lead to activation, proliferation, and differentiation of lymphocytes.

In the last decade, PACAP has clearly been identified as a potent anti-inflammatory factor, which acts by regulating the production of both anti- and proinflammatory mediators. In addition, PACAP regulates the expression of costimulatory

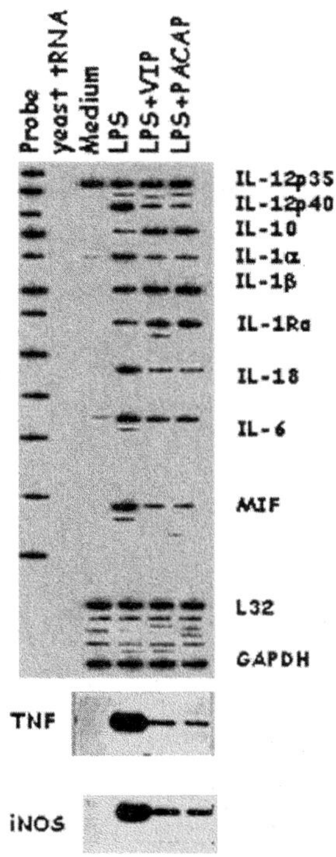

FIGURE 1. Effects of vasoactive intestinal peptide (VIP) and pituitary adenylate cyclase-activating polypeptide (PACAP) on the expression of macrophage-derived inflammatory mediators. Blots show RNase protection assays.

molecules, being an action that may be related to the modulation of Th1/Th2 differentiation.

Effects of PACAP on Macrophages

Regulation of the Production of Macrophage-Derived Mediators

It has been shown that one of the ways by which PACAP modulates the immune response is the modulation of many macrophage functions. To this extent, PACAP has been shown to stimulate migration, adherence, phagocytosis, and superoxide production as well as the synthesis of IL-6 in resting macrophages.[42–44]

Microbial products such as lipopolysaccharide (LPS) induce macrophages to secrete several proinflammatory products such as TNF-α, IL-12, IL-1, IL-6, and nitric oxide (NO). PACAP inhibits the production of these proinflammatory mediators and stimulates the production of the anti-inflammatory cytokine IL-10 in macrophages activated by microbial products or IFN-γ[34,45–50] (FIG. 1). These effects are mediated by the presence of PAC1, VPAC1, and VPAC2 receptors on activated macrophages.

The stimulatory effect on IL-10 transcription is cAMP-dependent and mediated through an increase in CREB (cAMP-regulatory element binding proteins).[48] By contrast, the PACAP inhibition of TNF-α, iNOS, and IL-12 expression occurs through two transduction pathways, a cAMP-dependent and a cAMP-independent pathway. For TNF-α, the cAMP-independent pathway leads to a reduction in NF-κB binding and the cAMP-dependent pathway results in a change in the composition of the CRE-binding complex from high c-Jun/low CREB to high CREB/low c-Jun.[50] Optimal activation of iNOS and IL-12p40 requires both LPS and IFN-γ. For these two genes, PACAP inhibits IRF-1 binding in a cAMP-dependent manner and NF-κB binding in a cAMP-independent manner.[47,49] Recently, we showed that the inhibi-

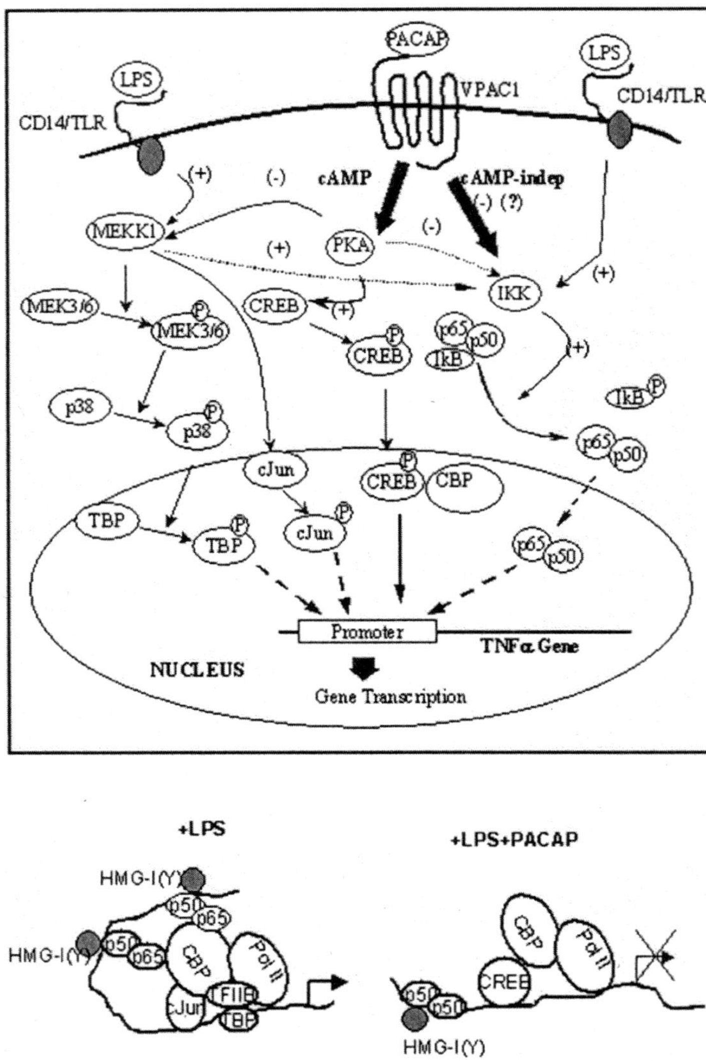

FIGURE 2. Pituitary adenylate cyclase-activating polypeptide (PACAP) exerts its effects through various molecular mechanisms.

tion of IRF-1 binding is due to a reduction in IRF-1 transcription mediated through the inhibition of Jak1/2-STAT1 phosphorylation/activation.[51] Also, we demonstrated that PACAP promotes JunB and inhibits c-Jun phosphorylation through effects on the MEKK1/MEK4/JNK pathway[52] (FIG. 2). Replacement of c-Jun with JunB in transcriptional complexes results in the transcriptional inactivation of various cytokine promoters. Finally, PACAP affects NF-κB at various levels (FIG. 2). A cAMP-independent pathway is responsible for the stabilization of I-κB, the cytoplasmic inhibitor complexed to NF-κB. The stabilization of I-κB is due to the inhibition of I-κB phosphorylation by IKKa, and results in the cytoplasmic sequestration of p65, a major component of the NF-κB complex.[40,49] In addition, PACAP promotes CREB phosphorylation through the cAMP/PKA pathway, and phosphorylated CREB translocates to the nucleus, where it competes for the coactivator CBP (CREB-binding protein). CBP, found in limiting amounts in the nucleus, is necessary for the stabilization of a transcriptionally active complex through interactions with several DNA bound transcriptional factors (FIG. 2). Removal of CBP by CREB prevents the transcriptional complex from acquiring the 'transcriptionally active' conformation. Finally, PACAP also affects the phosphorylation of TBP (the TATA-box binding protein) through inhibition of the MEKK1/MEK3/6/p38 MAPK pathway.[40] In the absence of phosphorylated TBP, there is an inefficient recruitment of the RNA polymerase II, which further weakens transcription. Although cAMP-inducing agents mimic several of the PACAP effects, the fact that this neuropeptide acts through both cAMP-dependent and cAMP-independent pathways allows them to function as an extremely efficient immunomodulator.

Of particular interest is the dual effect of PACAP on IL-6 production by macrophages, depending on the nature and dose of the inflammatory stimuli.[46,53] Whereas PACAP inhibits the release of IL-6 from macrophages stimulated by an LPS dose range from 100 pg/ml to 10 μg/ml, it enhances IL-6 secretion in unstimulated macrophages or macrophages stimulated with very low concentrations of endotoxin. Both stimulation and inhibition of IL-6 by PACAP are mediated by different receptors and intracellular signals. Whereas the inhibition of LPS-induced IL-6 production is mediated through PAC1 binding and PKC activation, stimulation of IL-6 release by PACAP is VPAC1/cAMP dependent.[46,53] A recent report has suggested that the inhibitory effect of PACAP on IL-6 production could be mediated through the inhibition of LPS binding to its receptor CD14 in macrophages by inducing the shedding of membrane-bound CD14.[54]

Because other molecules implicated in inflammatory responses such as chemokines and adhesion molecules are controlled by NF-κB, these molecules can also be targets for PACAP regulation. Chemokines are essential for leukocyte trafficking and inflammatory processes. Their involvement in such responses further suggests that the chemokines are important players in inflammatory disorders. The selective chemoattractant activities for macrophage and lymphocyte subsets make them ideal candidates to play a key role in leukocyte trafficking, getting the correct subpopulation of cells to migrate into the tissues.[55] PACAP has recently been shown to reduce chemokine production by activated macrophages.[56] The CXC chemokine MIP-2, which induces the migration of polymorphonuclear leukocytes, and the CC chemokines MIP-1a, MIP-1b, MCP-1, and RANTES, which are chemotactic for monocyte/macrophages and T cells, were inhibited in a long-lasting way. Inhibition has also been shown *in vivo*.[56,57] In a murine model of abdominal acute inflammation,

PACAP reduces the entry of polymorphonuclear leukocytes, macrophages, and lymphocytes to the peritoneal cavity, presumably through the inhibition of chemokine production.[56] The inhibition of cellular recruitment to sites of inflammation may also hamper the possible *in situ* antigen presentation that may contribute to exacerbation of clinical signs in chronic inflammation and reactivity to these antigens in autoimmune disorders.

Regulation of Macrophage Accessory Functions in Antigen-Specific Responses

Macrophages participate in the antigen-specific responses acting as antigen presenting cells, providing T lymphocytes with costimulatory molecules and a cytokine environment that influences the proliferation and differentiation of T cells. Among the costimulatory molecules, B7.1 and B7.2 play major roles. In macrophages, B7.1 and B7.2 are expressed only following activation, with B7.2 being induced earlier and at higher levels than B7.1.[58] PACAP is among the endogenous factors that regulate B7 expression in macrophages. Interestingly, this neuropeptide affects B7 expression in resting and activated macrophages in an opposite manner. In resting macrophages, PACAP upregulates B7.2, but not B7.1 expression at the mRNA and protein level both *in vivo* and *in vitro*. By contrast, PACAP downregulates both B7.1 and B7.2 expression in LPS/IFN-γ–activated macrophages. The effects of PACAP on B7 expression correlate with the effects on the stimulatory activity for T cells. The inhibition of B7.1/B7.2 expression in activated macrophages is in perfect agreement with the accepted role of PACAP as an endogenous anti-inflammatory agent. Moreover, since PACAP affects B7 but not MHC class II expression,[59,60] this neuropeptide could actually contribute to peripheral tolerance by inducing T cell anergy. By contrast, the upregulation of B7.2 in unstimulated macrophages could represent one of the mechanisms by which PACAP supports Th2 differentiation, which is to be discussed.

Effects of PACAP on Lymphocytes: T Cell Function, Survival, and Differentiation

Key players of the antigen-specific responses are the T cells that develop in the thymus, where they are subjected to positive and negative selection, enabling them to recognize an antigenic determinant associated with an MHC molecule. Clones not selected are eliminated by apoptosis. In the peripheral lymphoid organs, different subsets of cells play different roles in the immune response. Following initial TCR engagement, antigen-specific CD4 cells enter an activation and proliferative stage that is signaled by profound alterations in the cell surface expression of activation and adhesion molecules. Activation is accompanied by the onset of cytokine synthesis, IL-2, IL-3, IL-4, IFN-γ, etc., progressively more biased towards the Th1 or Th2 phenotypes and differentiate into clones of antigen-specific effector T cells. The end of an immune response requires the elimination of the vast majority of antigen-specific T cells through apoptosis in a phenomenon referred to as activation-induced cell death (AICD). Withdrawal of growth factors, such as IL-2, and surface molecules, such as Fas, induced on T cells after activation, participate in this process.

Its antiproliferative effects first evidenced the immunomodulatory properties of PACAP after mitogen stimulation. In concanavalin A–stimulated murine splenocytes, PACAP causes a dose-dependent inhibition of cell proliferation and inhibits IL-2 production.[61,62] PACAP also protects lymphocytes against apoptosis induced by different stimuli to inhibit certain cytotoxic mechanisms and to promote Th2 differentiation.

Firstly, PACAP acts as a survival factor for $CD4^+CD8^+$ thymocytes against glucocorticoid-induced apoptosis, suggesting the possible involvement of this neuropeptide in the control of positive selection of thymocytes and their differentiation.[63] On the other hand, it was recently described that PACAP protects activated CD4 T cells against AICD both *in vitro* and *in vivo*.[36] CD4 T cells undergo AICD primarily through Fas/Fas ligand (FasL) interactions.[64] Fas is expressed constitutively on CD4 T cells and upregulated following activation, whereas FasL expression is induced only following TCR restimulation.[65] The PACAP protection against AICD is actually the result of an inhibitory effect on FasL expression in restimulated CD4 T cells.[36] The inhibition of FasL expression is mediated through the effects on several transcription factors, that is, NF-κB, NF-ATp, and Egr2,3.[66] FasL/Fas interactions are involved not only in CD4 T apoptosis, but also in cytotoxicity against Fas-bearing targets. Cytotoxic CD8 T cells (CTL) kill targets through a calcium-dependent, perforin/granzyme-mediated mechanism and a calcium-independent, FasL-mediated mechanism.[67] PACAP does not affect perforin/granzyme-mediated cytotoxicity, but drastically inhibits FasL-mediated lysis of both allogeneic and syngeneic Fas-bearing targets. PACAP inhibits FasL-mediated cytotoxicity by preventing FasL expression on the cytotoxic T cells both *in vivo* and *in vitro*.[68] CD4 T effector cells also express cytotoxic activity. However, in contrast to CD8 CTLs, CD4 lytic effectors kill targets only through FasL/Fas-mediated interactions.[64] Antigen-presenting cells activate CD4 T cells in an MHC II-restricted manner, leading to the upregulation of FasL, which then enables the CD4 T cells to lyse both cognate APCs (direct targets) and neighboring Fas-bearing cells (bystander targets) in an antigen-independent and MHC-nonrestricted manner.[69] PACAP inhibits FasL expression in allogeneic and antigen-specific CD4 effectors generated *in vivo* and their cytotoxicity for both direct and bystander targets.[70]

Following antigenic stimulation, CD4 T cells differentiate into Th1 and Th2 effector cells, characterized by specific cytokine profiles and functions. Determining factors for the differentiation include the nature of the APC and the expression of costimulatory molecules on them and the cytokine microenvironment.[71] Among cytokines, IL-12 and IL-4 appear to be the determinant factors for Th1 and Th2 differentiation, respectively. Regarding the immunomodulatory role of PACAP in Th1/Th2 differentiation, it has been shown that this neuropeptide induces Th2 responses *in vivo* and *in vitro*.[60] Macrophages treated *in vitro* with PACAP gain the ability to induce Th2-type cytokines (IL-4 and IL-5) and inhibit Th1-type cytokines (IFN–γ, IL-2) in Ag-primed CD4 T cells. *In vivo* administration of PACAP in Ag-immunized mice results in a decreased number of IFN-γ–secreting cells and an increased number of IL-4–secreting cells.[60] There are several possible nonexcluding mechanisms for the PACAP bias towards Th2. Inhibition of macrophage IL-12 production by PACAP is one possibility. Because IL-4 dominates over IL-12 driving naïve CD4 T cells towards the Th2 phenotype,[71] a reduction in IL-12 by PACAP even in the absence of an effect on IL-4 will result in Th2 differentiation. A second possibility is upregulation of B7.2 expression on macrophages by PACAP. Finally, PACAP may support Th2, but not Th1 proliferation *in vitro*, promoting the generation of memory Th2 cells *in vivo*. These effects correlate with a reduction in FasL expression and inhibition of apoptosis in Th2, but not Th1 cells.

ROLE OF PACAP ON INFLAMMATORY AND AUTOIMMUNE DISORDERS

From the preceding sections it can be concluded that PACAP modulates the function of inflammatory cells through specific receptors, affecting both innate and adaptive immunity. One of the major targets for PACAP activity is the stimulated macrophage. Through the release of cytotoxic molecules, including cytokines, oxygen radicals, and nitric oxide, macrophages decrease the pathogen load. The subsequent release of proinflammatory cytokines, the processing and presentation of the antigen, and the upregulation of costimulatory molecules position the macrophage as an important participant in the induction of adaptive immunity. Responding to stimulatory and costimulatory signals delivered by APCs (including dendritic cells, B cells, and macrophages), CD4 T cells proliferate and differentiate into effector Th1 and Th2 cells. At the conclusion of an immune response, both activated APCs and T cells have to be deactivated and/or eliminated. In the absence of deactivation/elimination of stimulated immune cells, excessive tissue and organ damage leads to pathological conditions and even death. A number of endogenous factors, particularly anti-inflammatory cytokines, contribute to the downregulation of the immune response. Neuropeptides, such as PACAP, can be added to the list of endogenous anti-inflammatory molecules. PACAP exerts its anti-inflammatory function in several ways: (1) direct inhibition of proinflammatory cytokine production (TNF-α, IL-6, IL-12) by activated macrophages; (2) upregulation of IL-10 production (a potent anti-inflammatory cytokine); (3) inhibition of B7.1/B7.2 expression in activated macrophages and subsequent inhibition of their stimulatory activity for antigen-specific T cells; (4) inhibition of IL-2 production and T cell proliferation; (5) inhibition of Th1 responses (reduction in both the amounts of Th1 cytokines and the number of cytokine-producing Th1 cells); and (6) inhibition of FasL/Fas-mediated cytotoxicity of CD8 and CD4 T cells against direct and bystander targets. In contrast to these well-defined anti-inflammatory functions, PACAP supports the generation and long-term survival of Th2 cells, representing the first neuropeptide, together with the structurally related peptide VIP, with a possible role in the generation of memory Th2 cells.

Because of these effects on the immune system, PACAP may be used to modulate inflammatory processes as well as autoimmune disorders. The appearance of inflammatory cells, antigen-specific Th1 cells, and bystander tissue destruction are common to pathological conditions such as rheumatoid arthritis (RA), experimental allergic encephalomyelitis, inflammatory bowel disease, and others. Because Th1 and Th2 populations cross-regulate each other, it may be feasible to convert an autoimmune disease mediated by inflammatory pathogenic Th1 cells to one in which protective Th2 populations predominate. The evidence supporting this possibility comes from animal models of pathologies such as RA, in which PACAP has been shown to reduce the incidence and severity of the disease.

Rheumatoid arthritis is a chronic inflammatory illness of unknown etiology but with autoimmune features characterized by chronic inflammation of synovial tissues. The principal symptoms are due to massive infiltration of immune cells (neutrophils, macrophages, and T cells) into the synovial membrane and fluid, releasing large quantities of chemokines that recruit cells to the site of inflammation, matrix metalloproteinases that destroy the joint tissues, and proinflammatory mediators produced by macrophages and fibroblasts (TNF-α, IL-1, and IL-6) and T lymphocytes (IFN-γ) that contribute to generate joint damage.[72] In this sense, there is polarization of the T cell response to a Th1 one, suggesting that an imbalance in the T response towards a self-Ag could also be important in the development of arthritis. As a result of all these facts, the synovium, which in normal conditions is a fragile bilayer membrane covering the joint cartilage and bone, is transformed into a thick invasive one that destroys joint structure, producing deformation of the tissue that explains the rigidity and paralysis of the patients in the last steps of the illness.

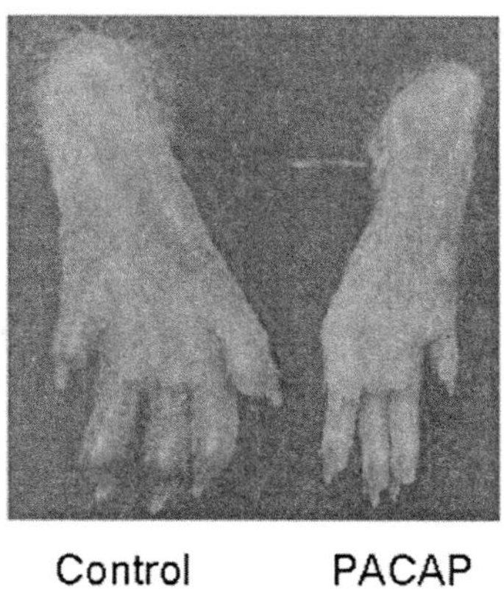

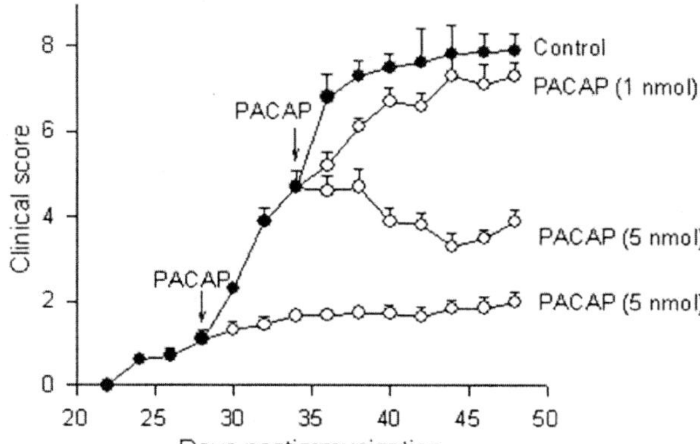

FIGURE 3. Pituitary adenylate cyclase-activating polypeptide (PACAP) prevents collagen-induced arthritis.[73] Controls are arthritic mice.

By using the experimental murine model of collagen-induced arthritis, which shares common clinical, histologic, and immunological features with human RA, we demonstrated that treatment of arthritic mice with PACAP produces a general beneficial improvement of the disease.[73] PACAP treatment decreases the frequency of arthritis, delaying the onset, reducing the severity of symptoms, and preventing joint damage (FIG. 3). The therapeutic effect of PACAP is due to a reduction of the two deleterious components of the disease, that is, the inflammatory and the autoimmune. Thus, PACAP not only acts directly to reduce the levels of proinflammatory mediators such as TNF-α, IL-6, IL-1β, IL-12, iNOS, and IL-18, but also increases the amounts of anti-inflammatory cytokines such as IL-10 and IL-1Ra. In this sense, the downregulation of TNF-α is crucial to explain the remission of the disease, because this cytokine is considered to have a critical role in arthritis, promoting the production of most other proinflammatory mediators. PACAP also reduces the levels of the chemokines RANTES, MCP-1, MIP-1α, MIP-1β, MIP-2, all of them are responsible for the infiltration and activation of various leukocyte populations in joint tissue, contributing to the pathology of arthritis. PACAP also downregulates the expression and activity of some matrix metalloproteinases, which have a crucial role in the depletion of proteoglycan that contributes to the destruction of both cartilage and bone. As a result of the levels of all of these harmful soluble factors in RA, a clear remission of the chronic inflammation of the joint of the affected mice is observed.

The action of PACAP is not restricted to the mediators produced by synoviocytes; it also affects the cytokines released by the infiltrated T cells. Strong evidence indicates that most T cells present in the inflamed tissues in RA show a Th1 cytokine pattern.[74] In addition, Ig isotype switching directed by Th1 or Th2 cytokines (i.e., IFN-γ and IL-4 induce IgG2a and IgG1 synthesis, respectively) is another marker of this disease, which shows high anti-collagen IgG2a circulating levels.[75] PACAP treatment reduces IFN-γ levels (a Th1 cytokine) and increases IL-4 levels (a Th2 cytokine) and results in a reduction of IgG2a and an increase of IgG1. These two facts confirm the Th2-inducing response of PACAP, which possibly contributes to remission of the disease, blocking its autoimmune component.

Moreover, PACAP-related peptide VIP was reported to have an important downregulative action on arthritis.[57] Therefore, as in other inflammatory diseases, these endogenously produced peptides are increased in arthritic mice, acting as a natural anti-arthritic attempt to reduce the excessive response of the immune system.

The beneficial effects of PACAP could also be extended to acute inflammatory conditions such as toxic shock syndrome. Sepsis is defined as a systemic inflammatory response syndrome induced by infection. Bacterial products such as endotoxins or LPS play a pivotal role in the initiation of the response that could lead to endotoxic shock, multiple organ dysfunction, and a high mortality rate. The mechanisms and temporal appearance of mediators in this process have been studied in several animal models.[76] Following systemic administration of LPS, high levels of circulating TNF-α, IL-1, IL-6, IL-12, and IFN-γ precedes hypotension, tissue damage, and organ dysfunction. Nitric oxide and other mediators are also involved in this process. Several attempts have been undertaken to control sepsis by neutralizing individual inflammatory components, but despite many efforts no improvement in the mortality rate has been achieved.[8,77] Because it is unlikely that blockade of a single mediator

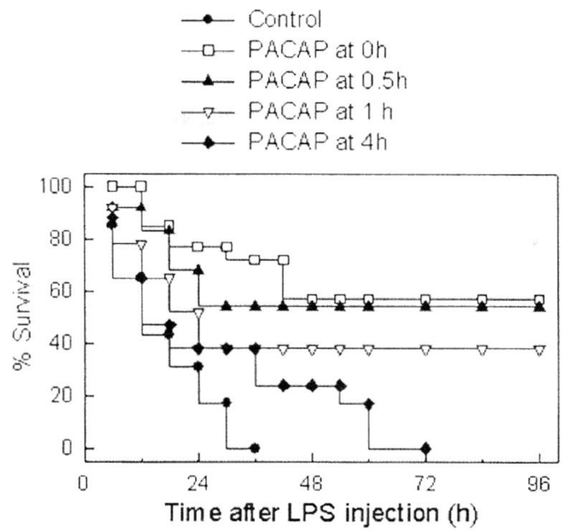

FIGURE 4. Pituitary adenylate cyclase-activating polypeptide (PACAP) prevents lethal endotoxic shock. PACAP was injected at different times after lipopolysaccharide (LPS) administration, and survival of mice was determined.

will be effective in controlling sepsis, modulators blocking several inflammatory agents should be an interesting focus of attention.

The anti-shock effect of PACAP on experimental endotoxin has been reported in different animal models. In a high-dose endotoxin murine model, the administration of PACAP inhibits the elevation of circulating levels of TNF-α, IL-6, IL-12, IFN-γ, and NO and also increases the circulating levels of the anti-inflammatory cytokine IL-10.[78,79] Unique in the protective effect of PACAP could be its effect on IL-6 reduction mediated by the PAC1 receptor, although the VPAC1 receptor is also implicated, and to a lesser degree, the VPAC2 receptor could participate in the protective effect.[78] Associated with the effect on cytokine circulating levels, PACAP protect mice from endotoxic shock even if the administration is delayed 2 hours after endotoxin injection (FIG. 4).

In conclusion, based on the protective effects of PACAP, the exogenous administration of this peptide and other related peptides, such as VIP and/or agonists, could offer an alternative to existing treatments for arthritis and other inflammatory/Th1-autoimmune diseases, such as multiple sclerosis, inflammatory bowel disease, or autoimmune diabetes, as well as for endotoxic shock.

REFERENCES

1. EBONG, S., D. CALL, J. NEMZEK, *et al.* 1999. Immunopathologic alterations in murine models of sepsis of increasing severity. Infect. Immun. **67:** 6603–6610.
2. FIGEN, J.W., A.C. MULLER KOBOLD, P. DE BOER, *et al.* 2000. Leukocyte activation and cytokine production during experimental human endotoxemia. Eur. J. Int. Med. **11:** 89–95.

3. Southey, A., S. Tanaka, T. Murakami, *et al.* 1997. Pathophysiological role of nitric oxide in rat experimental colitis. Int. J. Immunopharmacol. **19:** 669–676.
4. Marinova-Mutafchieva, L., R.O. Williams, L.J. Mason, *et al.* 1997. Dynamics of proinflammatory cytokine expression in the joints of mice with collagen-induced arthritis (CIA). Clin. Exp. Immunol. **107:** 507–512.
5. Stallmach, A., W. Strober, T.T. MacDonald, *et al.* 1998. Induction and modulation of gastrointestinal inflammation. Immunol. Today **19:** 438–441.
6. Martin, R., N.H. Ruddle, S. Reingold & D.A. Hafler. 1998. T helper cell differentiation in multiple sclerosis and autoimmunity. Immunol. Today **19:** 495–498.
7. Geissler, K. 1996. Current status of clinical development of interleukin-10. Curr. Opin. Hematol. **3:** 203–208.
8. Cain, B.S., D.R. Meldrum, A.H. Harken & R.C. McIntyre. 1998. The physiologic basis for anticytokine clinical trials in the treatment of sepsis. J. Am. Coll. Surg. **186:** 337–350.
9. Tilley, S.L., T.M. Coffman & B.H. Koller. 2001. Mixed messages: modulation of inflammation and immune responses by prostaglandins and thromboxanes. J. Clin. Invest. **108:** 15–23.
10. Tak, P.P. & G.S. Firenstein. 2001. NF-κB: a key role in inflammatory diseases. J. Clin. Invest. **107:** 7–11.
11. Klein, T.W., C. Newton & H. Friedman. 1998. Cannabinoid receptors and immunity. Immunol. Today **19:** 373–381.
12. Bijlsma, J.W.J., M. Cutolo, A.T. Masi & I.C. Chikanza. 1999. The neuroendocrine immune basis of rheumatic diseases. Immunol. Today **20:** 298–301.
13. Gomariz, R.P., C. Martinez, C. Abad, *et al.* 2001. Immunology of VIP: a review and therapeutical perspectives. Curr. Pharm. Des. **7:** 89–111.
14. Lechner, O., G.J. Wiegers, A. Oliveira-Dos-Santos, *et al.* 2000. Glucocorticoid production in the murine thymus. Eur. J. Immunol. **30:** 337–346.
15. Xing, L., J. Guo & X. Wang. 2000. Induction and expression of beta-calcitonin gene-related peptide in rat T lymphocytes and its significance. J. Immunol. **165:** 4359–4366.
16. Gaytan, F., A.J. Martinez-Fuentes, F. Gracia-Navarro, *et al.* 1994. Pituitary adenylate cyclase activating peptide (PACAP) immunolocalization in lymphoid tissue of rat. Cell Tissue Res. **276:** 233–237.
17. Abad, C., C. Martinez, J. Leceta, *et al.* 2002-2003. Pituitary adenylate-cyclase-activating polypeptide expression in the immune system. Neuroimmunomodulation **10:** 177–186.
18. Miyata, A., A. Arimura, R.R. Dahl, *et al.* 1989. Isolation of a novel 38 residue-hypothalamic polypeptide which stimulates adenylate cyclase in pituitary cells. Biochem. Biophys. Res. Commun. **164:** 567–574.
19. Arimura, A. 1992. Pituitary adenylate cyclase activating polypeptide (PACAP): discovery and current status of research. Regul. Pept. **37:** 287–303.
20. Vaudry, D., B.J. Gonzalez, M. Basille, *et al.* 2000. Pituitary adenylate cyclase-activating polypeptide and its receptors: from structure to functions. Pharmacol. Rev. **52:** 269–324.
21. Harmar, A.J., A. Arimura, I. Gozes, *et al.* 1998. International Union of Pharmacology. XVII. Nomenclature of receptors for vasoactive intestinal peptide and pituitary adenylate cyclase-activating polypeptide. Pharmacol. Rev. **50:** 265–270.
22. Guerrero, J.M., J.C. Prieto, F.L. Elorza, *et al.* 1981. Interaction of vasoactive intestinal peptide with human blood mononuclear cells. Mol. Cell. Endocrinol. **21:** 151–160.
23. Wiik, P., P.K. Opstad & A. Boyum. 1985. Binding of vasoactive intestinal polypeptide (VIP) by human blood monocytes: demonstration of specific binding sites. Regul. Pept. **12:** 145–163.
24. Ottaway, C.A. & G. Greenberg. 1984. Interaction of vasoactive intestinal peptide with mouse lymphocytes: specific binding and the modulation of mitogen responses. J. Immunol. **132:** 417–423.
25. Calvo, J.R., J.M. Guerrero, P. Molinero, *et al.* 1986. Interaction of vasoactive intestinal peptide (VIP) with human peripheral blood lymphocytes: specific binding and cyclic AMP production. Gen. Pharmacol. **17:** 185–189.

26. SAKAKIBARA, H., K. SHIMA & S.I. SAID. 1994. Characterization of vasoactive intestinal peptide receptors on rat alveolar macrophages. Am. J. Physiol. **267:** L256–L262.
27. SEGURA, J.J., J.M. GUERRERO, R. GOBERNA & J.R. CALVO. 1991. Characterization of functional receptors for vasoactive intestinal peptide (VIP) in rat peritoneal macrophages. Regul. Pept. **33:** 133–143.
28. CALVO, J.R., J.M. GUERRERO, M.A. LÓPEZ-GONZALEZ, *et al.* 1994. Characteristics of receptors for VIP in rat peritoneal macrophage membranes. Peptides **15:** 309–315.
29. GOMARIZ, R.P., E. GARRIDO, J. LECETA, *et al.* 1994. Gene expression of VIP receptor in rat lymphocytes. Biochem. Biophys. Res. Commun. **203:** 1599–1604.
30. DELGADO, M., C. MARTINEZ, J. LECETA, *et al.* 1996. Differential VIP and VIP_1 receptor gene expression in rat thymocyte subsets. Peptides **17:** 803–807.
31. DELGADO, M., D. POZO, C. MARTINEZ, *et al.* 1996. Characterization of gene expression of VIP and VIP1-receptor in rat peritoneal lymphocytes and macrophages. Regul. Pept. **62:** 161–166.
32. ROBBERECHT, P., P. DE NEEF, P. GOURLET, *et al.* 1989. Pharmacological characterization of the novel helodermin/VIP receptor present in human SUP-T1 lymphoma. Regul. Pept. **26:** 117–126.
33. DELGADO, M., C. MARTINEZ, M.C. JOHNSON, *et al.* 1996. Differential expression of vasoactive intestinal peptide receptors 1 and 2 (VIP-R1 and VIP-R2) mRNA in murine lymphocytes. J. Neuroimmunol. **68:** 27–38.
34. DELGADO, M., E.J. MUÑOZ-ELIAS, R.P. GOMARIZ & D. GANEA. 1999. VIP and PACAP inhibit IL-12 production in LPS-stimulated macrophages. Subsequent effect on IFNγ synthesis by T cells. J. Neuroimmunol. **96:** 167–181.
35. KALTREIDER, H.B., S. ICHKAWA, P.K. BYRD, *et al.* 1997. Upregulation of neuropeptides and neuropeptides in a murine model of immune inflammation in lung parenchyma. Am. J. Respir. Cell. Mol. Biol. **16:** 133–144.
36. DELGADO, M. & D. GANEA. 2000. Vasoactive intestinal peptide and pituitary adenylate cyclase-activating polypeptide inhibit antigen-induced apoptosis of mature T lymphocytes by inhibiting Fas ligand expression. J. Immunol. **164:** 1200–1210.
37. JABRANE-FERRAT, N., D. BLOOM, A. WU, *et al.* 1999. Enhancement by vasoactive intestinal peptide of γ-interferon production by antigen-stimulated type 1 helper T cells. FASEB J. **13:** 347–353.
38. USDIN, T.B., T.I. BONNER & E. MEZEY. 1994. Two receptors for vasoactive intestinal polypeptide with similar specificity and complementary distribution. Endocrinology **135:** 2662–2680.
39. POZO, D., M. DELGADO, C. MARTINEZ, *et al.* 1997. Functional characterization and mRNA expression of pituitary adenylate cyclase activating polypeptide (PACAP) type I receptors in rat peritoneal macrophages. Biochim. Biophys. Acta **1359:** 250–262.
40. DELGADO, M. & D. GANEA. 2001. Vasoactive intestinal peptide and pituitary adenylate cyclase-activating polypeptide inhibit NF-κB-dependent gene activation at multiple levels in the human monocytic cell line THP1. J. Biol. Chem. **276:** 369–380.
41. SPENGLER, D., C. WAEBER, C. PANTALONI, *et al.* 1993. Differential signal transduction by five splice variants of the PACAP receptor gene. Nature **365:** 170–175.
42. DELGADO, M., E. GARRIDO, M. DE LA FUENTE & R.P. GOMARIZ. 1996. Pituitary adenylate cyclase-activating polypeptide (PACAP38) stimulates rat peritoneal macrophage functions. Peptides **17:** 1097–1105.
43. GARRIDO, E., M. DELGADO, C. MARTINEZ, *et al.* 1996. Pituitary adenylate cyclase-activating polypeptide (PACAP38) modulates lymphocyte and macrophage functions: stimulation of adherence and opposite effect on mobility. Neuropeptides **30:** 583–595.
44. ICHINOSE, M., M. ASAI, K. IMAI & M. SAWADA. 1995. Enhancement of phagocytosis in mouse macrophages by pituitary adenylate cyclase-activating polypeptide (PACAP) and related peptides. Immunopharmacology **30:** 217–224.
45. DELGADO, M., D. POZO, C. MARTINEZ, *et al.* 1999. Vasoactive intestinal peptide and pituitary adenylate cyclase-activating polypeptide inhibit endotoxin-induced TNF-α production by macrophages: *in vitro* and *in vivo* studies. J. Immunol. **162:** 2358–2367.

46. MARTINEZ, C., M. DELGADO, D. POZO, *et al.* 1998. Vasoactive intestinal peptide and pituitary adenylate cyclase-activating polypeptide modulate endotoxin-induced IL-6 production by murine peritoneal macrophages. J. Leuk. Biol. **63:** 591–601.
47. DELGADO, M., E.J. MUÑOZ-ELIAS, R.P. GOMARIZ & D. GANEA. 1999. Vasoactive intestinal peptide and pituitary adenylate cyclase-activating polypeptide prevent inducible nitric oxide synthase transcription in macrophages by inhibiting NF-κB and IFN regulatory factor 1 activation. J. Immunol. **162:** 4685–4696.
48. DELGADO, M., E.J. MUÑOZ-ELIAS, R.P. GOMARIZ & D. GANEA. 1999. Vasoactive intestinal peptide and pituitary adenylate cyclase-activating polypeptide enhance IL-10 production by murine macrophages: *in vitro* and *in vivo* studies. J. Immunol. **162:** 1707–1716.
49. DELGADO, M. & D. GANEA. 1999. Vasoactive intestinal peptide and pituitary adenylate cyclase-activating polypeptide inhibit interleukin-12 transcription by regulating nuclear factor κB and Ets activation. J. Biol. Chem. **274:** 31930–31940.
50. DELGADO, M., E.J. MUÑOZ-ELIAS, Y. KAN, *et al.* 1998. Vasoactive intestinal peptide and pituitary adenylate cyclase-activating polypeptide inhibit tumor necrosis factor a transcriptional activation by regulating nuclear factor-kB and cAMP response element-binding protein/c-jun. J. Biol. Chem. **273:** 31427–31436.
51. DELGADO, M. & D. GANEA. 2000. Inhibition of IFN-γ-induced janus kinase-1-STAT1 activation in macrophages by vasoactive intestinal peptide and pituitary adenylate cyclase-activating polypeptide. J. Immunol. **165:** 3051–3057.
52. DELGADO, M. & D. GANEA. 2000. Vasoactive intestinal peptide and pituitary adenylate cyclase activating polypeptide inhibit the MEKK1/MEK4/JNK signaling pathway in LPS-stimulated macrophages. J. Neuroimmunol. **110:** 97–105.
53. MARTINEZ, C., D. DELGADO, D. POZO, *et al.* 1998. VIP and PACAP enhance IL6 release and mRNA levels in resting peritoneal macrophages: *in vitro* and *in vivo* studies. J. Neuroimmunol. **85:** 155–167.
54. DELGADO, M., J. LECETA, C. ABAD, *et al.* 1999. Shedding of membrane-bound CD14 from lipopolysaccharide-stimulated macrophages by vasoactive intestinal peptide and pituitary adenylate cyclase-activating polypeptide. J. Neuroimmunol. **99:** 61–71.
55. SCHALL, T.J. & K.B. BACON. 1994. Chemokines, leukocyte trafficking, and inflammation. Curr. Opin. Immunol. **6:** 865–873.
56. DELGADO, M. & D. GANEA. 2001. Inhibition of endotoxin-induced macrophage chemokine production by vasoactive intestinal peptide and pituitary adenylate cyclase-activating polypeptide: in vitro and in vivo. J. Immunol. **167:** 966–975.
57. DELGADO, M., C. ABAD, C. MARTINEZ, *et al.* 2001. Vasoactive intestinal peptide prevents experimental arthritis by downregulating both autoimmune and inflammatory components of the disease. Nat. Med. **7:** 563–568.
58. LENSCHOW, D.J., T.L. WALUNAS & J.A. BLUESTONE. 1996. CD28/B7 system of T cell costimulation. Annu. Rev. Immunol. **14:** 233–258.
59. DELGADO, M., W. SUN, J. LECETA & D. GANEA. 1999. VIP and PACAP differentially regulate the costimulatory activity of resting and activated macrophages through the modulation of B7.1 and B7.2 expression. J. Immunol. **163:** 4213–4223.
60. DELGADO, M., J. LECETA, R.P. GOMARIZ & D. GANEA. 1999. VIP and PACAP stimulate the induction of Th2 responses by upregulating B7.2 expression. J. Immunol. **163:** 3629–3635.
61. TANG, H., L. SUN, Z. XIN & D. GANEA. 1996. Down-regulation of cytokine expression in murine lymphocytes by PACAP and VIP. Ann. N.Y. Acad. Sci. **805:** 768–778.
62. TATSUNO, I., P.E. GOTTSCHALL & A. ARIMURA. 1991. Inhibition of mitogen-stimulated proliferation of murine splenocytes by a novel neuropeptide, pituitary adenylate cyclase-activating polypeptide: a comparative study with vasoactive intestinal peptide. Endocrinology **128:** 728–734.
63. DELGADO, M., E. GARRIDO, C. MARTINEZ, *et al.* 1996. Vasoactive intestinal peptide and pituitary adenylate cyclase-activating polypeptide (PACAP27 and PACAP38) protect CD4+CD8+ thymocytes from glucocorticoid-induced apoptosis. Blood **87:** 5152–5161.
64. JU, S.T., D.J. PANKA, H. CUI, *et al.* 1995. Fas (CD95)/FasL interactions required for programmed cell death after T-cell activation. Nature **373:** 444–448.

65. SUDA, T., T. OKAZAKI, Y. NAITO, *et al.* 1995. Expression of the Fas ligand in cells of the T cell lineage. J. Immunol. **154:** 3806–3813.
66. DELGADO, M. & D. GANEA. 2001. Vasoactive intestinal peptide and pituitary adenylate cyclase activating polypeptide inhibit expression of Fas ligand in activated T lymphocytes by regulating c-Myc, NFκB, NF-AT, and early growth factors 2/3. J. Immunol. **166:** 1028–1040.
67. BERKE, G. 1995. The CTL kiss of death. Cell **81:** 9–12.
68. DELGADO, M. & D. GANEA. 2000. Vasoactive intestinal peptide and pituitary adenylate cyclase activating polypeptide inhibit T cell-mediated cytotoxicity by inhibiting Fas ligand expression. J. Immunol. **165:** 114–123.
69. SMYTH, M.J. 1997. Fas ligand-mediated bystander lysis of syngeneic cells in response to an allogeneic stimulus. J. Immunol. **158:** 5765–5772.
70. DELGADO, M. & D. GANEA. 2001. VIP and PACAP inhibit Fas ligand-mediated bystander lysis by CD4+ T cells. J. Neuroimmunol. **112:** 78–88.
71. O'GARRA, A.O. 1998. Cytokines induce the development of functionally heterogeneous T helper cell subsets. Immunity **8:** 275–283.
72. FELDMANN, M., F.M. BRENNAN & R.N. MAINI. 1996. Role of cytokines in rheumatoid arthritis. Ann. Rev. Immunol. **14:** 397–440.
73. ABAD, C., C. MARTINEZ, J. LECETA, *et al.* 2001. Pituitary adenylate cyclase-activating polypeptide inhibits collagen-induced arthritis: an experimental immunomodulatory therapy. J. Immunol. **167:** 3182–3189.
74. MAURI, C., R.O. WILLIAMS, M. WALMSLEY & M. FELDMANN. 1996. Relationship between Th1/Th2 cytokine patterns and the arthriogenic response in collagen-induced arthritis. Eur. J. Immunol. **26:** 1511–1520.
75. SEKI, N., Y. SUDO, T. YOSHIOKA, *et al.* 1988. Type II collagen-induced murine arthritis induction and perpetuation of arthritis require synergy between humoral and cell-mediated immunity. J. Immunol. **140:** 1477–1484.
76. KARIMA, R., S. MATSUMOTO, H. HIGASHI & K. MATSUSHIMA. 1999. The molecular pathogenesis of endotoxic shock and organ failure. Mol. Med. Today **5:** 123–132.
77. VINCENT, J. & R. CHAMLOU. 1996. Sepsis trials. Curr. Opin. Anaesthesiol. **9:** 146–156.
78. DELGADO, M., R.P. GOMARIZ, C. MARTINEZ, *et al.* 2000. Anti-inflammatory properties of the type 1 and type 2 vasoactive intestinal peptide receptors: role in lethal endotoxic shock. Eur. J. Immunol. **30:** 3236–3246.
79. DELGADO, M., C. MARTINEZ, D. POZO, *et al.* 1999. Vasoactive intestinal peptide (VIP) and pituitary adenylate cyclase-activating polypeptide (PACAP) protect mice from lethal endotoxemia through the inhibition of TNF-α and IL-6. J. Immunol. **162:** 1200–1205.

Sympathetic Abnormalities during Autoimmune Processes

Potential Relevance of Noradrenaline-Induced Apoptosis

ADRIANA DEL REY, ALEXA KABIERSCH, SIGRID PETZOLDT, AND HUGO O. BESEDOVSKY

Department of Immunophysiology, Institute of Physiology, Medical Faculty, 35037, Marburg, Germany

ABSTRACT: The sympathetic nervous system is one of the major pathways involved in immune-neuroendocrine interactions. Disturbances in these interactions are likely to have consequences during lymphoproliferative diseases. Work derived from our group as well as from several others led us to the hypothesis that the overstimulation of the immune system that characterizes this type of pathology results in decreased sympathetic nerve activity in lymphoid organs. To explore this possibility, we used as a model lpr/lpr mice, which develop a genetically determined autoimmune, lupus-like lymphoproliferative disease. We show that 18-week-old female C57Bl/6J lpr/lpr mice, which do not show overt symptoms of the disease but already have increased IgM and IgG2a levels in the blood, have decreased noradrenaline (NA) concentration and content in the spleen, but not in the kidney, as compared to normal C57Bl/6J littermates. Lpr/lpr mice do not express normal Fas, and therefore apoptosis cannot be triggered through this receptor. The defects in sympathetic innervation in the spleen of lpr/lpr mice prompted us to evaluate whether NA could influence lymphoid cell mass by inducing apoptosis. We found that NA can directly induce apoptosis in normal lymphoid cells via β-adrenergic receptors. From the reported results we propose that reduction in sympathetic nerve function in lpr/lpr mice contributes to aggravation of the disease and suggest that in addition to the incapacity to mount Fas-mediated apoptosis, a second proapoptotic mechanism, namely, that triggered by NA, is defective in these animals because of reduced availability of the neurotransmitter.

KEYWORDS: apoptosis; noradrenaline; autoimmune disease; sympathetic nervous system

INTRODUCTION

The existence of immunoregulatory circuits based on interactions between sympathetic nerves and immune cells has been proposed on the basis of abundant

Address for correspondence: Adriana del Rey, Department of Immunophysiology, Institute of Physiology, Medical Faculty, Deutschhausstrasse 2, 35037, Marburg, Germany. Voice: +49-6421-2862175; fax: +49-2868925.
delrey@mailer.uni-marburg.de

Ann. N.Y. Acad. Sci. 992: 158–167 (2003). © 2003 New York Academy of Sciences.

evidence showing that sympathetic mediators can modulate immune processes and that, conversely, the functioning of the sympathetic nervous system is affected during changes in the activity of the immune system (for a review, see Refs. 1–5). For example, we have shown that surgical denervation of the spleen results in enhanced immune responses to innocuous antigens.[6] More recently, we reported that general sympathetic denervation at the time of antigen priming impedes the clonal deletion of the specific CD4Vb cells that proliferate in response to stimulation with staphylococcal enterotoxin B, a process that characterizes the late phase of the *in vivo* immune response to superantigens in normal animals.[7] Regarding the afferent branch of sympathetic nervous system-immune interactions, we found that activation of the immune system by innocuous antigens results in decreased sympathetic nerve activity and turnover rate in the spleen[6] and that splenic noradrenaline (NA) concentration changes biphasically during the immune response to superantigens.[7]

Interactions of this type are likely to have a consequence for the course of lymphoproliferative diseases. The just evidence mentioned, together with the work of several other groups, led us to the hypothesis that the overstimulation of the immune system that characterizes lymphoproliferative diseases would result in decreased sympathetic nerve activity in lymphoid organs. This decrease would, in turn, relieve immune cells from the inhibitory effect of NA and thus favor expression of the disease. To explore this possibility, we used as a model mice homozygous for the lpr mutation (lpr/lpr mice). These mice develop a genetically determined autoimmune lymphoproliferative disease that resembles certain characteristics of systemic lupus erythematosus in humans (for a review, see Refs. 8 and 9). A characteristic of lpr/lpr mice is that they carry a mutation within the Fas gene; therefore, apoptosis cannot be triggered through this receptor. As just mentioned, we found that denervation impedes the deletion of those CD4+ T cells that proliferate in response to superantigens.[7] Because apoptosis is currently considered the main mechanism that leads to such deletion,[10] we also investigated whether NA can directly induce apoptosis of lymphoid cells with the aim of identifying a mechanism by which the sympathetic neurotransmitter could control the expansion of lymphoid cells.

MATERIAL AND METHODS

Animals

Normal C57Bl/6J and C57Bl/6J animals homozygous for the lpr mutation (lpr/lpr) (kindly provided by Dr. K. Hartmann, Institute for Experimental Immunology, Philipps University, Marburg, Germany) were permanently housed in temperature-, humidity-, and light (12-h cycles)-controlled rooms and fed *ad libitum*.

Reagents

L-noradrenaline hydrochloride (L-arterenol-hydrochloride) and S-propranolol (β-blocker) were obtained from Fluka Chemie AG, Buchs, Switzerland. Isoproterenol (β-adrenergic agonist), methoxamine (α-adrenergic agonist), and propidium iodide were obtained from Sigma-Aldrich Chemie Gmbh, Steinheim, Germany. Dexamethasone was from Serva GmbH, Heidelberg, Germany, and FITC-labeled

Annexin V was obtained from Bender MedSystems, Vienna, Austria. RPMI 1640 was purchased from GIBCO; fetal calf serum (FCS), penicillin, streptomycin, glutamine, and HEPES were from Biochrom/Seromed, Berlin, and 2-mercaptoethanol from Merck, Darmstadt.

Immunoglobulin Determinations

Eighteen-week-old C57Bl/6J and C57Bl/6J lpr/lpr female mice were killed by cervical dislocation, blood was collected in EDTA-coated tubes, and the spleen and kidney were weighted and immediately frozen. IgM levels in plasma were determined by ELISA using a commercially available kit (Bethyl Laboratories Inc., Texas, USA). In the case of the IgG2a isotype, the Igh-1b allotypic variant (the one of the C57Bl/6J mice) is not detectable by the classic anti-IgG2a xenoantibodies provided in commercially available kits (Refs. 11 and 12 and own observations). We therefore developed a quantitative ELISA immunoassay to detect IgG2a in the plasma of C57Bl/6J mice. Briefly, microtiter plates were coated with mouse-anti-mouse IgG2a^b (PharMingen, Heidelberg, Germany) for 16 hours at 40°C and washed with phosphate-buffered saline solution (PBS) containing 0.05% Tween. After blocking unspecific binding sites with PBS containing 0.5% bovine serum albumin for 1 hour at room temperature, 50 µl of different concentrations of purified mouse IgG2a b allotype (PharMingen, Heidelberg, Germany) used as standards or dilutions of plasma samples were added. After 2 hours of incubation at room temperature and washing with PBS-Tween, biotinylated anti-mouse IgG2a^b (PharMingen, Heidelberg, Germany) was added, and the plates were incubated for 1 hour. Streptavidin-horseradish peroxidase (PharMingen), 3,4',5,5'-tetramethyl benzidine (TMB, Kirkegaard and Perry, Gaithersburg, Maryland, USA), and H_2O_2 were usedas the detection system; previous washing was done with PBS-Tween. The reaction was stopped by the addition of 50 µl of 1 M H_2SO_4, and evaluation was done at 450 nm with the reference filter at 570 nm using an automatic ELISA reader.

Noradrenaline Determinations

Noradrenaline determinations in the spleen and left kidney were performed by HPLC, as previously described.[13] Briefly, tissue samples were homogenized in 0.4 M perchloric acid and centrifuged, and aliquots of the supernatant were injected into an HPLC system with electrochemical detection. Peaks were quantified by peak height evaluation and by area integration with an evaluation software (Millennium Session Manager, Millipore Corp.).

Evaluation of Apoptosis

Cell suspensions were freshly prepared from the thymus of 8- to 10-week-old C57Bl/6J mice. Thymuses were collected in cold PBS containing 0.1% BSA and gently pressed through a metal grid, filtered through a 100-µm nylon mesh (Nybolt, Schweizerische Seidengazefabrik AG, Zürich, Switzerland,), washed, resuspended in complete medium (RPMI 1640 containing FSC 5%, penicillin-streptomycin, 2 mM L-glutamine, 1% HEPES, and 5×10^{-5} M 2-ME), and cell concentration and viability was determined. Then, 2×10^5 cells in a final volume of 0.5 ml were cultured for 4 hours with or without the addition of the various compounds. The percentage of apoptotic cells was evaluated by assessment of membrane phopholipid asymmetry (exposure of phosphatidylserine) with FITC-labeled Annexin V. Briefly, after the incubation period, cells were washed with binding buffer (BB, 10 mM Hepes/NaOH pH 7.4, 140 mM NaCl, 2.5 mM $CaCl_2$) and resuspend in BB containing 0.4 μg/ml Annexin-FITC and 2 μg/ml propidium iodide. After incubation for 10 min in the dark at 4 °C, 1 ml cold BB was added, the cells were washed twice with BF, resuspend in 500 μl BB and analyzed by flow cytometry on a FACScan® (Becton Dickinson & Co.).

Statistical Analysis

Results are expressed as mean ± SE. Data were analyzed using one-way analysis of variance (ANOVA) followed by Fischer's test for multiple comparisons. Differences were considered significant at $P < 0.05$.

RESULTS AND DISCUSSION

Splenic Noradrenaline Concentration Is Reduced in lpr/lpr Mice

It has long been known that females are more susceptible to the development of autoimmune diseases; therefore, the studies reported here were performed in female mice. MRL is the strain most commonly selected as genetic background for the lpr mutation; however, the MRL strain itself (without carrying the lpr mutation) is predisposed to autoimmune disease and subsequently also develops lymphoproliferative autoimmune disease.[14] We have therefore used C57Bl/6J lpr/lpr for these studies because the only difference with the normal strain used for comparison (C57Bl/6J) is that it carries the mutated Fas gene. In the C57 background, the lymphoproliferative disease induced by the lpr mutation develops later than in the MRL background.[15] The studies were performed in 18-week-old mice. No overt symptoms of the disease were detected at this age in C57Bl/6J lpr/lpr mice, as indicated by normal body weight and the absence of palpable lymphoadenopathies. However, IgM and IgG2a levels in blood of C57Bl/6J lpr/lpr mice were markedly increased compared to values determined in normal C57Bl/6J animals, showing that a pathological state was already expressed (FIG. 1). The NA content in the spleen of lpr/lpr mice was markedly reduced compared to that of control mice. This reduction was also significant when NA values were calculated per whole organ despite the fact that the spleen was clearly enlarged (FIG. 1). No significant alterations in NA content and concentration were detected in the kidney, another abdominal organ used as control.

These results are in line with those of a previous report also showing a decrease in NA concentration in the spleen of MRL lpr/lpr mice[16] and with our studies demonstrating that the sympathetic activity in lymphoid organs depends on the degree of immunological activity.[6,17–19] For example, the NA content in lymphoid organs of specific-pathogen–free animals but those otherwise kept under conventional conditions is significantly lower than that of animals bred under germ-free conditions and that consequently have an underdeveloped immune system.[17] Another example is that in mice that are immunoincompetent because of the lack of T cells, NA content

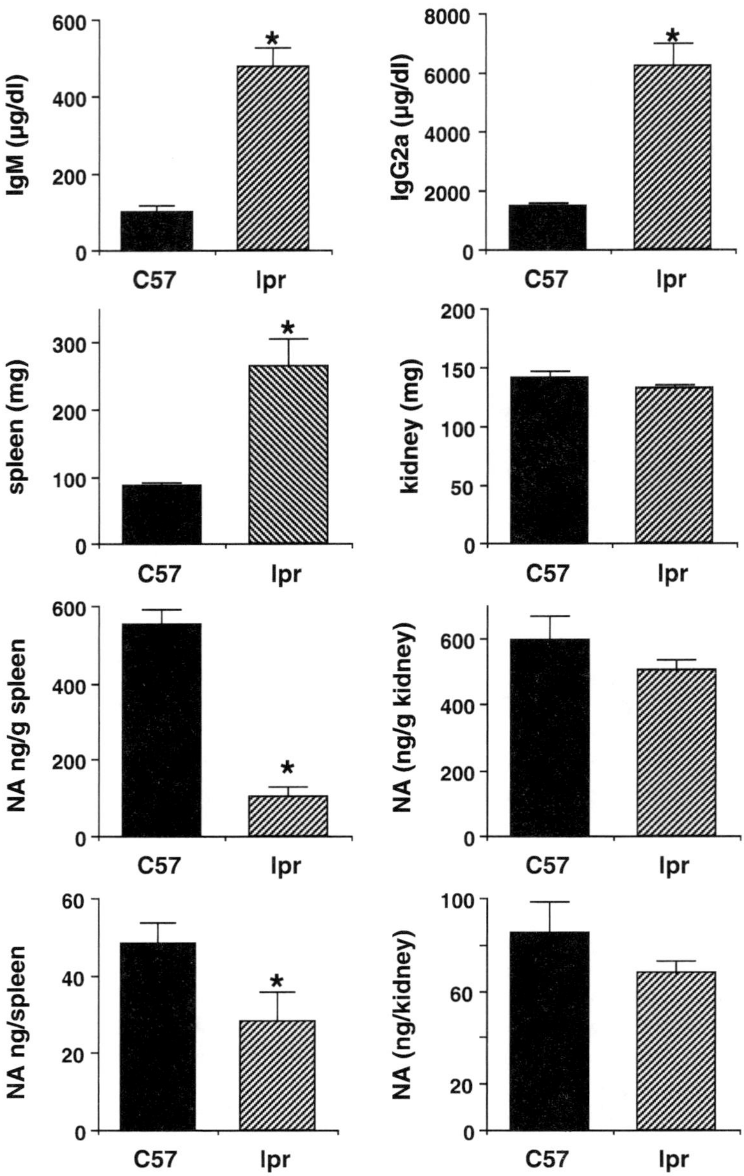

FIGURE 1. Immunoglulin levels in plasma and noradrenaline (NA) concentration and content in the spleen and kidney of 18-week-old C57Bl/6J (C57) and C57Bl/6J lpr/lpr (lpr) female mice were evaluated, as described in **Material and Methods**. Each column represents the mean ± SE. **P* <0.05 as compared to the corresponding parameter of the control mice.

in lymphoid organs is increased. When immunocompetence is reestablished either by thymus transplantation or T cell inoculation, NA levels decrease and the pattern of sympathetic innervation is normalized.[18] We have also shown that the decrease in splenic NA content during an *in vivo* induced specific immune response is more sustained in immunologically high responder animals.[19]

Noradrenaline Induces Apoptosis in Lymphoid Cells

The major immunological deficit in lpr/lpr mice is uncontrolled lymphoproliferation associated so far with a Fas gene mutation. The defects in sympathetic innervation in the spleen of lpr/lpr mice just described prompted us to evaluate whether NA could influence lymphoid cell mass by inducing apoptosis. If so, this would indicate a potential relevance of the decreased endogenous NA concentration in lpr/lpr mice for expression of the disease.

The capacity of NA to induce apoptosis in lymphoid cells was tested using thymocytes freshly obtained from C57Bl/6J adult mice. Cells were cultured for 4 hours with different concentrations of NA. Dexamethasone was used as positive control for comparison. The combination of annexin V and propidium iodide allows apoptotic cells to be distinguished from dead cells. As shown in FIGURE 2A, the percentage of apoptotic thymocytes in cultures treated with 1 mM NA was significantly increased compared with control cultures, but it was somewhat lower than that in cultures incubated with 1 μM dexamethasone. The percentage of dead cells that cumulated during the culture period was also increased when 1 μM NA was added (FIG. 2B). FIGURE 2C shows the additive percentages of apoptotic and dead cells under this culture condition. Both concentrations of NA used (1 μM and 1 mM) induced a significant increase in apoptotic and dead cells, the higher NA concentration being comparable to the apoptosis induced by 1 μM dexamethasone.

To study whether the proapoptotic effect of NA is mediated via α- or β-adrenergic receptors, two different approaches were followed. First, the capacity of the α-adrenergic agonist methoxamine and of the β-agonist isoproterenol to induce apoptosis in thymocytes was determined. Only isoproterenol could induce apoptosis to a degree comparable to that of NA (FIG. 3A). These results agree with those reported by Anderson *et al.*[20] and Gu *et al.*[21] using the synthetic β-agonist and other methods for detection of apoptosis. However, since NA stimulates both α- and β-adrenergic receptors, it was necessary to determine if β-blockade interferes with the apoptotic effect of the endogenous sympathetic mediator. Therefore, as a second approach, thymic cells were incubated simultaneously with NA and the β-blocker propranolol. This treatment resulted in significant inhibition of NA-induced apoptosis (FIG. 3B). These results agree in part with those of Stevenson *et al.*,[22] showing that prolonged administration of NA results in significantly more apoptotic cells in lymphoid organs, but they reported that the effect is α-adrenergic mediated.[22] However, the experimental design used does not allow a definitive conclusion that the effects observed are directly mediated by NA. For example, α-adrenergic stimulation *in vivo* can cause a decrease in blood flow in lymphoid organs,[23] thus decreasing oxygen supply, a situation that may favor the induction of apoptosis. In any case, the results of the *in vitro* experiments shown here provide the first conclusive evidence that the proapoptotic effect of the natural sympathetic mediator NA can be exerted directly on lymphoid cells.

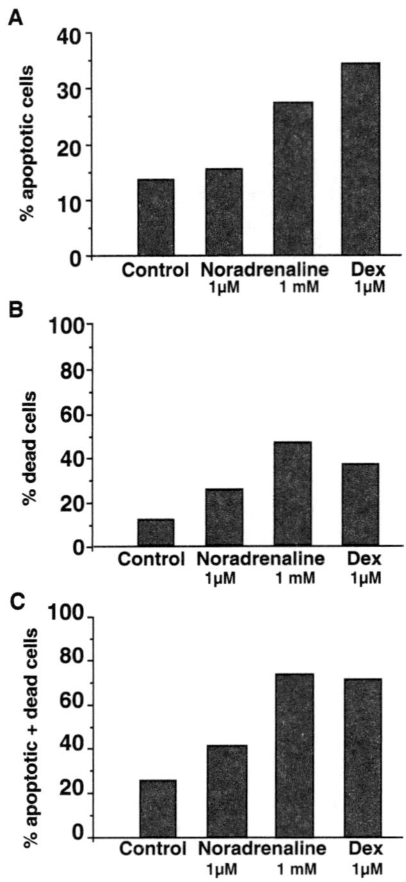

FIGURE 2. Thymocytes freshly obtained from C57Bl/6J mice were incubated for 4 hours in the absence or the presence of different noradrenaline (NA) concentrations or dexamethasone (Dex). (**A**) Percentage of apoptotic cells; (**B**) percentage of dead cells; and (**C**) sum of both apoptotic and dead cells determined after these treatments.

Apoptosis is the main mechanism involved in the control of immune cell mass and turnover. We therefore hypothesize that NA-induced apoptosis of lymphoid cells may either interfere with or delay the expression of autoimmune lymphoproliferative diseases. A defect in sympathetic innervation would be of particular relevance in lpr/lpr mice, because we recently found that NA-induced apoptosis is independent of the Fas-FasL pathway (manuscript in preparation).

The proapoptotic effect of NA shown here has to be added to the other multiple immunoregulatory effects of sympathetic neurotransmitters that have previously been reported.[1–5] Although some studies indicate that catecholamines are immunostimulatory whereas others indicate that they are inhibitory, there is certainly no lack of reports showing that sympathetic neurotransmitters can affect the immune

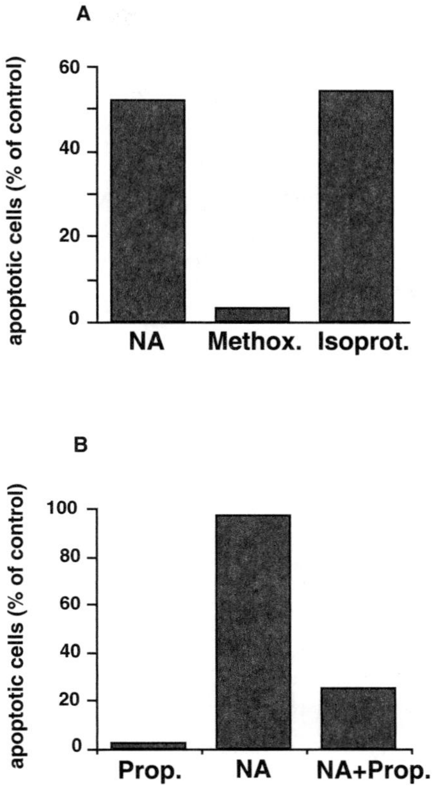

FIGURE 3. Thymocytes freshly obtained from C57Bl/6J mice were incubated for 4 hours in the presence of 0.1 mM noradrenaline (NA), or the same concentration of the α-agonist methoxamine (Methox.) or the β-agonist isoproterenol (Isoprot.) (**A**); or 10 μM propranolol (Prop.), 1 mM NA, or both (NA + Prop.) (**B**). Results are expressed as percentage of the values obtained in simultaneous control cultures (no NA, agonist, or antagonist added).

response, The evidence available is only apparently contradictory, because the experimental models used to approach this problem differ considerably regarding the antigenic stimulus, the immune parameter evaluated, the doses of the agonists and antagonists applied, the type of α- or β-receptor involved, and particularly during which step of an immune response are lymphoid and/or accessory cells exposed to sympathetic neurotransmitters. As a unifying concept, it was proposed that NA is permissive during the early steps of an immune response but inhibitory in later steps.[24] This view would predict that during prolonged immune processes, sympathetic nerves restrain the activity of immune cells. This restraint is expected to be less expressed in lpr/lpr mice because, as shown here, noradrenergic nerves in lymphoid organs are either less active or destroyed even at early stages of the lymphoproliferative disease that develops in these mice.

In summary, the reported results lead to the proposal that a reduction in sympathetic nerve function in lpr/lpr mice contributes to aggravation of the disease and may reveal that in addition to the incapacity to mount Fas-mediated apoptosis, a second proapoptotic mechanism, namely, that triggered by NA, is defective in these animals because of reduced availability of the neurotransmitter.

ACKNOWLEDGMENT

This work was supported by the Deutsche Forschungsgemeinschaft (SFB 297).

REFERENCES

1. Besedovsky, H. O., M. Da Prada, A. Del Rey & E. Sorkin. 1981. Immunoregulation by sympathetic nervous system. Trends Pharmacol. Sci. **2:** 236–238.
2. Madden, K.S. & D.L. Felten. 1995. Experimental basis for neural-immune interactions. Physiol. Rev. **75:** 77–106.
3. Besedovsky, H.O. & A. Del Rey. 1996. Immune-neuro-endocrine interactions: facts and hypotheses. Endocr. Rev. **17:** 64–102.
4. Kohm, A.P. & V.M. Sanders. 2000. Norepinephrine: a messenger from the brain to the immune system. Immunol. Today **21:** 539–542.
5. Elenkov, I.J., R.L. Wilder, G.P. Chrousos & E.S. Vizi. 2000. The sympathetic nerve: an integrative interface between two supersystems: the brain and the immune system. Pharmacol. Rev. **52:** 595–638.
6. Besedovsky, H.O., A. Del Rey, E. Sorkin, *et al.* 1979. Immunoregulation mediated by the sympathetic nervous system. Cell. Immunol. **48:** 346–355.
7. Del Rey, A., A. Kabiersch, S. Petzoldt & H.O. Besedovsky. 2002. Involvement of noradrenergic nerves in the activation and clonal deletion of splenic T cells stimulated by superantigen *in vivo*. J. Neuroimmunol. **127:** 44–53.
8. Nagata, S. & T. Suda. 1995. Fas and Fas ligand: lpr and gld mutations. Immunol. Today **16:** 39–43.
9. Nose, M., M. Nishihara, J. Kamogawa, *et al.* 2000. Genetic basis of autoimmune disease in MRL/lpr mice: dissection of the complex pathological manifestations and their susceptibility loci. Rev. Immunogenet. **2:** 154–164.
10. Wahl, C., T. Miethke, K. Heeg. & H. Wagner. 1993. Clonal deletion as direct consequence of an *in vivo* T cell response to bacterial superantigen. Eur. J. Immunol. **23:** 1197–1200.
11. Klein-Schneegans, A.S., L. Kuntz, S. Trembleau, *et al.* 1990. Serum concentrations of IgM, IgG1, IgG2b, IgG3 and IgA in C57BL/6 mice and their congenics at the nu (nude) locus. Thymus **16:** 45–54.
12. Klein-Schneegans, A.S., L. Kuntz, P. Fonteneau & F. Loor. 1989. An indirect asymmetrical sandwich ELISA using anti-allotype antibodies for the specific and quantitative measurement of mouse IgG2a of IgH-1b allotype. J. Immunol. Methods **125:** 207–213.
13. Kabiersch, A., A. Del Rey, C.G. Honegger & H.O. Besedovsky. 1988. Interleukin-1 induces changes in norepinephrine metabolism in the rat brain. Brain Behav. Immun. **2:** 267–274.
14. Kono, D.H. & A.N. Theofilopoulos. 2000. Genetics of systemic autoimmunity in mouse models of lupus. Int. Rev. Immunol. **19:** 367–387.
15. Kelley, V.E. & J.B. Roths. 1985. Interaction of mutant lpr gene with background strain influences renal disease. Clin. Immunol. Immunopathol. **37:** 220–229.
16. Breneman, S.M., J.A. Moynihan, L.J. Grota, *et al.* 1993. Splenic norepinephrine is decreased in MRL-lpr/lpr mice. Brain Behav. Immun. **7:** 135–143.
17. Del Rey, A., H.O. Besedovsky, E. Sorkin, *et al.* 1981. Immunoregulation mediated by the sympathetic nervous system II. Cell. Immunol. **63:** 329–334.

18. BESEDOVSKY, H.O., A. DEL REY, E. SORKIN, *et al.* 1987. T lymphocytes affect the development of sympathetic innervation of mouse spleen. Brain Behav. Immun. **1:** 185–193.
19. DEL REY, A., H.O. BESEDOVSKY, E. SORKIN, *et al.* 1982. Sympathetic immunoregulation: difference between high- and low-responder animals. Am. J. Physiol. **242:** R30–R33.
20. ANDERSON, K.L., G. ANDERSON, R.H. MICHELL, *et al.* 1996. Intracellular signaling pathways involved in the induction of apoptosis in immature thymic T lymphocytes. J. Immunol. **156:** 4083–4091.
21. GU, C., Y.C. MA, J. BENJAMIN, *et al.* 2000. Apoptotic signaling through the beta-adrenergic receptor. A new Gs effector pathway. J. Biol. Chem. **275:** 20726–20733.
22. STEVENSON, J.R., J. WESTERMANN, P.M. LIEBMANN, *et al.* 2001. Prolonged alpha-adrenergic stimulation causes changes in leukocyte distribution and lymphocyte apoptosis in the rat. J. Neuroimmunol. **120:** 50–57.
23. ROGAUSCH, H., A. DEL REY, A. KABIERSCH, *et al.* 1997. Endotoxin impedes vasoconstriction in the spleen: role of endogenous interleukin-1 and sympathetic innervation Am. J. Physiol. **272:** R2048–R2054.
24. MADDEN, K.S. & S. LIVNAT. 1991. Catecholamine action and immunologic reactivity. *In* Psychoneuroimmunology. R. Ader, D.L. Felten & N. Cohen, Eds. :283–310. Academic Press, Inc. San Diego, CA.

Antimicrobial Chromogranins and Proenkephalin-A–Derived Peptides

Antibacterial and Antifungal Activities of Chromogranins and Proenkephalin-A–Derived Peptides

M.H. METZ-BOUTIGUE, Y. GOUMON, J.M. STRUB,
K. LUGARDON, AND D. AUNIS

INSERM Unité 575, IFR37 "Physiopathologie du Système Nerveux," Strasbourg, France

Laboratoire de Spectrometrie de Masse Bio-Organique, Universite Louis Pasteur, CNRS UMR 7509, ECPM, Strasbourg, France

ABSTRACT: The secretory granules from adrenal medullary chromaffin cells contain a complex mixture of low-molecular mass constituents such as catecholamines, ascorbate, nucleotides, calcium, peptides, and several high-molecular mass water-soluble proteins including chromogranins and proenkephalin-A. These proteins are sequestered into secretory granules in which processing yields a large variety of peptides. These fragments are released into the extracellular space upon cell stimulation and are recovered in blood, lymph, cerebrospinal fluid, and synovial fluid. Some of them have biological activity on cells in an autocrine, paracrine, or endocrine fashion. In addition, we have shown that peptides with antimicrobial activity are present with the secretory chromaffin granules and demonstrated that they are released from stimulated chromaffin cells. We have shown that posttranslational modifications modulate the antimicrobial activities. For some peptides, using confocal laser microscopy, we have examined the interaction of the rhodaminated peptides with biological membranes. In addition, we have shown that chromofungin, the antifungal peptide corresponding to chromogranin $A_{47\text{-}66}$, can bind calmodulin in the presence of calcium and induce inhibition of calcineurin, a calmodulin-dependent enzyme. Because these antibacterial peptides are colocalized with catecholamines, they may be activated during stress, playing a role as a first protective barrier against bacterial infection, and thus act as factors of the innate immunity shortly after infection and before the induction and mobilization of an adaptative immune system.

KEYWORDS: chromogranin A and B; proenkephalin-A, vasostatin-I; neuropeptide; neuroimmunity; innate immunity; antibacterial and antifungal peptide

Address for correspondence: M.H. Metz-Boutigue, INSERM Unité 575, IFR37 "Physiopathologie du Système Nerveux," 5 rue Blaise Pascal 67084, Strasbourg, France. Voice: 33-3-88-45-66-09; fax: 33-3-88-60-08-06.
metz@neurochem.u-strasbg.fr

Ann. N.Y. Acad. Sci. 992: 168–178 (2003).

TABLE 1. Composition of the soluble material present in the matrix of the secretory granules of chromaffin cells from the bovine adrenal medulla

Catecholamines: 0.6–0.8 M
Nucleotides: ATP, AMP, ADP, GDP, and UDP
Enzymes and cofactors
Ions: Ca^{2+}, Mg^{2+}, Na^{+}, and PO_4^{2-}
Peptides: NPY, substance P, VIP, CRF, enkephalins, somatostatin, neurotensin, etc.
Proteins: chromogranins, proenkephalin-A, etc.

INTRODUCTION

Secretory granules from adrenal medullary chromaffin cells contain a complex mixture of molecules including catecholamines, low-molecular mass constituents, and numerous water-soluble peptides and proteins (TABLE 1). All of these components are released into the circulation in response to splanchnic nerve stimulation. Large amounts of chromogranins (CGs) and proenkephalin-A (PEA) are present in the adrenal medullary chromaffin granules,[1,2] and we have used these organelles as a model to study their processing.[3–5] In addition, we have established the post-translational modifications of bovine CGA,[6] human CGA,[7] and bovine CGB.[8] Since 1995, we have found that antibacterial and antifungal peptides are present in the intragranular matrix and are released in the extracellular medium of stimulated chromaffin cells.[4,9–12] These peptides, derived from CGs and PEA, are active against gram-positive and gram-negative bacteria and can also prevent fungal growth. Interestingly, we have identified these peptides in secretions of immune cells (polynuclear neutrophils), indicating that these peptides established a communication between the neuroendocrine and the immune systems.[10,11]

NATURAL ANTIMICROBIAL PEPTIDES AND INNATE IMMUNITY

From the perspective of the microbe, the tissues of living multicellular organisms are rich sources of nutrients. Therefore, to avoid being parasitized and digested, all living multicellular organisms have developed a rapid and effective response to challenge pathogens. Among the different mechanisms that have evolved to act efficiently, the production of a large variety of natural antimicrobial peptides is attracting increasing attention. The importance of these molecules is clearly established in the immune defense of invertebrates,[13,14] whereas in vertebrates, they act as a first line of defense against pathogens and in the control of natural flora.[13,15] These antimicrobial peptides are located at sites exposed to microbial invasion such as the epithelia of amphibians, mammals, and insects. They are present in the hemolymph of insects and stored in the secretory granules of immune cells in mammals and birds. In addition, human intestinal Paneth cells, which are secretory epithelial cells located at the bottom of the crypts in the small intestine, express defensins[16] also produced in various epithelia such as psoriatic skin[17] and trachea.[18,19] Because these host defenses are present at birth, they are grouped under the heading "innate immunity," an evolutionary ancient defense mechanism. Surveys of antimicrobial peptides have revealed links between the antimicrobial peptides in vertebrates and those in invertebrates.[20–22] Recently, new data have highlighted similarities between pathogen recognition, signaling pathways, and effector mechanisms of innate immunity in *Drosophila* and mammals.[23] As the need for new antimicrobial agents has rapidly been increasing in recent years due to the fast growing number of antibiotic-resistant bacteria, interest in antibacterial peptides is expanding. Their therapeutic potential in immunodeficient patients, chemotherapy, organ grafting, and antibiotic-resistant bacterial infections is currently under intensive investigation.

In the present review, after a short presentation of the various antimicrobial peptides secreted during stress by stimulated chromaffin cells from the adrenal medulla, we focus on vasostatin-I (CGA1-76),[11,12] the highly conserved N-terminal fragment resulting from the natural processing of CGA. This CGA-derived peptide, predominantly generated after processing, displays antibacterial and antifungal activities. The second antibacterial peptide presented here is enkelytin,[10] corresponding to the bisphosphorylated form of $PEAP^{209\text{-}237}$.

ANTIBACTERIAL AND ANTIFUNGAL CHROMAFFIN GRANULE PEPTIDES

In 1995, we initially reported the presence of antimicrobial peptides with the matrix of secretory granules from the adrenal medulla.[4] These natural peptides, which inhibit the growth of bacteria and fungi, are processed from the N-terminal (vasostatin-I) and the C-terminal (secretolytin, enkelytin) ends of the precursors (FIG. 1). These peptides are released from stimulated chromaffin cells, but also as a novel product from stimulated polynuclear neutrophils. Interestingly, in these secretory fluids the concentration of antimicrobial peptides falls in the micromolar range,[10] that is, close to the concentration necessary for the antimicrobial activity. In addition, the antimicrobial activities of some CG- and PEA-derived peptides

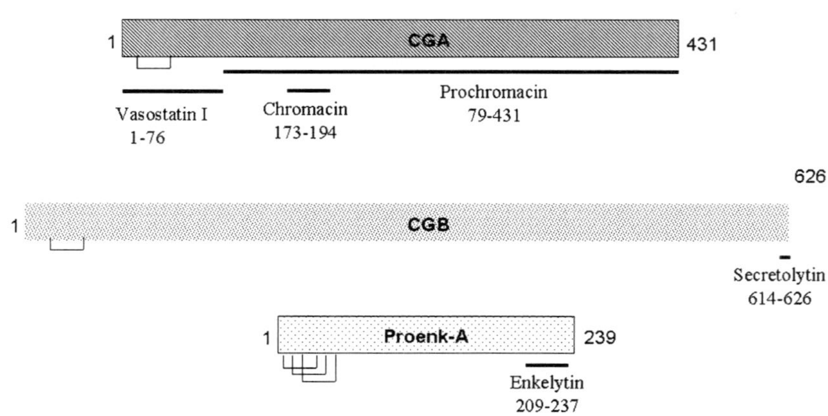

FIGURE 1. Location of the antimicrobial peptides isolated from the intragranular matrix of bovine chromaffin granules in the sequences of chromogranin A (CGA), chromogranin B (CGB), and proenkephalin-A (PEA).

depends on posttranslational modifications such as *O*-glycosylation and phosphorylation.[9,10] These modifications occur at an early stage within the pre-secretory granules and may represent regulatory steps related to still unknown physiological and pathological conditions. As previously reported, vasostatin-I and enkelytin correspond to the most highly conserved domains in their precursors. Therefore, the antimicrobial activities displayed by these peptides are likely to have occurred early in evolution. Furthermore, CGs and PEA are widely distributed not only in endocrine, neuroendocrine, and nerve cells, but also in immune cells. Their liberation from these cells indicates that these peptides are likely to play a role in inflammatory processes. Therefore, we suggest that in stress situations, these peptides might act by raising an immediate protective barrier against infection. Hence, the antibacterial and antifungal activities might provide a highly beneficial strategy against pathogenic invasion.

VASOSTATIN-I: A MULTIFUNCTIONAL ANTIMICROBIAL PEPTIDE

The N-terminal natural bovine CGA1-76 corresponds to a conserved domain, showing a high yield of identity with human, pig, rat, equine, and frog, respectively (FIG. 2). In all species examined so far, the disulfide bridge C17-C38 is conserved and the sequence SILRHQNLLKELQ (CGA50-62) is strictly unchanged (FIG. 2). Vasostatins are multifunctional peptides. The vasoinhibitory effect has been reproduced with recombinant and synthetic vasostatin-I. In addition, vasostatin-I exhibits other biological activities such as the autocrine inhibition of parathyroid hormone secretion,[24] regulation of cell adhesion,[25] and neurotoxic effects in neuronal/microglial cell cocultures.[26] All of these biological properties indicate that vasostatins are likely to have important biological functions, yet to be more extensively elucidated.

Natural bovine vasostatin-I was isolated from soluble material included in granular matrix from chromaffin bovine cells (FIG. 3). This peptide is selectively active against *Micrococcus luteus* and *Bacillus megaterium*, completely inhibiting their growth at 2 μM and 0.2 μM (TABLE 2). By contrast, no activity is detectable at 10 μM against other gram-positive bacteria. To complete the spectrum of activity of

```
               1        10        20        30        40        50        60        70    76
bCGA 1-76 :  LPVNSPMNKGDTEVMKCIVEVISDTLSKPSPMPVSKECFETLRGDERILSILRHQNLLKELQDLALQGAKERTHQQ
hCGA 1-76 :  -----------------------------------Q------------------------------------A---
pCGA 1-76 :  -----------------------------------Q------------------------------------S---
rCGA 1-76 :  -------T----K----VL-----S----------P--L---Q----V------------------------AQ--
mCGA 1-76 :  ------T----K---VL-----S----------P--L---Q------------------------------A--P
oCGA 1-76 :  ---TNN------K----------------N-L-IIE--L---------I-------------EI-V---N---Q--
eCGA 1-76 :  -------DT----------------------V---Q------------------------------------AP--
fCGA 1-76 :  ---SSLEGEDNTK----------------N-V-ITQD-L---------I-------------E--A---M--LQKA
```

FIGURE 2. Alignment of the vasostatin-I sequences from different species: b, bovine; h, human; p, pig; r, rat; m, mouse; o, ostrich; e, equine; f, frog.[11]

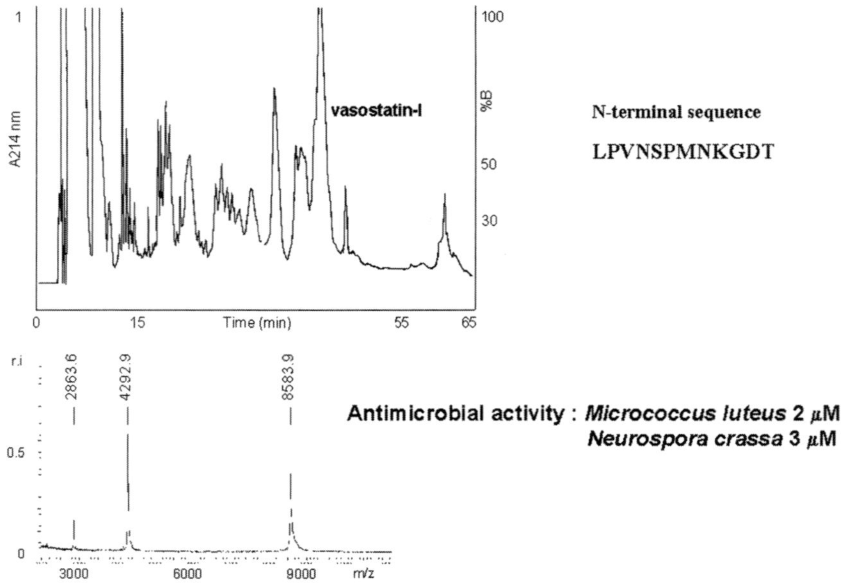

FIGURE 3. Isolation of natural vasostatin-I present with soluble intragranular matrix from bovine chromaffin cells. Analysis by sequencing and mass spectrometry (MALDI-TOF). The antibacterial and antifungal activities are indicated.

TABLE 2. The antimicrobial activity of vasostatin-I against gram-positive bacteria, filamentous fungi, and yeasts[11]

Gram-positive bacteria	*Bacillus megaterium*	*Micrococcus luteus*
	0.2 µM	2 µM
Filamentous fungi	*Neurospora crassa*	*Fusarium culmorum*
	Alternaria brassicola	*Fusarium oxyporum*
	Nectria haematococca	*Aspergillus fumigatus*
	1–10 µM	
Yeasts	*Saccharomyces cerevisiae*	*Candida albicans*
	10 µM	

vasostatin-I, its ability to affect the growth of filamentous fungi and yeast cells was examined (TABLE 2). Interestingly, in the concentration range of 1–10 µM, this peptide is strongly active against a variety of filamentous fungi. The specificity towards bacteria and fungi is remarkable, because vasostatin-I is inactive against bovine erythrocytes.

To characterize the active domain of vasostatin-I, this natural peptide is digested with endoproteinase Glu-C. The generated fragments are isolated with reverse phase HPLC. In one major peak, a peptide corresponding to CGA47-70 was active against

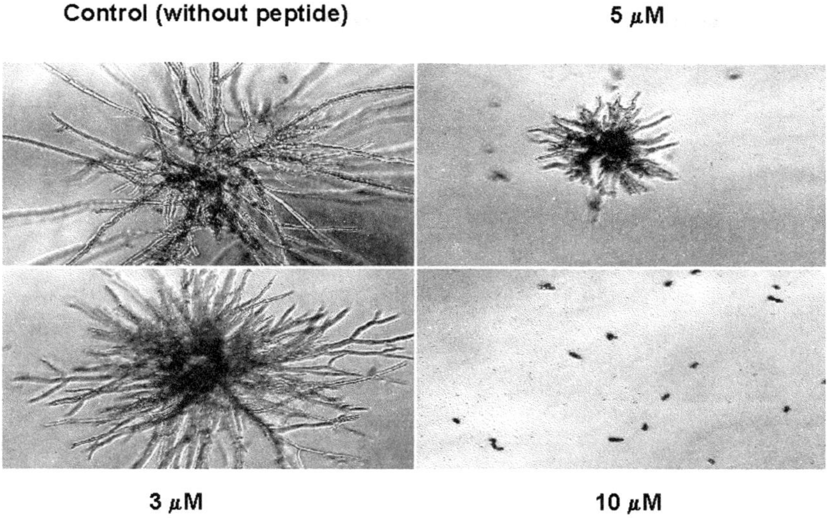

FIGURE 4. Inhibition of fungal growth of *Alternaria brassicola* by synthetic peptide CGA47-66 (chromofungin).

Neurospora crassa with a MIC100 of 7 μM. To illustrate this antifungal activity the inhibition of fungal growth (*Alternaria brassicola*) by CGA47-70 was reported (FIG. 4). To investigate the structural features involved in the antifungal activity of the highly conserved C-terminal moiety of vasostatin-I, we tested the activity of different synthetic peptides (CGA41-60, CGA41-70, and CGA47-70) to examine the role of the tripeptide RGD (position 43-45) and the length of the peptide. CGA41-60 displays weak activity, suggesting that the tripeptide RGD may confer some hindrance for the antifungal activity; CGA41-70 can kill several fungi, suggesting the importance of the C-terminal end of this fragment to counteract the inhibitory effect of the tripeptide RGD (position 43-45); fragments CGA41-60 and CGA41-70 are active, showing a relation between their activities and the peptide chain length. Because the shortest active peptide, CGA47-66, displayed the highest antifungal activity, it was used to investigate the molecular mechanism implicated in the antimicrobial activities. This peptide was named chromofungin.

STRUCTURAL AND BIOLOGICAL ANALYSIS OF CHROMOFUNGIN (CGA47-66)

The first step of this study was to determine the three-dimensional structure of chromofungin in water/trifluoroethanol solution (50/50) using ^{1}H NMR spectroscopy. This analysis indicates that the peptide adopts an alphahelical structure in solution and that the region CGA53-66 is crucial for the amphipathic character. To examine the importance of this amphipatic C-terminal sequence, we tested the antifungal activity of the chromofungin-derived peptide with two proline residues, which disrupt the helical structure and the amphipathic character, in place of Leu61 and Leu64. This modified peptide was inactive at 5 μM, but it inhibits the growth of *N. crassa* by 81% at 100 mM, showing that the amphipathic helix is crucial for the antifungal activity.[12]

Studies of the penetration of chromofungin into lipid monolayers were performed at peptide concentrations ranging from 5×10^{-9} to 2×10^{-8} Mres.[12] When ergosterol, the main sterol in yeast and fungus plasma membrane, was included in the lipid monolayer, we observed an increase in the penetration of the peptide.

We then examined with confocal laser microscopy the interaction of rhodamine-labeled chromofungin with *Aspergillus fumigatus*, *A. brassicola,* and *Candida albicans.*[12] Fungal spores were incubated at 30°C first for 24 or 40 hours and then for 1, 16, or 21 hours with 10 μM of fluorescent peptides (chromofungin and an inactive control peptide, CGB602-626). Fluorescent chromofungin was visible at the level of the cell wall, where it seemed to accumulate, but also in the inner part of *A. fumigatus*. By contrast, the inactive peptide was undetectable at any treatment time. Futhermore, we showed that chromofungin penetrated the cell wall at the fungus weakest point and then invaded the numerous hyphaes, inducing distortion of the wall and formation of numerous vacuoles. Interestingly, treatment of *A. fumigatus* or *C. albicans* for 1 hour with higher concentrations of unlabeled chromofungin (100 mM) together with the inactive CGB revealed an intense fluorescence in *A. fumigatus* and *C. albicans*. This new data indicated that chromofungin at high concentrations destabilizes the cell wall, allowing inert peptide to penetrate in microorganisms.

Besides destabilization of the microorganism cell wall, chromofungin may also exert activity on intracellular targets. It was previously shown that CGA can interact with CaM and that the domain responsible for this interaction is probably located in the N-terminal region.[27] CaM bonds a variety of peptides that can form positively

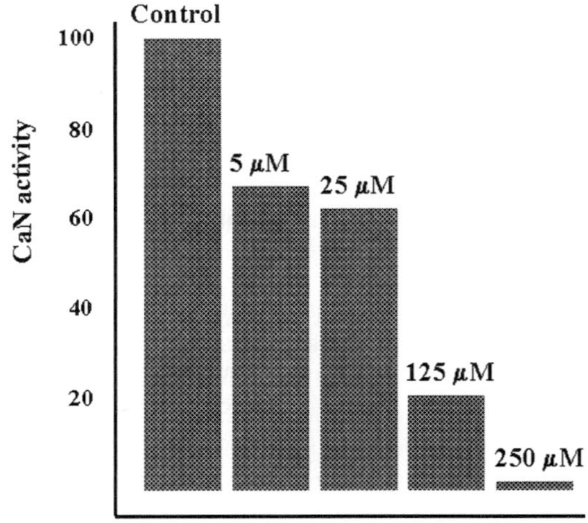

FIGURE 5. Calcineurin phosphatase activity in the presence of CGA47-66 (calcineurin).[12]

charged amphiphilic helices. The sequences of the binding domains have been mapped and revealed a model peptide. The comparison of this sequence with chromofungin revealed high 60% analogy.[12] This alignment suggests that chromofungin may represent the CGA domain able to bind CaM. This possibility was then tested by measuring the effect of chromofungin on the activity of calcineurin (CaN), a CaM-dependent enzyme. Recently, it was established that CaN plays a crucial role in hyphal growth, morphology, and maintenance of the apical Ca^{2+} gradient in the filamentous fungi *N. crassa*. Therefore, we examined the effect of chromofungin on CaN phosphatase activity.[12] At a concentration of 5 μM, corresponding to the minimal inhibitory concentration against the filamentous fungi growth, inhibition of CaN was evaluated to be 32% (FIG. 5).

To conclude, vasostatin-I contains a highly conserved region of 14 amino acids; the corresponding peptides possess potent antifungal activity due to its ability to cross microorganism cell membranes and perhaps to target and inhibit CaM-binding enzymes (CaN and chitin synthase), crucial for fungal growth.

ENKELYTIN, THE ANTIMICROBIAL PEPTIDE DERIVED FROM PROENKEPHALIN-A

Different PEA-derived peptides have been isolated from the complex mixture of intragranular matrix from chromaffin cells, and among them the natural potent antibacterial peptide named enkelytin[10] has been characterized as the bisphosphorylated form of PEA209-237. Enkelytin is active on gram-positive bacteria including *Staphylococcus aureus* in the micromolar range. With the use of sequencing and mass spectrometry analysis, the antibacterial activity was related with the presence of phosphate groups on serine residues 221 and 223.

Three-dimensional ^{1}HNMR analysis of PEA209-237 shows that enkelytin was structured as an L-shape conformation and that residue P227 is responsible for conformational Cis-Trans isomerization changes. In addition, the synthetic peptide with 3 glutamic residues in place of the 3 putative phosphorylated serine residues in position 215, 221, and 223 inhibits by 20% the bacterial growth at 10 μM, suggesting the importance of negative charges in the expression of the antibacterial activity of enkelytin. In addition, to correlate the antimicrobial activity of enkelytin with structural features, different enkelytin-derived peptides were tested. At the conclusion of these experiments we show that the activity is directly related to three parameters[10]: the length of the peptide, the natural conformational constraints induced by the proline residues in position 212, 214, and 227, and the phosphorylation of serine in position 221 and 223.

To further characterize the biological function of enkelytin, a major released PEA-derived peptide, we looked for its presence in biological fluids involved in defense mechanisms. Using a combination of Western blot, sequencing, and mass spectrometry, antibacterial C-terminal PEA-derived fragments were identified in numerous bovine and rabbit infectious fluids and in secretions of stimulated polynuclear neutrophils.[10]

The involvement of opioids in the regulation of interactive events between the nervous and the immune system appears to have a long evolutionary history. The relation between the immune and the nervous system also exists in invertebrates, and

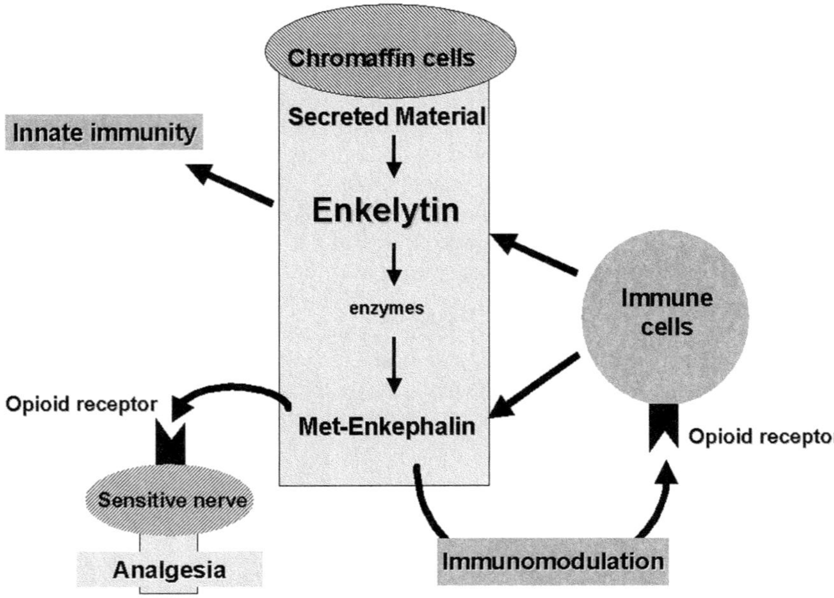

FIGURE 6. A model of interaction and communication between the nervous, endocrine, and immune systems is proposed for enkelytin (the bisphosphorylated form of PEA209-237).

the co-release of enkelytin and enkephalin represents a unified neuroimmune protective response to stress situations that may be accompanied by infectious diseases (FIG. 6).

CONCLUSIONS

The identification of different antibacterial and antifungal peptides, derived from neuropeptides, with the secretions of chromaffin and immune cells, suggests that these molecules play a role in the communication between the neuroendocrine and the immune system acting in innate immunity for the host defense. Although some important questions concern the expression of their activities in physiological and pathological situations, these different peptides may represent prototypic molecules useful for the development of new therapeutic agents.

ACKNOWLEDGMENTS

This work was funded by INSERM and supported by grants from the Meiji Institute of Health Science (Odawara, Japan), the Direction des Recherches, Etudes et Techniques (Grant DRET 96-099 to D.A.), the University Louis Pasteur (Strasbourg,

France) (Contrats PPF 1997-2000 to D.A.), the Ligue contre le Cancer (to M.H.M.B. and D.A.), the Association Recherche et Partage (Ph.D. grant to K.L.), and the Fondation pour la Recherche Médicale (Ph.D. grant to K.L.). We express our gratitude to all our collaborators who contributed to this work.

REFERENCES

1. SIMON, J.P. & D. AUNIS. 1989. Biochemistry of chromogranin A family. Biochem. J. **262:** 1–13.
2. DILLEN, L. *et al.* 1993. Post-translational processing of proenkephalin-A and chromogranins/secretogranins. Neurochem. Int. **22:** 315–352.
3. METZ-BOUTIGUE, M.H. *et al.* 1993. Intracellular and extracellular processing of chromogranin A. Determination of cleavage sites. Eur. J. Biochem. **217:** 247–257.
4. STRUB, J.M. *et al.* 1995. Processing of chromogranin B in bovine adrenal medulla. Identification of secretolytin, the endogenous C-terminal fragment of residues 614-626, with antibacterial activity. Eur. J. Biochem. **229:** 356–368.
5. GOUMON, Y. *et al.* 2000. Processing of proenkephalin-A in bovine chromaffin cells. J. Biol. Chem. **275:** 38355–38362.
6. STRUB, J.M. *et al.* 1997. Phosphorylation and O-glycosylation sites of bovine chromogranin A from adrenal medullary chromaffin granules and their relationship with biological activities. J. Biol. Chem. **272:** 11928–11936.
7. GADROY, P. *et al.* 1998. Phosphorylation and O-glycosylation sites of human chromogranin A (CGA79-439) from urine of patients with carcinoid tumors. J. Biol. Chem. **273:** 34087–34097.
8. LUGARDON, K. 2000. Implication des chromogranines A et B dans l'immunité innéé. Activité antifongique de la vasostatine-I: découverte et développements. Thèse de l'Université Louis Pasteur de Strasbourg, France.
9. STRUB, J.M. *et al.* 1996. Antibacterial activity of glycosylated and phosphorylated chromogranin A-derived peptide 173-194 from bovine adrenal medullary chromaffin granules. J. Biol. Chem. **271:** 28533–28540.
10. GOUMON, Y. *et al.* 1998. Characterization of antibacterial COOH-terminal proenkephalin-A-derived peptides (PEAP) in infectious fluids. Importance of enkelytin the antibacterial PEAP209-237 secreted by stimulated chromaffin cells. J. Biol. Chem. **273:** 29847–29856.
11. LUGARDON, K. *et al.* 2000. Antibacterial and antifungal activities of vasostatin-I, the N-terminal fragment of chromogranin A. J. Biol. Chem. **275:** 10745–10753.
12. LUGARDON, K. *et al.* 2001. Structural and biological characterization of chromofungin, the antifungal chromogranin A-(47-66)-derived peptide. J. Biol. Chem. **276:** 35875–35882.
13. BOMAN, H. 1995. Peptide antibiotics and their role in innate immunity. Annu. Rev. Immunol. **13:** 61–92.
14. HOFFMANN, J.A. *et al.* 1996. Innate immunity in higher insects. Curr. Opin. Immunol. **8:** 8–13.
15. ZASLOFF, M. *et al.* 1992. Antibiotic peptides as mediators of innate immunity. Curr. Opin. Immunol. **4:** 3–7.
16. OUELLETTE, A.J. & M.E. SELSTED. 1996. Paneth cell defensins: endogenous peptides components of intestinal host defence. FASEB J. **10:** 1280-–289.
17. HARDER, J. *et al.* 1997. A peptide antibiotic from human skin. Nature **387:** 861.
18. DIAMOND, G. *et al.* 1996. Inducible expression of an antibiotic peptide gene in lipopolysaccharide-challenged tracheal epitehelial cells. Proc. Natl. Acad. Sci. USA **93:** 5156–5160.
19. RUSSELL, J.P. *et al.* 1996. Coordinate induction of two antibiotic genes in tracheal epithelial cells exposed to the inflammatory mediators lipolysaccharide and tumor necrosis factor alpha. Infect. Immun. **64:** 1565–1568.
20. CHARLET, M. *et al.* 1996. Innate immunity. Isolation of several cysteine-rich antimicrobial peptides from the blood of a mollusc, *Mytilus edulis*. J. Biol. Chem. **271:** 21808–21813.

21. LEE, I.H. *et al.* 1997. Clavanins, alpha-helical antimicrobial peptides from tunicate hemocytes. FEBS Lett. **400:** 158–162.
22. ZHAO, C.Q. *et al.* 1997. cDNA cDNA cloning of three cecropin-like antimicrobial peptides (Styelins) from the tunicate, *Styela clava*. FEBS Lett. **412:** 144–148.
23. HOFFMANN, J. *et al.* 1999. Phylogenetic perspective in innate immunity. Science **284:** 1313–1318.
24. RUSSELL, J. *et al.* 1994. Inhibition of parathyroid hormone secretion by amino terminal chromogranin peptides. Endocrinology **135:** 337–342.
25. GASPARRI, A. *et al.* 1997. Chromogranin A fragments modulate cell adhesion. Identification and characterization of a pro-adhesive domain. J. Biol. Chem. **272:** 20835–20843.
26. CIESIELSKI-TRESKA, J. *et al.* 1998. Chromogranin A induces a neurotoxic phenotype in brain microglial cells. J. Biol. Chem. **273:** 14339–14346.
27. YOO, S.H. 1992. pH-dependent association of chromogranin A with secretory vesicle membrane and a putative membrane binding region of chromogranin A. Biochemistry **31:** 6134–6140.

In Vivo Effects of Growth Hormone on Thymic Cells

WILSON SAVINO,[a-c] SALETE SMANIOTTO,[a,d] NADINE BINART,[c] MARIE CATHERINE POSTEL-VINAY,[c] AND MIREILLE DARDENNE[b]

[a]*Laboratory on Thymus Research, Department of Immunology, Oswaldo Cruz Institute, Oswaldo Cruz Foundation, Rio de Janeiro, Brazil*

[b]*CNRS FRE 2444, Université Paris V, Hôpital Necker, Paris, France*

[c]*Inserm U-344, Université Paris V, Hôpital Necker, Paris, France*

[d]*Department of Morphology, Federal University of Alagoas, Maceió, Brazil*

ABSTRACT: Increasing evidence has placed the thymus as a target for neuroendocrine control. Herein we review the pleiotropic effects of growth hormone (GH) on this primary lymphoid organ, with emphasis on data derived from *in vivo* experiments. A series of results strongly indicate that GH enhances thymocyte proliferation in both rodents and humans. Moreover, *in vivo* treatment with GH enhances interleukin (IL)-6 production by mouse thymocytes, and *ex vivo* experiments show that production of other cytokines, such as IL-1 and GM-CSF, is also augmented. In a second vein, GH exerts a modulatory role on thymic hormone production, particularly the secretion of thymulin. In GH-treated animals as well as GH-transgenic mice, thymulin secretion is enhanced. In acromegalic patients we found higher levels of thymulin secretion, whereas the opposite was seen in dwarf mice and GH receptor knockout animals. Developing T cell migration is also under GH influence. Recombinant GH was found to increase human T cell engraftment in the thymus of SCID mice. Moreover, *ex vivo* thymocyte traffic into and out of thymic nurse cell complexes is enhanced after GH treatment. Lastly, we show that thymocyte export *in vivo* is modulated by GH, which favors the homing of CD4$^+$ recent thymic emigrants towards lymph nodes. In conclusion, the possibility that GH improves *in vivo* thymic functions, including thymocyte proliferation and migration, points to this molecule as a potential therapeutic adjuvant in T cell associated immunodeficiencies.

KEYWORDS: growth hormone; thymus; thymocytes; thymic epithelial cells; thymic nurse cells; thymulin; cytokines; extracellular matrix; integrins; insulin-like growth factors

Address for correspondence: Wilson Savino, Laboratory on Thymus Research, Department of Immunology, Oswaldo Cruz Institute, Oswaldo Cruz Foundation, Ave. Brasil 4365, Manguinhos 21045-900 - Rio de Janeiro, Brazil. Voice: 55 21 2588-4557; fax: 55 21 2280 1589.
savino@gene.dbbm.fiocruz.br

Ann. N.Y. Acad. Sci. 992: 179–185 (2003). © 2003 New York Academy of Sciences.

INTRODUCTION

In the context of the growth hormone (GH)-mediated cross-talk between the neuroendocrine and immune systems, increasing evidence shows that the physiology of the thymus is modulated by GH. Herein we review examples of such control, emphasizing the *in vivo* effects of GH on thymic cells. To facilitate the comprehension of the data discussed, we will first provide a brief overview of the process of intrathymic T cell differentiation within the thymic microenvironment.

The thymus is the primary lymphoid organ in which bone marrow-derived T cell precursors undergo a process of maturation, resulting in the migration of positively selected thymocytes to T cell-dependent areas of peripheral lymphoid organs. Importantly, although thymocyte proliferation and differentiation persist throughout life, they diminish with aging: older thymuses are significantly atrophied with fewer thymocytes than younger ones and with a reduced capability of exporting T cells to the periphery.[1,2]

Thymocyte differentiation involves expression of membrane markers and rearrangements of T cell receptor (TCR) genes, as well as migration within the thymic lobules. The most immature thymocytes, located in the outer cortex, express neither the TCR/CD3 complex nor the accessory molecules CD4 or CD8, being termed double-negative thymocytes. Maturation progresses with migration towards the inner cortex and acquisition of the CD4 and CD8, generating the $CD4^+CD8^+$ double-positive thymocytes, which comprise 80% of thymocytes. At this stage, TCR genes are rearranged, and thymocytes expressing productive TCR will react with peptides presented by molecules of the major histocompatibility complex, expressed on the membranes of the thymic microenvironment, a tridimensional network consisting of thymic epithelial cells (TECs), macrophages, dendritic cells, fibroblasts, and extracellular matrix (ECM) components. This interaction, essentially occurring in the cortex, determines the positive and negative selection events, crucial for normal thymocyte differentiation. Positive selection allows $CD4^+CD8^+$ thymocytes to be rescued from death and to become mature, $CD4^+$ or $CD8^+$ single-positive cells, both expressing high densities of the CD3/TCR complex and now located in the medulla of the thymic lobules. In principle, these cells will leave the organ to form the majority of the T cell repertoire in the periphery of the immune system.[2,3]

MOLECULAR BASES FOR THE ROLE OF GROWTH HORMONE ON THYMIC CELLS

This first point related to the action of GH on thymic cells concerns the expression of GH receptor, which was first demonstrated in human TECs by ligand-specific binding assay and was further confirmed *in situ* and *in vitro* by immunocytochemistry and RT-PCR.[4,5] Additionally, GH receptor expression has been demonstrated in murine and human thymocytes, particularly in the $CD4^-CD8^-$ immature subset.[5,6]

Various intracellular signaling pathways can be triggered by activation of the GH receptor, as reported in a variety of nonimmune cell types.[7] GH acts by binding to a membrane receptor that belongs to the cytokine receptor superfamily.[8] This binding results in dimerization of the receptor and activation of the Jak2/Stat cascade,[9,10] a general pathway that seems to occur in GH-treated TECs (unpublished data).

Another aspect related to the molecular basis is the notion that IGF-1 is involved in several effects of GH in the thymus. For example, incubating GH-treated TECs with anti-IGF-1 or anti-IGF-1 receptor antibodies[11,12] can abrogate the *in vitro* effects of GH on TECs in terms of endocrine function and the ability to adhere to thymocytes. Accordingly, both thymocytes and TECs can produce IGF-1 and express the respective receptor, and we recently presented evidence of a GH-controlled IGF-1/IGF-1 receptor circuitry.[13]

Finally, to better understand the intrathymic GH/IGF-1 circuitry we must keep in mind that in addition to the pituitary gland, the thymus itself should be included as a source of GH: both thymocytes and TECs can express and secrete the hormone.[6]

MODULATORY EFFECTS OF GROWTH HORMONE ON PROLIFERATION OF THYMIC CELLS

It is well established that GH enhances TEC proliferation *in vitro,*[11] an effect that occurs in the context of cyclin upregulation (our unpublished data). Interestingly, the GH releasing inhibitor somatostatin, as well as its analogue octreotide, significantly blocks human cultured TEC proliferation, as ascertained by ^{3}H-thymidine incorporation.[14] Nevertheless, whether GH stimulates TEC growth *in vivo*, particularly during thymus ontogeny, remains to be determined.

The enhancing effects of GH on thymocyte proliferation were first proposed when injections of GH3 (pituitary adenoma cells able to produce GH) to old rats were found to reverse age-dependent thymic atrophy, with a consequent increase in thymocyte numbers.[15] This finding was in keeping with data showing that transgenic mice overexpressing GH or GH-releasing hormone exhibit overgrowth of the thymus.[16] In fact, even when we normalize the number of thymocytes per gram of body weight, GH-transgenic animals have higher thymocyte numbers than do the corresponding age/sex-matched counterparts (Smaniotto *et al*, manuscript in preparation). In humans, HIV-induced thymic atrophy has been shown to be partially restored by daily injections of GH, clearly suggesting a thymopoietic effect of the hormone.[17]

GROWTH HORMONE UPREGULATES HORMONAL AND CYTOKINE PRODUCTION BY THYMIC CELLS

Few data concern the *in vivo* effects of GH on the intrathymic production of cytokines. We showed that injection of GH in aging animals induced an upregulation of IL-6 production by thymocytes.[18] Although *in vivo* GH treatment can augment IL-2 secretion by peripheral T cells,[19] data on thymocytes are lacking. In a second vein, fetal calf thymocytes treated *ex vivo* with GH exhibited increased transcript levels of IL-1α, IL-1β, IL-6, and GM-CSF.[20]

As regards GH effects on cytokine production by microenvironmental cells, again only *in vitro* data have been reported. An increase in the secretion of IL-1α, IL-1β, and IL-6 by bovine microenvironmental cell cultures under GH treatment has been documented.[18] Whether or not GH modulates chemokine production by the thymic microenvironment needs to be investigated.

Much more data are available on the *in vivo* modulatory effect of GH on thymic hormone production, particularly the secretion of thymulin by TEC. In general, high circulating levels of GH result in increased thymulin serum levels, whereas low levels of GH decrease circulating thymulin, as summarized in TABLE 1. (For a review, see Ref. 3.) These data are in keeping with recent findings that GH-transgenic mice exhibit high thymulin serum levels, the opposite being observed in GH receptor knockout mice (FIG. 1).

TABLE 1. *In vivo* effects of growth hormone upon thymulin secretion

Thymulin serum levels in pathological or experimental condition	References
Dwarf mice exhibit a precocious decay in thymulin	23
Hypophysectomy in rats yields a transient decrease in thymulin	24
Deficient GH production in children is paralleled by low thymulin production, which is restored after exogenous GH treatment	25
Acromegalic patients exhibit elevated thymulin serum levels	26
Injection of GH in aging animals increases thymulin levels	18

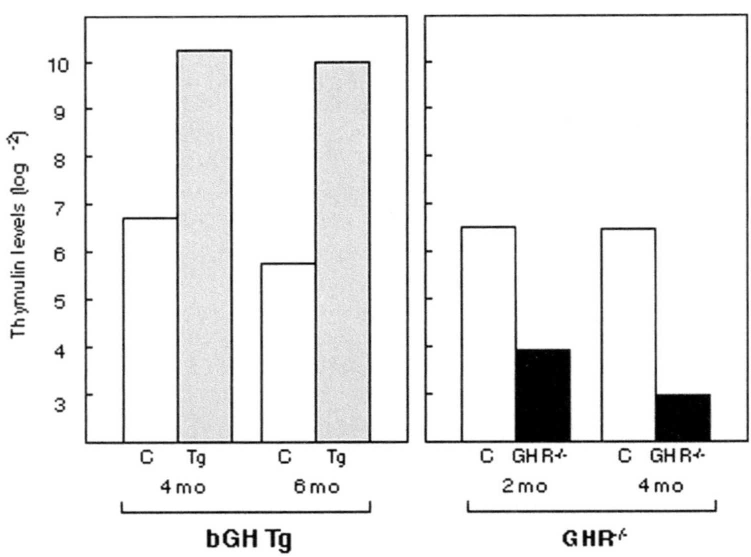

FIGURE 1. Thymulin levels in genetically engineered mice, either transgenic for the bovine growth hormone (bGH-Tg) or knockout for the growth hormone receptor ($GHR^{-}/^{-}$). As compared to corresponding age-matched controls (*open bars*), bGH-Tg animals exhibit significantly higher circulating levels of thymulin, the opposite being observed in $GHR^{-}/^{-}$ mice (P <0.01). Results are shown in two different ages for each type of animal. Data express the mean ± standard error of 5–7 animals.

In any case, it is noteworthy that the enhancing effects of GH on thymulin secretion derive from the direct action of GH on the thymic epithelium, because this effect can be obtained *in vitro* by treating TEC cultures with GH.[11]

GROWTH HORMONE MODULATES THYMOCYTE MIGRATION

Although relatively few studies have been conducted to determine if GH modulates developing T cell migration, this is a likely issue. Pioneer studies by Taub and coworkers[21] have shown that recombinant GH increases human T cell engraftment in the thymus of SCID mice and that such an effect could be abrogated with anti-β1 or anti-β2 integrin antibodies, a finding that strongly suggests the involvement of adhesion molecules and extracellular matrix.

As regards intrathymic cell traffic, data based on *in vivo* experiments unfortunately are still lacking. In any case, using *in vitro* systems we showed that GH was able to upregulate adhesion of thymocytes on TEC cultures, an effect that was prevented by pretreating TECs with anti-ECM or anti-ECM receptor antibodies.[22] Moreover, *ex vivo* thymocyte traffic into and out of the thymic nurse cell complexes was enhanced after GH treatment.[22]

Recent data strongly indicate that thymocyte export *in vivo* can be modulated by GH. In one study conducted in mice, we injected intrathymically fluorescein isothiocyanate (FITC) and traced recent thymic emigrants (i.e., $FITC^+$ cells) in peripheral organs 16 hours post-FITC injection. We noted that a single intrathymic injection of GH resulted in modulation in recent thymic emigrant homing, with higher numbers of $CD4^+ FITC^+$ cells in the lymph nodes as compared to those in controls,[23] a finding that was confirmed in GH transgenic animals (Smaniotto *et al.*, in preparation).

Similar results were reported in AIDS patients. In a recent study in which five HIV-1 patients were subjected to long-term (3–12 months) treatment with GH, not only reversal of the thymic atrophy, but also an increase in $CD4^+$ naïve T cells was seen, likely corresponding to recent thymic emigrants.[17]

CONCLUDING REMARKS

Although it is certain that our knowledge of the role of GH in thymus physiology is far from complete, the data just discussed clearly indicate the pleiotropic effects of this hormone on thymic cells. In this regard, the use of genetically engineered mice will hopefully shed more light on relevant aspects of thymic functions, such as thymocyte proliferation, shaping the T cell repertoire within the organ, and exporting to the periphery of the immune system. Such knowledge, once acquired, will be important for designing protocols of GH-based immunotherapy in various immunodeficiencies.

ACKNOWLEDGMENTS

We thank Anne Bachelot for handling the colony of growth hormone receptor knockout mice and Marie-Claude Gagnerault for thymulin measurements. This work was partially supported with grants from Inserm/Fiocruz and Capes/Cofecub France/ Brazil conjoint Programmes, CNPq, and Capes (Brazil).

REFERENCES

1. ANDERSON, G. & E.J. JENKINSON. 2001. Lymphostromal interactions in thymic development and function. Nat. Rev. Immunol. **1:** 31–40.
2. BERZINS, S.P., A.P. ULDRICH, J.S. SUTHERLAND, *et al.* 2002. Thymic regeneration: teaching an old immune system new tricks. Trends Mol. Med. **8:** 469–476.
3. SAVINO, W. & M. DARDENNE. 2000. Neuroendocrine control of the thymus. Endocrine Rev. **21:** 412–443.
4. BAN, E., M.-C. GAGNERAULT, H. JAMMES, *et al.* 1991. Specific binding sites for growth hormone in cultured mouse thymic epithelial cells. Life Sci. **48:** 2141–2148.
5. MELLO-COELHO, V., M.-C. GAGNERAULT, J.C. SOUBERBIELLE, *et al.* 1998. Growth hormone and its receptor are expressed in human thymic cells. Endocrinology **139:** 3837–3842.
6. GAGNERAULT, M.-C., M.-C. POSTEL-VINAY & M. DARDENNE. 1996. Expression of growth hormone receptors in murine lymphoid cells analyzed by flow cytofluorometry. Endocrinology **137:** 1719–1726.
7. HERRINGTON, J. & C. CARTER-SU. 2001. Signaling pathways activated by the growth hormone receptor. Trends Endocrinol. Metab. **12:** 252–257.
8. BAZAN, F. 1990. Structural design and molecular evolution of a cytokine receptor superfamily. Proc. Natl. Acad. Sci. USA **87:** 6934–6938.
9. ARGETSINGER, L.S., G.S. CAMPBELL, X. YANG, *et al.* 1993. Identification of JAK2 as a growth hormone receptor-associated tyrosine kinase. Cell **74:** 237–244.
10. RAM, P.A., S. PARK, H.K. CHOI & D.J. WAKMAN. 1996. Growth hormone activation of Stat1, Stat3 and Stat5 in rat liver. J. Biol. Chem. **271**: 5929–5940.
11. TIMSIT, J., W. SAVINO, B. SAFIEH, *et al.* 1992. Growth hormone and insulin-like growth factor-I stimulate hormonal function and proliferation of thymic epithelial cells. J. Clin. Endocrinol. Metabol. **75:** 183–188.
12. MELLO-COELHO, V., D.M.S. VILLA-VERDE, M. DARDENNE & W. SAVINO. 1997. Pituitary hormones modulate cell-cell interactions between thymocyte and thymic epithelial cells. J. Neuroimmunol. **76:** 39–49.
13. MELLO-COELHO, V., D.M.S. VILLA-VERDE, D.A. FARIAS-DE-OLIVEIRA, *et al.* 2002. Functional growth hormone-controlled IGF-1/IGF-1 receptor autocrine/ paracrine circuit in human and murine thymic epithelial cells. Neuroendocrinology **75:** 139–150.
14. FERONE, D., P. MARTIN-VAN-HAGEN, P.M. VAN-KOETSVELD, *et al.* 1999. *In vitro* characterization of somatostatin receptors in the human thymus and effects of somatostatin and octreotide on cultured thymic epithelial cells. Endocrinology **140:** 373–380.
15. KELLEY, K.W., S. BRIEF, H.J. WESTLY, *et al.* 1986. GH3 pituitary adenoma cells can reverse thymic aging in rats. Proc. Natl. Acad. Sci. USA **83:** 5663–5667.
16. DIALYNAS, E., H. BROWN-BORG & A. BARTKE. 1999. Immune function in transgenic mice overexpressing growth hormone (GH) releasing hormone, GH or GH antagonist. Proc. Soc. Exp. Biol. Med. **221:** 178–183.
17. NAPOLITANO, L.A., J.C. LO, M.B. GOTWAY, *et al.* 2002. Increased thymic mass and circulating naïve CD4 T cells in HIV-1-infected adults treated with growth hormone. AIDS **16:** 1103–1111.
18. GOYA, R.G., M.C. GAGNERAULT, M.C. LEITE-DE-MORAES, *et al.* 1992. *In vivo* effects of growth hormone on thymus function in aging mice. Brain Behav. Immun. **6:** 341–354.
19. KELLEY, K.W., S. BRIEF, H.J. WESTLY, *et al.* 1987. Hormonal regulation of the age-associated decline in immune function. Ann. N. Y. Acad. Sci. **496:** 91–97.
20. CHEN, H.T., L.A. SCHULER & R.D. SCHULTZ. 1998. Growth hormone receptor and regulation of gene expression in fetal lymphoid cells. Mol. Cell. Endocrinol. **137:** 21–29.
21. TAUB, D.D., G. TSARFATY, A.R. LLOYD, *et al.* 1994. Growth hormone promotes human T cell adhesion and migration to both human and murine matrix proteins in vitro and directly promotes xenogeneic engraftment. J. Clin. Invest. **94:** 293–300.

22. SAVINO, W., S. SMANIOTTO, V. MELLO-COELHO & M. DARDENNE. 2000. Is there a role for growth hormone upon intrathymic T cell migration? Ann. N.Y. Acad. Sci. **917:** 749–754.

23. PELLETIER, M., S. MONTPLAISIR, M. DARDENNE & J.-F. BACH. 1976. Thymic hormone activity and spontaneous autoimmunity in dwarf mice and their littermates. Immunology **30:** 783–788.

24. DARDENNE, M. & W. SAVINO. 1990. Neuroendocrine control of the thymic epithelium: modulation of thymic endocrine function, cytokeratin expression and cell proliferation by hormones and neuropeptides. Prog. Neuroendocrineimmunol. **3:** 18–25.

25. MOCCHEGIANI, E., A. SARTORIO, L. SANTARELLI, *et al.* 1996. Thymulin, zinc and insulin-like growth factor-I (IGF-1) activity before and during recombinant growth hormone (rec-GH) therapy in children and adults with GH deficiency. J. Endocrinol. Invest. **19:** 630–637.

26. TIMSIT, J., B. SAFIEH, M.-C. GAGNERAULT, *et al.* 1990. Increase of circulating levels of thymulin in hyperprolactinemia and acromegaly. C.R. Acad. Sci. (Paris) Serie III **310:** 7–13.

Role of the Thymus in the Development of Tolerance and Autoimmunity towards the Neuroendocrine System

VINCENT GEENEN AND FABIENNE BRILOT

Liege University Center of Immunology, Institute of Pathology CHU-B23, B-4000 Liege-Sart Tilman, Belgium

ABSTRACT: The thymus is the unique lymphoid organ inside which a confrontation occurs throughout life between neuroendocrine self-antigens and a recently evolved system with original recombination machinery driving random generation of immune response diversity. Through transcription of neuroendocrine genes in the thymus stromal network and expression of cognate receptors by immature T cells, the neuroendocrine system regulates early T cell differentiation. In addition and more specifically, intrathymic presentation of neuroendocrine self-antigens by, or in close association with, major histocompatibility complex (MHC) proteins is responsible for the establishment of central immune self-tolerance of neuroendocrine principles. All members of the insulin gene (*INS*) family are expressed in the thymus stroma according to a precise hierarchy and cell topography: *IGF2* (thymic epithelial cells) > *IGF1* (thymic macrophages) >> *INS* (thymic medullary epithelial cells and/or dendritic cells). Given this hierarchical pattern in gene expression, the protein IGF-2 is more tolerated than INS. *Igf2* transcription is defective in the thymus of bio-breeding (BB) rat, one animal model of type 1 diabetes (T1DM). This thymus-specific defect in *Igf2* expression may explain both the absence of central tolerance to INS-secreting ß cells and the lymphopenia (including lack of regulatory RT6$^+$ T cells) in diabetes-prone BB rats. INS B:9-23 and the homologous sequence of IGF-2 compete for binding to DQ8, an MHC class II allele conferring major susceptibility to T1DM. In young DQ8$^+$ T1DM patients, INS B:9-23 presentation by DQ8 elicits a dominant IFN-γ secretion by isolated PBMCs, whereas presentation of the IGF-2 self-antigen promotes a dominant regulatory interleukin-10 secretion. These data demonstrate that opposite immune responses are driven by MHC presentation of a self-antigen (here, IGF-2) and an autoantigen (INS, as "altered" self). The important tolerogenic properties of thymic self-antigens deserve now to be exploited for prevention and/or cure of devastating autoimmune diseases such as T1DM.

KEYWORDS: **thymus; type 1 diabetes, insulin; IGF-2**

Address for correspondence: Dr. Vincent Geenen, Liege University Center of Immunology, Institute of Pathology CHU-B23, B-4000 Liege-Sart Tilman, Belgium.

Ann. N.Y. Acad. Sci. 992: 186–195 (2003). © 2003 New York Academy of Sciences.

INTRODUCTION

The thymus is crucially located at the crossroad between the immune and the neuroendocrine systems, and among all lymphoid structures, only the thymus ensures the generation of a diverse repertoire of T cell receptors that are self-tolerant. This central self-tolerance is extremely powerful, because only 1–2% of T cell progenitors will leave the thymus as mature T cells that are self-tolerant but competent against non-self-antigens presented at the periphery. Molecular mechanisms involved in thymic clonal deletion of self-reactive T cells have been extensively described. However, little attention has been paid to the self-antigens that are effectively presented to thymocytes (pre-T cells) by the thymic major histocompatibility complex (MHC) machinery. Intrathymic expression of genes encoding peripheral tissue-specific autoantigens is more and more being documented.[1–11] Consequently, a defect in central self-tolerance as a crucial factor in pathogenesis of organ-specific autoimmune diseases has become a major topic of contemporary research in autoimmunity. Hierarchical patterns exist in intrathymic transcription of neuroendocrine-related genes so that one dominant self-antigen precursor for each family is expressed in the thymus stroma. Thymic neuroendocrine self-antigens are homologous, but not identical, to peripheral neuroendocrine autoantigens. Such biochemical difference led us to investigate that opposite immune responses might be driven by related homologous self-antigens and autoantigens. This hypothesis appeared to be correct after preliminary investigation of the cytokine profile elicited by the presentation of antigens derived from members of the insulin family.

DUAL ROLE OF THYMIC NEUROENDOCRINE SELF-ANTIGEN PRECURSORS

The intrathymic synthesis of the neurohypophysial peptide oxytocin (OT) was reported in 1986.[12] Subsequent studies to elucidate the physiological role of thymic OT have indicated that thymic OT does not behave as a secreted neurohormone, but as the self-antigen of the neurohypophysial peptide family.[13,14] OT presentation to immature T cells involves a 55-kDa protein that is expressed in thymic epithelial cell (TEC) plasma membrane and that is labeled by both antibody to neurophysin (OT-binding 10-kDa protein) and an antibody directed to the 45-kDa heavy chain of MHC class I proteins.[15] The precise biochemical mechanisms responsible for the synthesis of this chimeric protein remain to be elucidated, but a similar neurophysin-MHC class I protein has been identified in cell membranes of small cell lung carcinoma.[16] Neurotensin (NT) and somatostatin were the first neuropeptides detected by immunocytochemistry in the thymic parenchyme.[17] Further studies conclusively demonstrated that NT (and NT-derived peptides) are presented by MHC class I proteins purified from TEC plasma membrane.[18]

Genes encoding specific neurohypophysial receptors are transcribed by thymic T cell subsets: OT receptor (OTR) is expressed by CD4–8–, CD4+8+, CD4+, and CD8+ thymic T cells, whereas V3R expression is restricted to CD4+8+ and CD8+ thymic T cells. Neither V1R nor V2R expression can be detected in the thymus.[19] Thymocyte OTR and V3R can transduce neurohypophysial peptides, in particular OT, according to the rules established for those receptors in other cellular systems (increase of phosphoinositide turnover coupled to mitogenic action).[20] In addition, OT markedly increases the phosphorylation of kinases implicated in focal adhesion ($p125^{FAK}$, $p130^{Cas}$).[21] Such an early event in the process of T cell differentiation could be crucial for the establishment of immunological synapses between immature T cells and thymic antigen-presenting cells (APCs), namely, TECs, dendritic cells (DCs), and macrophages. During ontogeny in Balb/c mice, *OT* transcripts are detected on E13 in both brain and thymus, whereas *VP* transcription starts on E14 in the brain and is clearly detected in the thymus only on E15 (unpublished data). *OT* precocious transcription in the thymus further concords with the role of thymic OT in the induction of central self-tolerance of the neurohypophysial peptides before their expression by hypothalamic neurons. Based on these two roles of thymic OT acting both as a self-antigen and as a ligand for neurohypophysial receptors expressed by pre-T cells, a model was elaborated transposing at the peptide level the dual role of the thymus in T cell differentiation.[22] Such model applies to other neuroendocrine-related self-antigen precursors expressed in the thymic stroma, and a definition of neuroendocrine self was proposed as follows: (1) neuroendocrine self-antigens correspond to peptide sequences highly conserved throughout evolution of one given family; (2) a hierarchy characterizes their expression pattern in the thymus; (3) the intrathymic processing of neuroendocrine self-antigen precursors is not coupled to the classic model of (neuro)secretion but to pathways of antigen presentation by MHC proteins; and (4) some differences exist in the processing between thymic APCs and dedicated peripheral APCs. For some neuroendocrine self-antigens (OT and NT), those differences imply that their presentation by thymic APCs is not restricted by MHC alleles.[23]

THYMIC EXPRESSION OF INSULIN-RELATED GENES

While searching for a precursor able to represent the whole insulin peptide family in front of T cells during their differentiation in the thymus, insulin-like growth factor 2 (IGF-2) was found to be the dominant insulin-related peptide expressed by TECs from different species.[24] Immunoreactive (Ir) IGF-1 was also detected in thymic cells with a macrophage-like morphology and topography, whereas Ir insulin could not be clearly identified within human thymic lobules. Again, IGF-2 secretion was not evidenced in human TEC primary cultures, although Ir IGF-2 could be detected by confocal microscopy at the outer surface of TEC plasma membranes (data not published). By reverse transcription-polymerase chain reaction (RT-PCR) and *in situ* hybridization (ISH), *IGF2* transcription by human TECs was further demonstrated and found to be under the control of the same promoters as in extrahepatic fetal and adult tissues.[25] *IGF1R* was found to be expressed in Jurkat T cells, and *IGF1* transcripts were also identified by ISH in thymic macrophages. Functional significance of the thymic IGF axis was evaluated by using murine fetal thymic organ cultures (FTOCs). FTOC treatment with an anti-IGF-2 monoclonal antibody induced an inhibition of the transition from CD4−8− T cells to CD4+8+ T cells as well as an increase in CD8+ cells. A similar inhibition of early T cell differentiation was observed when FTOCs were treated with anti-IGF-1R monoclonal antibody or anti-IGF-2R polyclonal antibody. In addition, anti-IGF-1R and anti-IGF-2R induced an 81% and a 34% decrease in FTOC total T cell number, respectively. In the same model, treatment with a specific antibody directed to (pro)insulin did not exert any significant effect on either T cell cellularity or T cell differentiation.[26]

From 1994, studies have repeatedly reported that the insulin gene (*INS*) is also transcribed in the thymus.[27] A debate recently raised about the precise nature of the thymic cell type responsible for *INS* transcription, that is, medullary TECs[28] or DCs.[29] Compared to IGF-2 (± 100 ng/g wet weight), the thymic content in INS protein is very low, ranging from 98–1,200 fmol/g wet weight in one study to 0.437 ± 0.218 pmol/mg protein in another.[30,31] Those studies did not investigate the functional effect of thymic INS on T cell differentiation, but evidenced a correlation between thymic *INS* mRNA levels and the presence of alleles conferring genetic susceptibility to type 1 diabetes (T1DM).

THYMIC INSULIN-RELATED PEPTIDES, CENTRAL TOLERANCE OF ISLET β CELLS, AND TYPE 1 DIABETES

As just discussed, a precise hierarchy and cell topography exist in the intrathymic expression of *INS*-related genes: *IGF2* (TEC) > *IGF1* (macrophages) ≫ *INS* (thymic DCs and/or medullary TECs). Such hierarchy is important since it is known that immune tolerance of a protein or a protein family primarily involves dominant epitopes of this protein or this family.[32,33] Theoretically according to this observation, IGF-2 should be more tolerated than IGF-1, and much more than INS. This assumption is indirectly verified by immunization, that is, active experimental breakdown of immune tolerance, with INS-related peptides. Following immunization, the titers and frequency of antibodies to INS are higher than those against IGF-1 and much higher than those against IGF-2. Also, the high prevalence of autoantibodies against INS (±40%) in the population could be related to the very low expression of *INS* in the thymus.[34] Finally, a number of studies recently failed to indicate any significant tolerogenic activities of INS administered either orally or subcutaneously.[35–37]

To gain further insight into the central tolerance mediated by thymic INS-related proteins, we advanced the hypothesis that thymus dysfunction could be involved in T1DM pathophysiology. This hypothesis was investigated through analysis of *Ins*, *Igf1,* and *Igf2* expression in the thymus of biobreeding (BB) rats, an animal model of human T1DM. *Ins*, *Igf1*, and *Igf2* transcripts were detected in the thymus of all diabetes-resistant BB rats (BBDR). By contrast, while *Ins* and *Igf1* transcripts were detected in the thymus of all diabetes-prone BB rats (BBDP), a defect in *Igf2* transcription was observed in 11 of 15 thymuses from BBDP rats, in close accordance with the diabetes incidence in this strain (86%).[38] This defect was thymus-specific since *Igf2* transcription was detected in the brain and liver of BBDP rats. The correlation between percentage of *Igf2*-deficient thymuses and incidence of autoimmune diabetes in BBDP rats, on the one hand, and the functional properties of IGF-2-mediated signaling on T cell proliferation/differentiation, on the other hand, may both contribute to the absence of central self-tolerance of islet β cells and to lymphopenia in BBDP rats.

A number of genetic loci conferring susceptibility or resistance to type 1 diabetes have been identified.[39] Recent studies support the hypothesis that genetically determined thymic INS levels play a critical role in INS-specific autoreactive T cell selection. Using an elegant model of graded *INS* transcription in the thymus, Chentoufi and Polychronakos[40] found that specific T cell reactivity to INS was inversely correlated with *INS* intrathymic expression. Expression of the transcription factor autoimmune regulator *Aire* is maximal in murine medullary TECs and is absent in the thymus epithelium of diabetic NOD mice.[41,42] The use of $Aire^{-/-}$ mice helped in demonstrating that the Aire protein promotes thymic transcription of tissue-specific genes,[43] in particular genes that are known to be expressed in the thymus and to intervene in central self-tolerance such as *OT, IGF2, INS,* and *NPY.*[44] These findings are important in view of the fact that thymic expression of autoantigens correlates with a higher level of self-tolerance and resistance to autoimmune diseases.[4,45] Finally, a defect in central self-tolerance of NOD mice has been demonstrated since Fas-dependent and independent apoptosis pathways are defective in the thymus of these mice.[46]

Thus, increasingly more studies indicate that a defect in thymus central self-tolerance could be involved as a crucial factor in the development and pathophysiology of autoimmune T1DM. Through such thymus dysfunction, self-reactive T cells will continuously leave the thymus, and the peripheral T cell pool will gradually be enriched with T cells equipped with a TCR directed towards epitopes specific for the

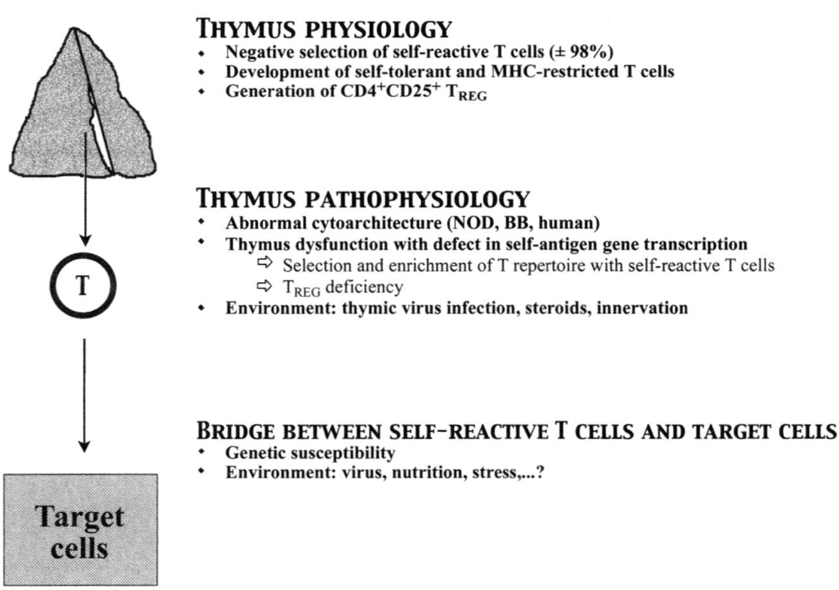

FIGURE 1. Thymus dysfunction in the pathophysiology of organ-specific autoimmune diseases. A defect in central self-tolerance results from a failure or a marked decrease in thymic transcription of genes encoding self-antigen precursors. This defect is responsible for a permanent thymic output and progressive enrichment of the peripheral T cell repertoire with self-reactive T cells. The impact of thymic self-antigens on the generation of specific T_{REG} lymphocytes is plausible but has not been demonstrated. The development of self-reactive T cells is not sufficient to induce autoimmune disease, and a molecular bridge must be established between self-reactive T cells and tissue autoantigens.

INS family. The hypothesis that thymic dysfunction could follow an infection by the diabetogenic strain B4 of coxsackie (CVB4) is currently being explored in our laboratory. From this perspective, a persistent and productive infection by CVB4 of cultured human TECs has been demonstrated.[47] The immunological effects induced by CVB4 thymus infection are currently investigated in depth. A thymus dysfunction resulting from CVB4 infection could intervene in intimate conjunction with the bystander effect evidenced by CVB4 infection of islet β cells.[48]

The presence of self-reactive lymphocytes is not a sufficient condition to develop T1DM. A bridge must be installed between self-reactive T cells and target β cell autoantigens depending on the influence of some external factors and a genetic background determined by the balance between susceptible and protective alleles (FIG. 1).

THYMUS SELF-ANTIGENS AS A WAY FOR THE DEVELOPMENT OF A NEW TYPE OF VACCINE

Increasingly more studies are documenting the highly immunogenic properties of INS, in particular the sequence INS B:9-23, which is the dominant epitope of the whole INS protein. Moreover, INS B:9-23 can be presented and has been co-crystallized with DQ8, an MHC class II allele conferring major genetic susceptibility to T1DM.[49] A cellular response to INS B:9-23 occurs in patients with T1DM. This CD4 response is MHC class II restricted and exhibits a proinflammatory profile with a high induction of IFN-γ in response to the presentation of INS B:9-23.[50] Following the "altered peptide ligand" strategy, the sequence B:9-23 of INS was modified by alanine substitutions introduced at different places. The peptide with alanine substitutions in positions 16 and 19 (NBI-6024) induced Th2 T cell responses in NBI-6024-derived T cell lines from NOD mice. Also, after administration to female NOD mice, NBI-6024 significantly delays but does not abolish the onset of autoimmune diabetes.[51] However, this strategy is based on INS B:9-23, and two recent studies have indicated that administration of INS-derived peptides to NOD mice can prime the autoimmune diabetogenic process or promote a fatal anaphylactic reaction.[52,53]

On the basis that IGF-2 is the dominant thymic peptide of the INS family and that IGF-2 is much more tolerated than INS, a novel type of vaccine could be developed for prevention and/or cure of T1DM. The immunogenic response in classic vaccination induces activated/memory T cells that are specific for antigen(s) shared by infectious agents. Analogously in T1DM, the presentation in the periphery of INS-derived autoantigen(s) activates specific CD4/CD8 T cells as well as memory T cells directed against these autoantigenic epitopes. In the novel type of tolerogenic vaccination, administration of a self-peptide derived of IGF-2 could anergize or even delete self-reactive T cells that have escaped thymus censorship because of thymic dysfunction in the establishment of β cell central self-tolerance. We are currently performing such studies with IGF-2 peptides that exhibit the same affinity and compete with INS B:9-23 for binding to DQ8. Preliminary data in DQ8+ T1DM adolescents show this hypothesis to be correct and that DQ8 presentation of INS B:9-23 and an IGF-2 derived peptide drives opposite immune responses with a dominant IL-10 response after DQ8 presentation of an IGF-2 self-antigen. Two mechanisms may be proposed to explain those findings. On the one hand, the peripheral T cell pool of

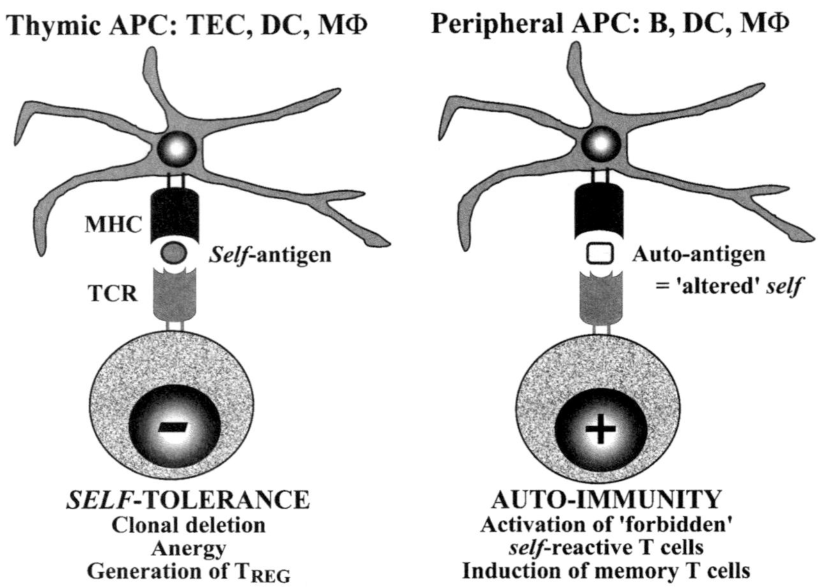

FIGURE 2. MHC presentation of self-antigen and autoantigen drives opposite immune responses. This novel concept proved to be valid for an IGF-2–derived self-antigen and the INS B:9-23 dominant immunogenic autoantigen. The tolerogenic properties of thymic self-antigens should lead to the development of a new generation of vaccines against organ-specific autoimmune diseases.

diabetic patients could contain only CD4 directed against INS-derived epitopes and the IGF-2 self-antigen would be recognized by those cells as a natural altered peptide ligand, eliciting a different response because of different transduction after binding to TCR specific for the DQ8-INS B:9-23 complex. On the other hand, the IGF-2 self-antigen could stimulate IGF-2–specific CD4+25+ T_{REG} cells. These preliminary data show that IGF-2 is a potent inducer of the secretion of IL-10, a major regulatory cytokine with potent immunosuppressive and anti-inflammatory properties.[54,55] They also document the potent tolerogenic properties of an IGF-2–derived peptide and may explain why it is so difficult to obtain antibodies to IGF-2 at high titers after active immunization with this peptide.

Most probably it is now time to distinguish an autoantigen and a self-antigen (FIG. 2). Although they are highly homologous and belong to the same family, they are not identical and this biochemical difference drives opposite immune responses (i.e., immunogenic vs tolerogenic, respectively). The powerful physiologic role of the thymus in self-tolerance induction should be further exploited to prevent and/or cure severe autoimmune diseases (such as T1DM) that constitute the tribute, paid mainly by mankind, for the complexity and efficiency of the immune system.

ACKNOWLEDGMENTS

This work was supported by Liège University, Fondation Leon Fredericq, Belgian NFSR and Belgian Federation against Cancer, Fondation Vaugrenier for Tolerance, European Association for the Study of Diabetes, European Union, and Juvenile Diabetes Research Federation. Our gratitude is due to Kai Wücherpfennig (Dana Farber Cancer Institute, Harvard University) who compared binding of INS B:9-23 and IGF-2 B:11-25 to human DQ8 MHC-II protein.

REFERENCES

1. PASCHKE, R. & V. GEENEN. 1995. Messenger RNA expression for a TSH receptor variant in the thymus of a two-year-old child. J. Mol. Med. **73:** 577–580.
2. MURAKAMI, M., Y. HOSOI, T. NEGISHI, *et al.* 1996. Thymic hyperplasia in patients with Graves' disease. Identification of thyrotropin receptors in human thymus. J. Clin. Invest. **98:** 2228–2234.
3. SMITH, K.M., D.C. OLSON, R. HIROSE & D. HANAHAN. 1997. Pancreatic gene expression in rare cells of thymic medulla: evidence for functional contribution to T cell tolerance. Intern. Immunol. **9:** 1355–1365.
4. EGWUAGU, C.E., P. CHARUKAMNOETKANOK & I. GERY. 1997. Thymic expression of autoantigens correlates with resistance to autoimmune disease. J. Immunol. **159:** 3109–3112.
5. FARR, A.G. & A. RUDENSKY. 1998. Medullary thymic epithelium: a mosaic of epithelial "self"? J. Exp. Med. **188:** 1–4.
6. HEATH, V.L., N.N. MOORE, S.M. PARNELL & D.W. MASON. 1998. Intrathymic expression of genes involved in organ specific autoimmune diseases. J. Autoimmunol. **11:** 309–318.
7. WERDELIN, O., U. CORDES & T. JENSEN. 1998. Aberrant expression of tissue specific proteins in the thymus: a hypothesis for the development of central tolerance. Scand. J. Immunol. **47:** 95–100.
8. SALMON, A.M., C. BRUAND, A. CARDONA, *et al.* 1998. An acetylcholine receptor alpha subunit promoter confers intrathymic expression in transgenic mice. Implications for tolerance of a transgenic self-antigen and autoreactivity in myasthenia gravis. J. Clin. Invest. **101:** 2340–2350.
9. SOSPEDRA, M., X. FERRER-FRANCESCH, O. DOMINGUEZ, *et al.* 1999. Transcription of a broad-range of self-antigens in human thymus suggests a role for central mechanisms in tolerance toward peripheral antigens. J. Immunol. **161:** 5918–5929.
10. KLEIN, L., M. KLUGMANN, K.-A. NAVE, *et al.* 2000. Shaping of the autoreactive T-cell repertoire by a splice variant of self protein expressed in thymic epithelial cells. Nat. Med. **6:** 56–61.
11. KYEWSKI, B., J. DERBINSKI, J. GOTTER & L. KLEIN. 2002. Promiscuous gene expression and central T-cell tolerance: more than meets the eye. Trends Immunol. **23:** 364–371.
12. GEENEN, V., J.J. LEGROS, P. FRANCHIMONT, *et al.* 1986. The neuroendocrine thymus: coexistence of oxytocin and neurophysin in the human thymus. Science **232:** 508–511.
13. ROBERT, F.R., H. MARTENS, N. CORMANN, *et al.* 1992. The recognition of hypothalamo-neurohypophysial functions by developing T cells. Dev. Immunol. **2:** 131–140.
14. MARTENS, H., B. MAGRANGE, F. ROBERT, *et al.* 1996. Cytokine production by human thymic epithelial cells: control by the immune recognition of the neurohypophysial self-antigen. Regul. Pept. **67:** 39–45.
15. GEENEN, V., E. VANDERSMISSEN, N. CORMANN-GOFFIN, *et al.* 1993. Membrane translocation and relationship with MHC class I of a human thymic neurophysin-like protein. Thymus **22:** 55–66.
16. NORTH, W.G. 2000. Gene regulation of vasopressin and vasopressin receptors in cancer. Exp. Physiol. **85:** 27s–40s.

17. SUNDLER, F., R.E. CARRAWAY, R. HAKANSON, *et al.* 1978. Immunoreactive neurotensin and somatostatin in the chicken thymus. Cell Tiss. Res. **194:** 367–376.
18. VANNESTE, Y., A. NTODOU THOME, E. VANDERSMISSEN, *et al.* 1997. Identification of neurotensin-related peptides in human thymic epithelial cell membranes and relationship with major histocompatibility complex class I molecules. J. Neuroimmunol. **76:** 161–166.
19. HANSENNE, I., G. RASIER, M.P. DEFRESNE, *et al.* 2003. Neurohypophysial receptor gene expression by thymic T cell subsets and thymic T cell lymphoma cell lines. Dev. Immunol. In press.
20. MARTENS, H., F. ROBERT, J.J. LEGROS, *et al.* 1992. Expression of functional neurohypophysial peptide receptors by immature and cytotoxic T cell lines. Prog. NeuroEndocrinImmunol. **5:** 31–39.
21. MARTENS, H., O. KECHA, C. CHARLET-RENARD, *et al.* 1998. Neurohypophysial peptides stimulate the phosphorylation of pre-T cell focal adhesion kinases. Neuroendocrinology **67:** 282–289.
22. MARTENS, H., B. GOXE & V. GEENEN. 1996. The thymic repertoire of neuroendocrine-related self-antigens: physiological implications in T-cell life and death. Immunol. Today **17:** 312–317.
23. GEENEN, V., F. BRILOT, I. HANSENNE, *et al.* 2003. Thymus and T cells. *In* Encyclopedia of Neuroscience, 3rd Ed. G. Adelman & B.H. Smith, Eds. Elsevier. New York. In press.
24. GEENEN, V., I. ACHOUR, F. ROBERT, *et al.* 1993. Evidence that insulin-like growth factor-2 (IGF-2) is the dominant thymic peptide of the insulin superfamily. Thymus **21:** 115–127.
25. KECHA, O., H. MARTENS, N. FRANCHIMONT, *et al.* Characterization of the insulin-like growth factor axis in the human thymus. J. Neuroendocrinol. **11:** 435–440.
26. KECHA, O., F. BRILOT, H. MARTENS, *et al.* 2000. Involvement of insulin-like growth factors in early T cell development: a study using fetal thymic organ cultures. Endocrinology **141:** 1209–1217.
27. JOLICŒUR, C., D. HANAHAN & K.M. SMITH. 1994. T-cell tolerance toward a transgenic beta-cell antigen and transcription of endogenous pancreatic genes in the thymus. Proc. Natl. Acad. Sci. USA **91:** 6707–6711.
28. DERBINSKI, J., A. SCHULTE, B. KYEWSKI & L. KLEIN. 2001. Promiscuous gene expression in medullary thymic epithelial cells mirrors the peripheral self. Nat. Immunol. **2:** 1032–1039.
29. PUGLIESE, A., D. BROWN, D. GARZA, *et al.* 2001. Self-antigen-presenting cells expressing diabetes-associated autoantigens exist in both thymus and peripheral lymphoid organs. J. Clin. Invest. **107:** 555–564.
30. VAFIADIS, P., S.T. BENNETT, J.A. TODD, *et al.* 1997. Insulin expression is modulated by *INS* VNTR alleles at the *IDDM2* locus. Nat. Genet. **15:** 289–292.
31. PUGLIESE, A., M. ZELLER, A. FERNANDEZ, JR., *et al.* 1997. The insulin gene is transcribed in the human thymus and transcription levels correlate with allelic variation at the *INS* VNTR-*IDDM2* susceptibility locus for type 1 diabetes. Nat. Genet. **15:** 293–297.
32. ADORINI, L., E. APPELLA, G. DORIA & Z.A. NAGY. 1988. Mechanisms influencing the immunodominance of T cell determinants. J. Exp. Med. **168:** 2091–2104.
33. CABANIOLS, J.P., R. CIBOTTI, P. KOURILSKY, *et al.* 1994. Dose-dependent T cell tolerance to an immunodominant self-peptide. Eur. J. Immunol. **24:** 1743–1749.
34. NAQUET, P., J. ELLIS, D. TIBENSKY, *et al.* 1988. T cell autoreactivity to insulin in diabetic and related non-diabetic individuals. J. Immunol. **140:** 2569–2578.
35. CHAILLOUS, L., H. LEFEVRE, C. THIVOLET, *et al.* 2000. Oral insulin administration and residual beta-cell function in recent-onset type 1 diabetes: a multicentre randomised controlled trial. Lancet **356:** 545–549.
36. POZZILLI, P., D. PITOCCO, N. VISALLI, *et al.* 2000. No effect of oral insulin on residual beta-cell function in recent-onset type 1 diabetes (the IMDIAB VII). Diabetologia **43:** 1000–1004.
37. DIABETES PREVENTION TRIAL-TYPE 1 DIABETES STUDY GROUP. 2002. Effects of insulin in relatives of patients with type 1 diabetes mellitus. N. Engl. J. Med. **346:** 1685–1691.

38. KECHA-KAMOUN, O., I. ACHOUR, H. MARTENS, *et al.* 2001. Thymic expression of insulin-related genes in an animal model of autoimmune type 1 diabetes. Diabetes/Metab. Res. Rev. **17:** 146–152.
39. TODD, J.A. 1995 Genetic analysis of type 1 diabetes using whole genome approaches. Proc. Natl. Acad. Sci. USA **92:** 8560–8565.
40. CHENTOUFI, A.A. & C. POLYCHRONAKOS. 2002. Insulin expression levels in the thymus modulate insulin-specific autoreactive T-cell tolerance. The mechanism by which the IDDM2 locus may predispose to diabetes. Diabetes **51:** 1383–1390.
41. HEINO, M., P. PETERSON, N. SILLANPAA, *et al.* 2000. RNA and protein expression of the murine autoimmune regulator gene (Aire) in normal, RelB deficient and in NOD mice. Eur. J. Immunol. **30:** 1884–1893.
42. ZUKLYS, S., G. BALCIUNAITE, A. AGARWAL, *et al.* 2000. Normal thymic architecture and negative selection are associated with Aire expression, the gene defective in the autoimmune-polyendocrinopathy-candidiasis-ectodermal dystrophy (APECED). J. Immunol. **165:** 1976–1983.
43. ANDERSON, M.S., E.S. VENANZI, L. KLEIN, *et al.* 2002. Projection of an immunological self-shadow within the thymus by the Aire protein. Science **298:** 1395–1401.
44. ERICSSON, A., V. GEENEN, F. ROBERT, *et al.* 1990. Expression of preprotachykinin A and neuropeptide Y mRNA in the thymus. Mol. Endocrinol. **4:** 1211–1218.
45. SEBZDA, E., V.A. WALLACE, J. MAYER, *et al.* 1994. Positive and negative thymocyte selection induced by different concentrations of a single peptide. Science **263:** 1615–1618.
46. KISHIMOTO, H. & J. SPRENT. A defect in central tolerance in NOD mice. Nat. Immunol. **2:** 1025–1031.
47. BRILOT, F., W. CHEHADEH, C. CHARLET-RENARD, *et al.* 2002. Persistent infection of human thymic epithelial cells by coxsackievirus B4. J. Virol. **76:** 5260–5265.
48. HORWITZ, M.S. & N. SARVETNICK. 1999. Viruses, host responses and autoimmunity. Immunol. Rev. **169:** 241–253.
49. LEE, K.H., K. WUCHERPFENNIG & D.C. WILEY. 2001. Structure of a human insulin peptide-HLA-DQ8 complex and susceptibility to type 1 diabetes. Nat. Immunol. **2:** 501–507.
50. ALLEVA, D.G., P.D. CROWE, L. JIN, *et al.* 2001. A disease-associated cellular immune response in type 1 diabetics to an immunodominant epitope of insulin. J. Clin. Invest. **107:** 173–180.
51. ALLEVA, D.G., A. GAUR, L. JIN, *et al.* 2002. Immunological characterization and therapeutic activity of an altered-peptide ligand, NBI-6024, based on the immunodominant type 1 diabetes autoantigen insulin B-chain (9-23) peptide. Diabetes **51:** 2126–2134.
52. LIU, E., H. MORIYAMA, N. ABIRU, *et al.* 2002. Anti-peptide autoantibodies and fatal anaphylaxis in NOD mice in response to insulin self-peptides B:9-23 and B:13-33. J. Clin. Invest. **110:** 1021–1027.
53. KARGES, W., K. PECHHOLD, S. AL DAHOUK, *et al.* 2002. Induction of autoimmune diabetes through insulin (but not GAD65) vaccination in non obese diabetic and in RIP-37.1 mice. Diabetes **51:** 3237–3244.
54. COOKE, A., J.M. PHILLIPS & N.M. PARISH. 2001. Tolerogenic strategies to halt or prevent type 1 diabetes. Nat. Immunol. **2:** 810–815.
55. YANG, Z., M. CHEN, R. WU, *et al.* 2002. Suppression of autoimmune diabetes by viral IL-10 gene transfer. J. Immunol. **168:** 6479–6485.

Integrating Systemic Information at the Molecular Level

Cross-Talk between Steroid Receptors and Cytokine Signaling on Different Target Cells

DAMIÁN REFOJO,[a,b] ANA C. LIBERMAN,[a,b] DAMIANA GIACOMINI,[a] ALBERTO CARBIA NAGASHIMA,[a,b] MARIANA GRACIARENA,[a] CARLOS ECHENIQUE,[a] MARCELO PAEZ PEREDA,[c] GÜNTER STALLA,[c] FLORIAN HOLSBOER,[c] AND EDUARDO ARZT[a,b]

[a]*Laboratorio de Fisiología y Biología Molecular, Departamento de Fisiología y Biología Molecular y Celular, Facultad de Ciencias Exactas y Naturales (FCEN), Universidad de Buenos Aires, Ciudad Universitaria, Pabellón II, C1428EHA, Buenos Aires, Argentina*

[b]*Members of the Argentine National Research Council (CONICET)*

[c]*Max-Planck Institute of Psychiatry, 80804 Munich, Germany*

ABSTRACT: An essential event in immune activation is the increase of cytokines in both plasma and immune tissues. Steroid hormones influence several adaptive responses in both health and disease. Cytokines and steroids have an intimate cross-communication in many systems, making possible a satisfactory adaptive response to environmental changes. The ultimate level of integration of the cytokine-steroids cross-talk is the molecular level. We have demonstrated this in four types of cross-talk mechanisms on different cells in which steroids have major roles: (1) The tumor necrosis factor (TNF)-glucocorticoid receptor (GR) transcriptional interaction in cellular targets of TNF-induced cytotoxicity. TNF potentiates the transactivation activity of GR and the priming with TNF increases the protective action of GR on TNF-induced cytotoxicity. (2) The GR-T cell receptor (TCR) antagonism in GR-TCR–induced T cell apoptosis and its modulation by cAMP. cAMP inhibits the TCR-induced apoptosis through a PKA-CREB–dependent mechanism and potentiates glucocorticoid-induced apoptosis by means of a CREB-independent mechanism. (3) The GR influence on Th1-Th2 cytokine expression and differentiation. Glucocorticoids inhibit the induction of GATA-3 and T-bet transcription factors. (4) The influence of ER/Smad-4 signaling cross-communication on prolactinoma pathogenesis. Physical and functional interactions between Smad-4 and estrogen receptors take place in prolactinoma cells, providing a molecular explanation to link the tumorigenic action of these two important players of prolactinoma pathogenesis. The molecular cross-talk between steroids and transcription factors is the mechanism that provides the basis for the outcome of adaptive responses integrating the systemic information provided by hormones and cytokines.

Address for correspondence: Dr Eduardo Arzt, Lab Fisiología y Biología Molecular, FCEN-Universidad de Buenos Aires, Ciudad Universitaria, Pabellón II (C1428EHA), Buenos Aires, Argentina. Voice: 54-11-4576-3368; fax: 54-11-4576-3321.
earzt@fbmc.fcen.uba.ar.

Ann. N.Y. Acad. Sci. 922: 196–204 (2003).

KEYWORDS: **glucocorticoid; tumor necrosis factor (TNF); cAMP; T cell receptor (TCR); apoptosis; GATA-3; T-bet; Th1-Th2 differentiation; BMP-4; prolactinoma; estrogen**

INTRODUCTION

When environmental changes such as infectious states occur, organisms need to develop an adequate adaptive biological response. Through cytokines, cells receive information about the quality and magnitude of the aggression. Meanwhile, hormones give information about the changes suffered by different systems as a result of the environmental alterations. Thus, cytokines and hormones act as messengers that send systemic information at all cellular effectors. The final outcome of an adaptive response will depend on the satisfactory integration of this information at the intracellular level, which occurs through a molecular cross-talk between cytokines and steroid receptor signaling.

A key event in the activation of the immune response is the synthesis and release of several cytokines that play different regulatory and effector functions on both innate or adaptive immunity and other nonimmune systems. In the classic concept, cytokines are proteins secreted by the cells of innate and adaptive immunity in response to microbes and others antigens. However, in recent years it was observed that cytokines can also be produced by nonimmune cells.[1,2] As a consequence of the elevation of cytokine levels, the homeostatic balance becomes in a new metabolic and hormone state that facilitates some features of the immune reaction at the same time that limits others.[3] Steroid hormones influence several metabolic, reproductive, immune, and neuroendocrine responses in both health and disease. Glucocorticoids (GC), specially, inhibit both cytokine gene expression and their pleiotropic action on target cells, acting as an immunosuppressive and anti-inflammatory agent that contains overreactions of the immune system.[3–5] As glucocorticoids, estrogens also play several roles not only on the reproductive system but also on other systems.

Cytokines and steroid hormones exert a direct and cross influence on many different cell types, allowing the regulation of both acute and chronic adaptive responses to environmental modifications. These actions and interactions take place in immune cells with different developmental stages, such as thymocytes, mature T and B cells, differentiated Th1-Th2 cells, macrophages, and others, and nonimmune cells such as fibroblasts, neurons, and pituitary cells.[2,4]

In some conditions, the regulatory loop whereby signals triggered by cytokines cross talk with steroid receptors may result in enhancement of the transcriptional activity of the nuclear hormone receptors. In other situations, stimulation of the immune system dampens steroid, especially glucocorticoid, response element-regulated genes.[5,6] Similarly, the interaction of glucocorticoid receptors (GRs) with different transcription factors activated by cytokine/T cell receptor (TCR) stimulation modifies the transcriptional rates of genes driven by cytokines.[5,6] Thus, the functional cross-talk at the molecular level between immune signals and steroid receptors is essential for the cell to develop an adequate final biological response to both mediators and constitutes the ultimate level of interaction between the immune and the neuroendocrine signals.

In this chapter, we show how these interactions play a key role in four distinct models where immune activators (cytokines or TCR activating antibodies) and steroids co-signalize: (1) The GR-induced inhibition of the tumor necrosis factor (TNF)-induced cytotoxicity and the influence of TNF priming on GR transactivation-mediated survival on fibroblastic cell lines; (2) the mutual inhibition of GR and TCR-induced T cell apoptosis and their dual modulation by cAMP; (3) the GR influence on Th1-Th2 cytokine expression and differentiation; and (4) the influence of ER/BMP-4 signaling cross-communication in the prolactinoma pathogenesis.

TNF-GR TRANSCRIPTIONAL INTERACTION IN CELLULAR TARGETS OF TNF-INDUCED CYTOTOXICITY

Inflammatory cytokines such as TNF and interleukin-1 (IL-1) potentiate the transcriptional activation induced by glucocorticoids. In L-929 fibroblasts transiently transfected with glucocorticoid response elements (GRE)-CAT reporter plasmid, treatment with low doses of TNF-α potentiates the transcriptional activation induced by dexamethasone, an effect dependent on GR as it is completely blocked by GR antagonist RU 38486. Although TNF-α treatment augments the GR number 12 hours after administration, TNF-α increases the DEX-induced binding of GR to the GRE in gel shift assays, at time points at which an increase in GR number is most probably negligible (e.g., 15 minutes).[7] In addition, in GR-deficient cell lines transiently cotransfected with GRE-CAT reporter and GR expression vector driven by TNF-insensible promoters, TNF-α induces the same potentiation of GR-mediated transcriptional activation that is exerted on endogenous GR. The inflammatory cytokine enhancement occurs on different cell types as such fibroblastic, neuroblastoma, glioblastoma, and corticotropic cells, indicating that the aforedescribed interaction is a general molecular mechanism.

Dexamethasone-mediated activation of GR inhibits TNF-α–induced apoptosis. In addition, priming with TNF-α increases the efficacy of glucocorticoids to inhibit TNF-α–induced cytotoxicity showing the biological relevance of TNF-α-GR molecular interaction.[7]

TNF-R1 is the main receptor on most cell types and initiates most TNF biological activities. After ligand binding, the intracellular domain of TNF-R1 is recognized by TRADD, which reclutes the additional adapters, Fas-associated death domain (FADD), receptor-interacting protein (RIP), and TNF-R–associated death domain (TRAF2).[8] TNF-R1–induced apoptosis requires FADD, and stimulation of gene expression mainly occurs through TRAF2-dependent pathways.[9] FADD activates caspases and apoptosis, and TRAF2 activates NF-κB and AP-1 transcription factors. As GR, NF-κB also has a protective action on apoptosis triggered by TNF. Both pharmacological inhibitors and overexpression of IκB superrepressor protein (ssIκB) allow apoptosis at low nonapoptotic-inducing doses of TNF and potentiate cytotoxicity of high apoptotic doses of the cytokine. Moreover, glucocorticoid protection of TNF-induced cytotoxicity occurs at the same ratio at either normal (cells transfected with empty vector) or low (cells transfected with ssIκB) induction levels of NF-κB, suggesting that although GR and NF-κB mutually antagonize, both trigger surviving signals in L-929 cells.[10] This is an interesting case in which GR supports an anti-TNF action, independently of NF-κB protective activity, which is exerted by GR itself.

GR/TCR ANTAGONISM IN GR/TCR-INDUCED T CELL APOPTOSIS AND ITS MODULATION BY CAMP-INDUCING SIGNALS

Cross-talk between steroids and immune receptors also takes place in the regulation of lymphocyte and T cell hybridoma apoptosis, where both glucocorticoids and TCR signals induce cytotoxicity, but simultaneous stimulation results in cell survival.[11,12] The TCR-induced death pathway, which can be mimicked by anti-CD3 treatment, involved FasL induction that interacts with its receptor Fas, which, in turn, activates caspase 8.[13] By contrast, GR-dependent transcription of unknown genes promotes caspase 9 activation and apoptosis.[14]

NF-κB activation pathways have been described that mediate FasL induction and the proapoptotic effects of TCR activation.[15] To study GR/TCR cross-talk, T cells were transfected with reporter plasmid where luciferase expression is under transcriptional control of GRE and κB binding sites. Thus, glucocorticoid-induced GR activation inhibited TCR-induced κB-Luc reporter activity.[16] This suggests that GR can promote protection most probably through NF-κB interference. In the TCR reciprocal pathway, dexamethasone-induced GRE-Luc activity is strongly blocked by anti-CD3 treatment, suggesting that TCR inhibition of glucocorticoid–induced apoptosis involves the inhibition of GRE-regulated genes.[16]

cAMP-mediated signals also have a role in different lymphocyte functions, but their involvement in T cell death is not completely understood. Interestingly, cAMP can enhance GR-induced and inhibit TCR-mediated apoptosis on the same T cell.[16] The TCR-induced apoptosis inhibition of cAMP is reverted by pharmacological inhibitors of protein kinase A (PKA) as H89, showing PKA mediation of this effect. This pathway can activate cAMP response element binding protein (CREB)-mediated transcription because cAMP activates cAMP response element (CRE)-driven transcription and Gal4-CREB-luciferase constructs. In addition, in electrophoretic mobility shift assays of cAMP-treated cells, bands corresponding to CRE-binding factors are supershifted by anti-CREB specific antibodies. To test the involvement of CRE-driven transcription in cAMP modulation of apoptosis, we carried out experiments in which T cells were transfected with a CRE decoy DNA oligomer and treated with anti-CD3, dexamethasone, and cAMP. The titration of CRE-binding factors with the DNA oligomer blocked the protection of TCR-induced apoptosis, whereas it did not modify the potentiation of GC-induced apoptosis.[16] These results suggest that cAMP inhibits TCR-mediated apoptosis through a PKA-CREB–dependent mechanism, whereas a CREB-independent pathway exerts the enhancement by cAMP on GG-mediated cell death.

GR INFLUENCE ON TH1-TH2 CYTOKINE EXPRESSION AND DIFFERENTIATION

The existence of at least two T helper (Th) 1 and Th2 subsets, their roles in the immune response, as well as new concepts about their ontogeny were reviewed in detail in past years.[17,18] After TCR activation, naive helper T cells secrete IL-2, enter the cycle, and proliferate. Progeny begin to differentiate and become capable of producing both the Th1 cytokines interferon-γ (IFN-γ) and IL-2 involved mainly in the cell-mediated immune response or the Th2 cytokines such as IL-4, IL-5, and IL-13 that mediate predominantly humoral and eosinophilic responses. IL-12 and IL-4 are the strongest inducers of Th1 and Th2 differentiation, respectively. Moreover, mutual inhibitory regulation occurs between Th1 and Th2 cytokines that avoids the simultaneous activation of these two types of host defense. Thus, IFN-γ and IL-12 decrease Th2 cytokine production and IL-4, IL-10, and IL-13 inhibit the Th1 response.[17,18]

The transcription factor GATA-3 is probably the master driver of Th2 differentiation.[19] This factor can induce a Th2 commitment, even under Th1 differentiation conditions, and can remodel the chromatin within the IL-4 locus independently of IL-4/Stat6 activation pathway.[18,19] With regard to Th1 differentiation, the transcription factor T-bet emerges as the master regulator of the Th1 response. Indeed, ectopic expression of T-bet in cells growing under Th2 polarizing conditions promotes Th1 differentiation.[20] T-bet also regulates chromatin changes at the IFN-γ locus and induces IL-12Rβ2 independently of IL-12/Stat4.[21]

Even though the glucocorticoid influence on Th1 and Th2 cytokine production has been described, nothing is known about the possible interactions between GR and Th1-Th2 transcription factors.

Expression of IL-4 and IFN-γ mRNAs is detected early in TCR activation in a mechanism independent of Stat4- and Stat6-mediated signals. In the same way, both GATA-3 and T-bet are expressed after cell activation in the absence of either IL-4 or IL-12.[21] Taking this into account and considering that, as was postulated, IL-4/IL-12-independent expression of GATA-3/T-bet in naive or slightly differentiated T cells could have a major selective influence in Th1-Th2 subsequent fate, we carried out experiments under undifferentiated conditions to establish the possible interference of glucocorticoid on GATA-3 and T-bet expression. We found that splenocytes activated with T cell mitogens such as concanavalin-A (Con-A) show strong expression of both GATA-3 and T-bet transcripts. Interestingly, T-bet mRNA expression is strongly inhibited by dexamethasone and reverted by IL-12, whereas GATA-3 mRNA levels are also inhibited, but less so, by dexamethasone and reverted by IL-4 exposure. The reversion of these effects by cytokines suggests that glucocorticoids could be acting indirectly through inhibition of cytokines. Although in acute treatment GC also inhibits IL-4 and IL-5 cytokine synthesis and expression,[12] in more long-term experimental designs GC exposure early in the activation phase shifts the cell phenotype towards the Th2 subset.[22] If we consider the influence that Th1-Th2 mutual inhibitory regulation would have on subsequent differentiation, the greater sensibility to GC inhibition of T-bet with respect to GATA-3 could explain the apparent Th2 facilitation exerted by GC.

INFLUENCE OF ER-BMP-4/SMAD-4 SIGNALING CROSS-COMMUNICATION IN PROLACTINOMA PATHOGENESIS

Hyperprolactinemia is the most frequent hypothalamic-pituitary alteration in clinical endocrinology, and prolactinomas are their more common cause. Estrogens as well as growth factors play a role in lactotroph cell proliferation, and experimental and clinical evidence demonstrates the tumorigenic property of estrogens in prolactinomas. Thus, the increase in adenoma size during pregnancy or estrogen administration is positively related to estrogen receptor (ER) expression.[23,24] Epidemiologic

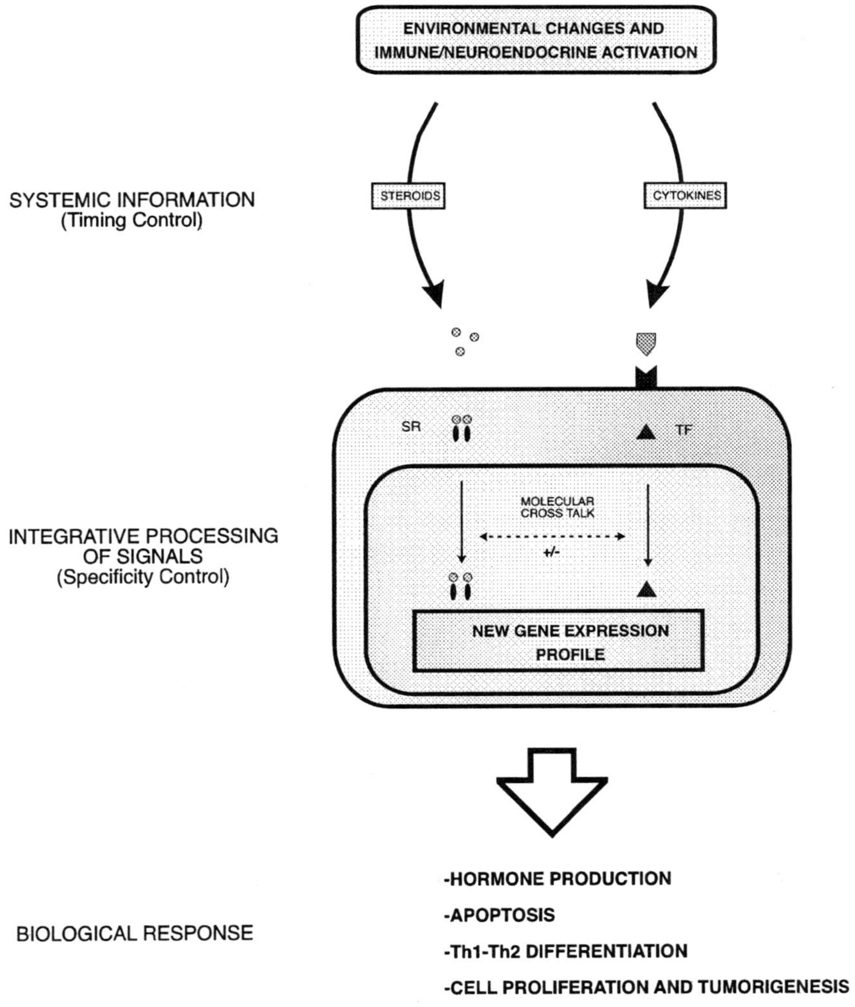

FIGURE 1. After environmental changes, such as infectious disease, cytokines are released by immune and nonimmune cells to favor an adaptive response. Hormones secreted by the neuroendocrine system give information about the changes that different organs undergo. To reach a biological response outcome, the neuroendocrine-immune system employs a systemic and an intracellular pathway. Hormones and cytokines act as the messengers of systemic information. The final intracellular processing of this information requires a molecular cross-talk between steroid receptors and transcription factors and promotes a specific biological response. TF, transcription factors; SR, steroid receptors.

study of these tumors shows that they are more frequent in women. In addition, dominant negative ER diminishes lactotroph cell growth in nude mice.[25]

Apart from hormones, pituitary cells can synthesize and release cytokines and growth factors. This capability constitutes the basis for the autoparacrine actions of cytokines in the control of pituitary hormone production and cell proliferation.[2]

Although transforming growth factor-β (TGF-β) exerts inhibitory actions on cell proliferation of lactosomatotropic cell lines,[26] bone morphogenetic protein-4 (BMP-4, a member of the TGF-β superfamily) has a stimulatory activity on cell growth both *in vitro* and *in vivo*. BMP-4 transduces signals through smad-4 protein, a signal cotransducer. In addition, either estradiol or BMP-4 enhanced cell proliferation, and additive effects are observed when both ligands are combined. Interestingly, treatment with antiestrogens blocks BMP-4–induced cell proliferation, whereas Smad-4 dominant negative expression inhibits estradiol effects, confirming that BMP-4 and estradiol act through overlapping signaling mechanisms.[27] Furthermore, ER coimmunoprecipitates with smad-4, showing that a physical interaction between Smad-4 and estrogen receptors takes place, constituting the demonstration of a ER-BMP-4/Smad-4 cross-talk relevant in a physiologic model.

GENERAL CONCLUSIONS

An adaptive cellular response is the consequence of context-dependent–integrative processing of signals triggered by cytokines, steroids, and other hormones, which results in a new gene activation/repression profile. This complex context depends on a cytokine-hormone milieu that provides systemic information to the cell. As shown in FIGURE 1 the neuroendocrine-immune response is composed by two branches, one systemic and the other intracellular, that allow integration of systemic information at the cellular level and generation of a time- and cell-specific pattern of response. The systemic pathway works as the messenger of the environmental changes and governs the temporal side of the response. The intracellular pathway, which is activated by the first and transduces its information, determines the tissue-specific side of the immunoendocrine processes. Molecular cross-talk is the mechanism that sustains integrative processing of systemic information at the intracellular level and therefore the variability and tissue specificity of responses as varied as TNF-induced cytotoxicity on fibroblasts, TCR-induced apoptosis on T cells, Th1-Th2 differentiation, and cytokine expression profiles, prolactinoma pathogenesis, and others.

A thorough advance in the knowledge of these molecular interactions will permit better understanding of not only the physiology but also the pathophysiology of steroid/cytokine cross-talk on different targets.

ACKNOWLEDGMENT

This work was supported by grants from the Volkswagen Foundation (I776 803), the Argentine Health Ministry (Beca Carillo-Oñativia), the Argentine National Research Council (CONICET), and the National Agency of Scientific and Technology Promotion (ANPCyT).

REFERENCES

1. SCHÖBITZ, B., E.R. DE KLOET & F. HOLSBOER. 1994. Gene expression and function of interleukin 1, interlukin 6 and tumor necrosis factor in the brain. Prog. Neurobiol. **44:** 397–432.
2. ARZT, E., M.P. PAEZ PEREDA, C. PEREZ CASTRO, *et al.* 1999. Pathophysiological role of the cytokine network in the anterior pituitary gland. Front. Neuroendocrinol. **20:** 71–95.
3. BESEDOVSKY, H.O. & A. DEL REY. 1996. Immune-neuro-endocrine interactions: facts and hypotheses. Endocr. Rev. **17:** 64–102.
4. MCEWEN, B., C. BIRON, K.W. BRUNSON, *et al.* 1997. The role of adrenocorticoids as modulators of immune function in health and disease: neural, endocrine and immune interactions. Brain Res. Rev. **23:** 79–133.
5. MCKAY, L.I. & J.A. CIDLOWSKI. 1999. Molecular control of immune/inflammatory responses: interactions between nuclear factor-kappa B and steroid receptor-signaling pathways. Endocr. Rev. **20:** 435–459.
6. REFOJO, D., A.C. LIBERMAN, F. HOLSBOER, *et al.* 2001. Transcription factor-mediated molecular mechanisms involved in the functional cross-talk between cytokines and glucocorticoids. Immunol. Cell. Biol. **79:** 385–394.
7. COSTAS, M., T. TRAPP, M. PAEZ PEREDA, *et al.* 1996. Molecular and functional evidence for *in vitro* cytokine enhancement of human and murine target cell sensitivity to glucocorticoids: TNF-α priming increases glucocorticoid inhibition of TNF-α-induced cytotoxicity/apoptosis. J. Clin. Invest. **98:** 1409–1416.
8. CHEN, G. & D.V. GOEDDEL. 2002. TNF-R1 signaling: a beautiful pathway. Science **296:** 1634–1635.
9. HSU, H., H.B. SHU, M.G. PAN, *et al.* 1996. TRADD-TRAF2 and TRADD-FADD interactions define two distinct TNF receptor 1 signal transduction pathways. Cell **84:** 299–308.
10. COSTAS, M.A., L. MULLER IGAZ, F. HOLSBOER, *et al.* 2000. Transrepression of NF-kappaB is not required for glucocorticoid-mediated protection of TNF-alpha-induced apoptosis on fibroblasts. Biochim. Biophys. Acta **1499:** 122–129.
11. ZACHARCHUK, C.M., M. MERCEP, P. CHAKRABORTI, *et al.* 1990. Programmed T lymphocyte death: cell activation and steroid-induced pathways are mutually antagonistic. J. Immunol. **145:** 4037–4045.
12. ASHWELL, J.D., F.W.M. LU & M.S. VACCHIO. 2000. Glucocorticoids in T-cell development and function. Ann. Rev. Immunol. **18:** 309–345.
13. KRAMMER, P.H. 2000. CD95's deadly mission in the immune system. Nature **407:** 789–795.
14. HAKEM, R., A. HAKEM, G.S. DUNCAN, *et al.* 1998. Differential requirement for caspase 9 in apoptotic pathways *in vivo*. Cell **94:** 339–352.
15. KASIBHATLA, S., L. GENESTIER & D.R. GREEN. 1999. Regulation of fas-ligand expression during activation-induced cell death in T lymphocytes via nuclear factor kappaB. J. Biol. Chem. **274:** 987–992.
16. MÜLLER-IGAZ, L., D. REFOJO, M. COSTAS, *et al.* 2002. CRE-mediated transcriptional activation is involved in cAMP protection of T-cell receptor-induced apoptosis but not in cAMP potentiation of glucocorticoid-mediated programmed cell death. Biochim. Biophys. Acta **1542:** 139–148.
17. GLIMCHER, L.H. & K.M. MURPHY. 2000. Lineage commitment in the immune system: the T helper lymphocyte grows up. Genes Dev. **14:** 1693–1711.
18. REINER, S.L. 2001. Helper T cell differetiation, inside and out. Curr. Opin. Immunol. **13:** 351–355.
19. ZHENG, W. & R.A. FLAVELL. 1997. The transcription factor GATA-3 is necessary and sufficient for Th2 cytokine gene expression in CD4 T cells. Cell **89:** 587–596.
20. SZABO, S.J., S.T. KIM, G.L. COSTA, *et al.* 2000. A novel transcription factor, T-bet, direct Th1 lineage commitment. Cell **100:** 655–669.
21. GROGAN, J.L. & R.M. LOCKSLEY. 2002. T helper cell differentiation: on again, off again. Curr. Opin. Immunol. **14:** 366–372.
22. RAMIREZ, F., D.J. FOWELL, M. PUKLAVEC, *et al.* 1996. Glucocorticoids promote a Th2 cytokine response by CD4 T cells *in vitro*. J. Immunol. **156:** 2406–2412.

23. GARCIA, M.M. & L.P. KAPCALA. 1995. Growth of a microprolactinoma to a macroprolactinoma during estrogen therapy. J. Endocrinol. Invest. **18:** 450–455.
24. STEFANEANU, L., K. KOVACS, E. HORVATH, *et al.* 1994. In situ hybridization study of estrogen receptor messenger ribonucleic acid in human adenohypophysial cells and pituitary adenomas. J. Clin. Endocrinol. Metab. **78:** 83–88.
25. LEE, E.J., W.R. DUAN, M. JAKACKA, *et al.* 2001. Dominant negative ER induces apoptosis in GH(4) pituitary lactotrope cells and inhibits tumor growth in nude mice. Endocrinology **142:** 3756–3763.
26. RAMSDELL, J.S. 1991. Transforming growth factor-alpha and -beta are potent and effective inhibitors of GH4 pituitary tumor cell proliferation. Endocrinology **128:** 1981–1990.
27. PAEZ PEREDA, M., D. GIACOMINI, D. REFOJO, *et al.* 2003. Involvement of bone morphogenetic protein Y (BMP-Y) in pituitary prolactinoma pathogenesis through a SMAD/ estrogen receptor crosstalk. Proc. Natl. Acad. Sci. USA **100:** 1034–1039.

Stress, Leukocyte Trafficking, and the Augmentation of Skin Immune Function

FIRDAUS S. DHABHAR

College of Dentistry & College of Medicine, The Ohio State University, Columbus, Ohio 43210, USA

ABSTRACT: Delayed type hypersensitivity (DTH) reactions represent cell-mediated immune responses that exert important immunoprotective (resistance to viruses, bacteria, and fungi) or immunopathologic (allergic or autoimmune hypersensitivity) effects. We have used the skin DTH response as an *in vivo* model to study neuro-endocrine-immune interactions. We hypothesized that just as an acute stress response prepares the cardiovascular and musculoskeletal systems for fight or flight, it may also prepare the immune system for challenges (e.g., wounding) that may be imposed by a stressor (e.g., an aggressor). Studies showed that acute (2 hours) stress experienced before primary or secondary cutaneous antigen exposure induces significantly enhanced skin DTH. This enhancement involves innate as well as adaptive immune mechanisms. Adrenalectomy eliminates the stress-induced enhancement of DTH. Acute administration of physiological concentrations of corticosterone and/or epinephrine to adrenalectomized animals enhances skin DTH. Compared with those in controls, DTH sites from acutely stressed or hormone-injected animals show significantly greater erythema and induration, numbers of infiltrating leukocytes, and levels of cytokine gene expression. In contrast to acute stress, chronic stress is immunosuppressive. Chronic exposure to corticosterone or acute exposure to dexamethasone significantly suppresses skin DTH. These results suggest that during acute stress, endogenous stress hormones enhance skin immunity by increasing leukocyte trafficking and cytokine gene expression at the site of antigen entry. Elucidation of mechanisms mediating a stress-induced enhancement of skin immune function is important because such immunoenhancement can have protective (wound healing, resistance to infection) or pathological (allergic or autoimmune hypersensitivity) consequences.

INTRODUCTION

"Stress" is a term that generally has a negative connotation. Yet, stress is a familiar aspect of life, being a stimulant for some individuals, but a burden for many others. We have defined stress as a constellation of events, comprised of a stimulus (*stressor*), that precipitates a reaction in the brain (*stress perception*), which subsequently activates physiologic fight or flight systems in the body (*stress response*).[1] The stress response results in the release of neurotransmitters and hormones that serve as the brain's messengers to the body. It is often overlooked that the conse-

Address for correspondence: Firdaus S. Dhabhar, 4179 Postle Hall, College of Dentistry & College of Medicine, The Ohio State University, 305 W. 12th Ave., Columbus OH 43210. Tel: 614-688-8562; fax: 614-247-6945.
dhabhar.1@osu.edu

Ann. N.Y. Acad. Sci. 992: 205–217 (2003). © 2003 New York Academy of Sciences.

quences of a stress response are adaptive in the short run,[2–4] although stress can be harmful when it is long-lasting.[1,5] An important distinguishing characteristic of stress is its duration. We define *acute stress* as stress that lasts minutes to hours, and *chronic stress* as stress that persists several hours a day for weeks or months. An important marker for deleterious amounts of chronic stress is a dysregulation of the circadian cortisol/corticosterone rhythm.[1,6]

It is important to recognize that an acute stress response is an evolutionarily adaptive psychophysiological survival mechanism and may have salubrious or health-promoting consequences.[7–9] Most natural selection pressures, the chisels of evolution, are stressors that may be loosely categorized as physiological (scarcity of food or water), physical (wounding, infection), or psychological (fear and aggression). One of the primary functions of the brain is to perceive stressors, warn of danger, and enable an organism to cope with the consequences. This is accomplished through the release of stress-responsive neurotransmitters and hormones. For example, when a gazelle sees a charging lion, the gazelle's brain detects a threat and orchestrates a physiologic response that prepares and enables the gazelle to flee. The stress response mounted under these conditions is of limited duration or "*acute.*" Under such conditions, immunoenhancement rather than immunosuppression would be adaptive, because wounding and infection are often the result of aggressive encounters in nature. It is unlikely that eons of evolution would select for a system capable of escaping the jaws of a lion only to have it succumb to the "jaws" of bacteria. Thus, whereas ovulation, copulation, or digestion may be put on hold during stress, an immune response may not be dispensable. In contrast to this idea, it is often suggested that stress-induced immunosuppression may confer a survival advantage by conserving energy. However, some proposed mechanisms for immunosuppression, such as leukocyte destruction, expend rather than conserve energy, and others, such as inhibition of cytokine production or leukocyte proliferation,[10,11] require a longer time course than that available during acute stress. Thus, while energy conservation may play a role in immunosuppression during chronic stress, it is unlikely to do so during acute stress.

It is also important to recognize that stress (mainly chronic or long-term) can also have detrimental immunosuppressive and health aversive effects.[5,12] In fact, stress has long been suspected to play a role in the etiology of many diseases, and numerous studies have shown that stress can be immunosuppressive and hence may be detrimental to health.[10,13] Moreover, glucocorticoid stress hormones are regarded widely as being immunosuppressive[14] and are used clinically as anti-inflammatory agents.[11] While endorsing the fact that stress and stress mediators can have potent immunosuppressive and health aversive effects, we have examined the potentially salubrious effects of stress and stress hormones in preparing the immune system for dealing with immunologic challenges (e.g., wounding or infection), which may be imposed by the actions of a stressor (e.g., a predator).

PARADOXICAL OBSERVATIONS ON THE EFFECTS OF STRESS ON IMMUNE FUNCTION

Three paradoxes present themselves from a review of the extensive literature examining the relation between stress, immune function, and health. First, as the preceding discussion suggests, it is paradoxical that organisms would have evolved to suppress immune function at a time when an active immune response may be critical for survival as, for example, under conditions of stress when an organism may be injured or infected by the actions of the stress-inducing agent (e.g., an attacking predator).

Second, on the one hand, stress is thought to suppress immunity and increase susceptibility to infection[12] and cancer.[15,16] However, on the other, it is thought to exacerbate inflammatory diseases such as psoriasis, asthma, arthritis, and lupus erythematosus (which should be ameliorated by suppressing immune function).[17,18]

Third, stress is known to exacerbate autoimmune and inflammatory diseases; however, stress hormones (glucocorticoids) are used clinically in the treatment of these diseases.[11]

In this chapter we present data to describe interactions between stress and immune function, which provides possible explanations for these paradoxical observations. We propose that two key parameters may influence the direction (enhancing versus suppressive) of the effects of stress on a given immune measure: (1) the effects of stress on leukocyte distribution in the body; and (2) the differential effects of acute versus chronic stress on immune function. It is important to recognize that factors such as gender, genetic background, age, route of administration, nature, and dose of the immunizing antigen, and time of day may also significantly affect the relation between stress and immune function.

STRESS-INDUCED REDISTRIBUTION OF IMMUNE CELLS WITHIN THE BODY

Stress and stress hormones induce significant changes in the distribution of leukocytes within the body. It has been suggested that an important function of endocrine mediators released under conditions of acute stress may be to ensure that appropriate leukocytes are present in the right place and at the right time to respond to an immune challenge that might be initiated by the stress-inducing agent (e.g., attack by a predator, invasion by a pathogen, etc.).[7,19,20] The modulation of immune cell distribution by acute stress may be an adaptive response designed to enhance immune surveillance and increase immune preparedness for potential (or ongoing) immune challenge. Such changes in immune cell distribution may also have significant implications for the way in which data on the effects of stress on immune function in a specific body compartment are interpreted.

Effects of Stress on Blood Leukocytes

Immune cells or leukocytes circulate continuously from the blood, into various organs, and back into the blood. This circulation is essential for the maintenance of an effective immune defense network.[21] The numbers and proportions of leukocytes in the blood provide an important representation of the state of the distribution of leukocytes in the body and of the state of activation of the immune system. Numerous studies have shown that stress and stress hormones induce significant changes in absolute numbers and relative proportions of blood leukocytes.[22–25] Studies have shown that a stress-induced increase in plasma corticosterone is accompanied by a significant decrease in numbers and percentages of lymphocytes and by an increase in numbers and percentages of neutrophils in the blood.[19] These changes in blood leukocyte distribution are apparent within 30 minutes of applying the stressor.[19] FACS analyses have revealed that absolute numbers of peripheral blood helper T cells (Th), cytolytic T cells (CTL), B cells, natural killer (NK) cells, and monocytes all show a rapid and significant decrease (40–70% lower than baseline) during stress.[19] Stress-induced decreases in blood leukocyte numbers are rapidly reversed, with leukocyte numbers returning to pre-stress baseline levels within 3 hours after the cessation of stress.[19]

Adrenal Stress Hormones Mediate Stress-Induced Changes in Blood Leukocyte Numbers

Dhabhar *et al.*[20,26] have shown that the stress-induced changes in leukocyte distribution are mediated by hormones released by the adrenal gland. Several studies have shown that glucocorticoid treatment induces changes in leukocyte distribution.[27–30] In rats, adrenalectomy (which eliminates the corticosterone and epinephrine stress response)[19,20,22] or cyanoketone treatment (which eliminates only the corticosterone stress reponse) has been shown to virtually eliminate the stress-induced redistribution of blood leukocytes.[20]

In apparent contrast to glucocorticoid hormones, catecholamine hormones have been shown to increase blood leukocyte numbers in rats[31] and humans.[32] On closer examination it was observed that following adrenaline or noradrenaline administration, neutrophil and NK cell numbers increase rapidly and dramatically, whereas T and B cell numbers decrease.[33,34] Carslon *et al.*[35] have shown that catecholamine pre-treatment results in increased accumulation of lymphocytes in the spleen and lymph nodes, which would be in agreement with a catecholamine-induced decrease in lymphocytes in the blood. By acutely administering epinephrine, norepinephrine, selective α- and β-adrenergic receptor agonists, or corticosterone to adrenalectomized animals, Dhabhar and McEwen[26] have shown that increases in blood granulocyte numbers may be mediated by the α_1- and β-adrenergic receptors and are counteracted by corticosterone acting at the Type II adrenal steroid receptor. Increases in lymphocytes may be mediated by the α_2 receptor, whereas decreases in lymphocytes may be mediated by β-adrenergic and Type II adrenal steroid receptors.[26]

Therefore, the absolute number of specific blood leukocyte subpopulations may be significantly affected by the ambient concentrations of epinephrine, norepinephrine, and corticosterone. Differences in concentrations and combinations of these hormones may explain reported differences in blood leukocyte numbers during different stress conditions (e.g., short- versus long-duration acute stress and acute versus chronic stress) and during exercise.[36]

Stress-Induced Redistribution of Blood Leukocytes: Functional Consequences

Dhabhar *et al.*[2–4,7,9,19,20] were the first to propose that a stress-induced decrease in blood leukocyte numbers may represent an adaptive response. Therefore, an acute stress response directs the body's "soldiers" (leukocytes) to exit their "barracks" (spleen and bone marrow), travel the "boulevards" (blood vessels), and take position at potential "battle stations" (skin, lining of gastrointestinal and urogenital tracts, lung, liver, and lymph nodes) in preparation for an immune challenge. In addition to "redeploying" leukocytes to potential battle stations, stress hormones may also better equip them for "battle" by enhancing processes such as antigen presentation, phagocytosis, and antibody production. In this manner, a hormonal alarm signal released by the brain upon detecting a stressor, "prepares" the immune system for potential challenges (wounding or infection) that may arise due to the actions of the stress-inducing agent (e.g., predator or attacker).

An important, but under-appreciated, function of endocrine mediators released under conditions of acute stress may be to ensure that appropriate leukocytes are present in the right place and at the right time to respond to an immune challenge that might be initiated by the stress-inducing agent (e.g., attack by a predator, invasion by a pathogen, etc.). The modulation of immune cell distribution by acute stress may be an adaptive response designed to enhance immune surveillance and increase the capacity of the immune system to respond to challenge in immune compartments (such as the skin and the epithelium of lung, gastrointestinal, and urogenital tracts), which serve as major defense barriers for the body. Therefore, endocrine mediators released during stress serve to enhance immune preparedness for potential (or ongoing) immune challenge. Studies showing stress-induced enhancements in immune parameters *in vivo* and *in vitro* are reviewed.

STRESS-INDUCED ENHANCEMENT OF IMMUNE FUNCTION

Whereas most studies in the field have focused on the immunosuppressive effects of stress, several studies have also revealed that stress can be immunoenhancing. In general, acute stress is found to be immunoenhancing, whereas chronic stress is immunosuppressive (provided the effects of stress on leukocyte numbers and proportions in the body compartment under examination are taken into consideration).

Stress-Induced Enhancement of Cell-Mediated Immunity

Because the skin is one of the targets to which leukocytes traffic during stress, it was hypothesized that a stress-induced leukocyte redistribution may increase immune surveillance in the skin and consequently enhance immune function should the skin be exposed to antigen following acute stress.[2] Initially, studies examined the effects of acute stress on skin immunity, using a rodent model for a skin delayed type hypersensitivity (DTH) response.[2] Acute restraint stress administered immediately before the challenge with antigen resulted in a large and long-lasting enhancement of skin DTH.[2] Histological analysis identified significantly larger numbers of leukocytes in the skin of stressed animals both before and after exposure to antigen and suggested that a stress-induced redistribution of leukocytes was one of the factors mediating the stress-induced enhancement of skin immunity.[2] Acute stress has similarly been shown to enhance skin DTH in mice,[8,37] hamsters,[38] and squirrel monkeys.[39]

Interestingly, acute stress administered at the time of sensitization also significantly enhances a skin DTH response following challenge.[40,41] In these studies, animals were stressed acutely (2-hour restraint) before the administration of the sensitizing antigen. Compared to control animals, stressed animals showed a significantly larger DTH response following challenge although no stress was applied at the time of challenge. These results showed that acute stress administered during either sensitization or challenge can significantly enhance a skin DTH response.[40,41] Such immunoenhancement was observed even 9 months after initial stress exposure at the time of immunization, showing that acute stress induces long-lasting enhancement of immunological memory.[41]

Stress-Induced Enhancement of Humoral Immunity

Wood *et al.* have shown that exposure to footshock stress enhances humoral as well as cell-mediated immunity to keyhole limpet hemocyanin (KLH).[42] These investigators administered a single acute footshock session on days –1, 0, 1, and 3 relative to sensitization (day 0). They observed that compared to non-stressed controls, animals stressed on days 0 or 1 showed enhanced immune responses with respect to serum anti-KLH IgG levels, splenocyte proliferation, and skin cell-mediated immunity to KLH antigen. Interestingly, non-stressed animals failed to show a significant increase in serum antibody titers and in KLH-stimulated splenocyte proliferation relative to non-immunized animals.[42] Similarly, Persoons *et al.* have shown that acute stress administered prior to intrathecal immunization with trinitrophenyl keyhole limpet hemocyanin (TNP-KLH) significantly enhanced the primary humoral response in rats.[43] They also showed that acute stress administered prior to antigen administration to previously immunized animals resulted in a significant enhancement of a secondary humoral response.[43] In another study, Carr *et al.* reported that cold stress enhanced IgG and IgM production by splenocytes and that this enhancement was mediated by the alpha-adrenergic receptor.[44]

Several other studies have reported stress-induced enhancement of humoral immune responses. For example, cold stress has been shown to accelerate antigen removal in mice.[45] Other stressors have been shown to increase antigen-specific antibody titers in rats, mice, and pigs.[42,43,46-49] It has also been proposed that glucocorticoids may shift the balance of an ongoing immune response in favor of humoral immunity,[50-53] and physiological doses of glucocorticoids have been shown to enhance immunoglobulin production by mitogen-[54] and IL-4-stimulated[55] human lymphocytes in culture.

Stress-Induced Enhancement of In Vitro *Immune Parameters*

Acute stressors such as handling,[56] restraint,[57] and footshock[58] have been shown to enhance mitogen-induced proliferation of blood and spleen leukocytes. Acute stress also enhances spleen macrophage phagocytic function,[59] blood polymorphonuclear leukocyte phagocytosis,[60] and blood NK cell activity,[57,61] Several studies have shown that *in vitro* administration of stress hormones to immune cells can enhance different aspects of immune function. In an important series of studies, Wiegers *et al.* have shown that low physiological concentrations of corticosterone have been shown to stimulate mitogen-[62] and anti-T cell receptor-induced[63] proliferation of splenocytes. Similarly, glucocorticoid hormones have been shown to enhance nitric oxide and interleukin (IL)-1β[64] and tumor necrosis factor-alpha (TNF-α) secretion by macrophages.[65] Interstingly, acute stress has been shown to induce acute phase proteins *in vivo.*[66–68]

Acute Stress Enhances Innate and Adaptive Immune Responses

It is important to bear in mind that most *in vivo* immune responses involve a combination of innate as well as adaptive cellular, humoral, and cytokine mechanisms.[69] It has been suggested that stress enhances innate immunity but suppresses adaptive immunity.[70] However, evidence shows that a stress response can enhance innate immunity[64,65,71] as well as the humoral and cellular[1,2,8,37,42] arms of an adaptive immune response.[72] The determining factor is whether the physiological conditions established during a stress response around the time of exposure to antigen, pathogen, or wounding favor immunoenhancement or immunosuppression. The mechanisms involving leukocyte trafficking and activation that are discussed above apply to neutrophils, monocytes, NK cells, T cells, and B cells. Thus, a stress-induced redistribution of monocytes and lymphocytes to the skin and lymph nodes would enhance an innate (role of monocytes or NK cells) or an adaptive immune response (role of monocyte antigen presentation, memory T or B cell function, effector monocyte, T cell, and NK cell function). Similarly, an acute stress-induced neutrophilia would favor immunoenhancement by mobilizing neutrophils into the blood stream and making them available in larger numbers for recruitment and activation at sites of inflammation. Because neutrophils are critical for most inflammatory reactions, an increase in neutrophil recruitment could enhance the inflammatory phase of both innate and adaptive immune responses. Mechanisms involving leukocyte activation are also enhanced during acute stress. For example, increased macrophage phagocytosis[71,73] would enhance innate immunity, whereas increased macrophage antigen presentation[74] would enhance adaptive immunity. Although we recognize that much work remains to be done, we propose that under conditions involving acute stress or exposure to acute physiologic concentrations of stress hormones, both innate as well as adaptive immune responses may be significantly enhanced.

STRESS-INDUCED SUPPRESSION OF IMMUNE FUNCTION

Numerous studies have shown that stress can be immunosuppressive and hence may be detrimental to health (for review see Refs. 10, 13, 14, and 75–77). Since these studies have been reviewed and discussed extensively, here we present only a few relevant examples of a stress-induced suppression of immune function and refer the reader to these excellent reviews and other chapters in this volume for a more detailed account of the subject.

It has been shown that in contrast to acute stress, chronic stress suppresses the skin DTH response.[1,78] A chronic stress-induced decrease in leukocyte mobilization from the blood to other body compartments is thought to be one of the mediators of this stress-induced suppression of skin DTH.[1] Similarly in human and animal studies, chronic stress has also been shown to suppress different immune parameters, examples of which include delayed type hypersensitivity,[78] antibody production,[79] NK activity,[13,80] leukocyte proliferation,[80] skin homograft rejection,[81] virus-specific T cell and NK cell activity,[82] and antimycobacterial activity of macrophages from susceptible mouse strains.[83]

THE STRESS SPECTRUM HYPOTHESIS

Dhabhar and McEwen have proposed that a stress response and its consequent effects on immune function may be viewed in the context of a Stress Spectrum.[1] One region of the stress spectrum is characterized by Acute Stress, that is, short-duration stress that may result in immunopreparatory or immunoenhancing physiological conditions. An important characteristic of acute stress is a rapid response mounted in the presence of the stressor followed by a rapid shut-off once the stress has subsided. The other end of the stress spectrum is characterized by Chronic Stress, that is, repeated or physiologically exhausting stress that may result in immunosuppression. An important characteristic of chronic stress is that the physiologic response either persists long after the stressor has subsided or is activated repeatedly to result in an overall integrated increase in exposure of the organism to stress hormones. The concept of "allostatic load" has been proposed to define the constant wear and tear that takes place while different physiologic systems respond to repeated or prolonged demands of internal and external stressors. (For a review see Refs. 5 and 84.) Conditions of high allostatic load would result in deleterious immunosuppression. Importantly, a disruption of the circadian corticosterone rhythm may be an indicator and/or mediator of the deleterious effects of chronic stress.[1,85] The stress spectrum model also proposes that between acute and chronic stress is an area that represents Resilience, that is, *the ability of physiologic systems to enable survival for extended periods of time under increasingly challenging conditions.*

CONCLUSIONS

Stress has long been suspected to play a role in the etiology of many diseases, and numerous studies have shown that stress can be immunosuppressive and hence may be detrimental to health. This chapter shows that under certain conditions, stress can exert immunoenhancing effects. The physiologic stress response may play a critical evolutionarily adaptive role. Stress hormones and neurotransmitters serve as messengers from brain to body. These messengers prepare the immune system for potential immunologic challenges (e.g., wounding or infection) that are perceived by the brain (e.g., the detection of predator or attacker).[3,4,9] However, it is important to recognize that while stress-induced enhancement of immune function may increase the rate of wound healing or resistance to infection, it may also exacerbate autoimmune and inflammatory disease. Therefore, there exists a Yin-Yang principle with respect to the effects of stress on immune function and perhaps on most physiologic parameters. Because these effects may potently influence the overall health of an organism, we might hypothesize that a physiologic equilibrium among these different systems would be most favorable for salubrity.

It is also important to recognize that humans as well as animals experience stress as an intrinsic part of life and in conjunction with many standard diagnostic, clinical, and experimental manipulations. Unintended stressors may significantly affect these diagnostic and clinical measures and overall health outcomes. Thus, when conducting clinical, diagnostic, or experimental manipulations, it may be important to account for the effects of stress on the specific physiologic parameter or health outcome being measured.

A determination of the physiologic mechanisms through which stress and stress hormones enhance or suppress immune responses may help our understanding and treatment of diseases thought to be affected by stress. The cellular and molecular mechanisms by which stress and stress hormones up- or downregulate an immune response merit further investigation. A greater understanding of these mechanisms would help in the development of biomedical treatments that could harness an individual's physiology to selectively enhance (during wounding, infections, or cancer) or suppress (during autoimmune or inflammatory disorders) the immune response depending on what would be most beneficial for the patient.

ACKNOWLEDGMENTS

Portions of the work described in this chapter were supported by grants from The Dana Foundation and by National Institutes of Health Grant RO1-48995. I am grateful for the advice, support, and friendship of Bruce McEwen. I would also like to thank Alison Saul, Jean M. Tillie, and Kavitha Viswanathan for their invaluable contributions to ongoing studies in the laboratory.

REFERENCES

1. DHABHAR, F.S. & B.S. MCEWEN. 1997. Acute stress enhances while chronic stress suppresses immune function *in vivo*: a potential role for leukocyte trafficking. Brain Beha. Immun. **11:** 286–306.
2. DHABHAR, F.S. & B.S. MCEWEN. 1996. Stress-induced enhancement of antigen-specific cell-mediated immunity. J. Immunol. **156:** 2608–2615.
3. DHABHAR, F.S. 2002. Enhancing versus suppressive effects of stress on immune function: the role of leukocyte trafficking and the kinetic and concentration conditions of exposure to stress hormones (New Investigator Award). Brain Behav. Immun. **16:** 785–798.
4. DHABHAR, F.S. 2002. A hassle a day may keep the doctor away: stress and the augmentation of immune function. Integr. Comp. Biol. **42:** 556–564.
5. MCEWEN, B.S. 1998. Protective and damaging effects of stress mediators: allostasis and allostatic load. N. Engl. J. Med. **338:** 171–179.
6. SEPHTON, S.E., R.M. SAPOLSKY, H.C. KRAEMER & D. SPIEGEL. 2000. Early mortality in metastatic breast cancer patients with absent or abnormal diurnal cortisol rhythms. J. Natl. Cancer Inst. **92:** 994–1000.
7. DHABHAR, F.S., A.H. MILLER, M. STEIN, *et al.* 1994. Diurnal and stress-induced changes in distribution of peripheral blood leukocyte subpopulations. Brain Behav. Immun. **8:** 66–79.
8. DHABHAR, F.S., A.R. SATOSKAR, H. BLUETHMANN, *et al.* 2000. Stress-induced enhancement of skin immune function: a role for IFNγ. Proc. Natl. Acad. Sci. USA **97:** 2846–2851.
9. DHABHAR, F.S. & B.S. MCEWEN. 2001. Bidirectional effects of stress and glucocorticoid hormones on immune function: possible explanations for paradoxical observations. *In* Psychoneuroimmunology, 3rd Ed. R. Ader, D.L. Felten & N. Cohen, Eds. Academic Press. San Diego.
10. ADER, R., D.L. FELTEN & N. COHEN. 2001. Psychoneuroimmunology, 3rd Ed. :1583. Academic Press. San Diego.
11. SCHLEIMER, R.P., H.N. CLAMAN & A. ORONSKY, Eds. 1989. Anti-inflammatory Steroid Action: Basic and Clinical Aspects, 1st Ed. :564. Academic Press. San Diego.
12. KIECOLT-GLASER, J.K., L. MCGUIRE, T.F. ROBLES & R. GLASER. 2002. Psychoneuroimmunology: psychological influences on immune function and health. J. Consult Clin. Psychol. **70:** 537–547.

13. IRWIN, M., T. PATTERSON, T.L. SMITH, *et al.* 1990. Reduction of immune function in life stress and depression. Biol. Psychiatry. **27:** 22–30.
14. MUNCK, A., P.M. GUYRE & N.J. HOLBROOK. 1984. Physiological functions of glucocorticoids in stress and their relation to pharmacological actions. Endocrine Rev. **5:** 25–44.
15. VALDIMARSDOTTIR, H.B., S.G. ZAKOWSKI, W. GERIN, *et al.* 2002. Heightened psychobiological reactivity to laboratory stressors in healthy women at familial risk for breast cancer. J. Behav. Med. **25:** 51–65.
16. BEN-ELIYAHU, S., G.G. PAGE, Y. RAZ & S. GUY. 1999. Evidence that stress and surgical interventions promote tumor development by suppressing natural killer cell activity. Int. J. Cancer **80:** 880–888.
17. HART, A. & M.A. KAMM. 2002. Mechanisms of initiation and perpetuation of gut inflammation by stress. Aliment. Pharmacol. Ther. **16:** 2017–2028.
18. SOLOMON, G.F. & R.H. MOOS. 1964. Emotions, immunity and disease. Arch. Gen. Psychiat. **11:** 657–669.
19. DHABHAR, F.S., A.H. MILLER, B.S. MCEWEN & R.L. SPENCER. 1995. Effects of stress on immune cell distribution: dynamics and hormonal mechanisms. J. Immunol. **154:** 5511–5527.
20. DHABHAR, F.S., A.H. MILLER, B.S. MCEWEN & R.L. SPENCER. 1996. Stress-induced changes in blood leukocyte distribution: role of adrenal steroid hormones. J. Immunol. **157:** 1638–1644.
21. SPRENT, J. & D.F. TOUGH. 1994. Lymphocyte life-span and memory. Science **265:** 1395–1400.
22. JENSEN, M.M. 1969. Changes in leukocyte counts associated with various stressors. J. Reticuloendothelial. Soc. **8:** 457–465.
23. MORROW-TESCH, J.L., J.J. MCGLONE & R.L. NORMAN. 1993. Consequences of restraint stress on natural killer cell activity, behavior, and hormone levels in Rhesus macaques (*Macaca mulatta*). Psychoneuroendocrinology **18:** 383–395.
24. HERBERT, T.B. & S. COHEN. 1993. Stress and immunity in humans: a meta-analytic review. Psychosom. Med. **55:** 364–379.
25. SCHEDLOWSKI, M., R. JACOBS, G. STRATMAN, *et al.* 1993. Changes of natural killer cells during acute psychological stress. J. Clin. Immunol. **13:** 119–126.
26. DHABHAR, F.S. & B.S. MCEWEN. 1999. Changes in blood leukocyte distribution: interactions between catecholamine and glucocorticoid hormones. Neuroimmunomodulation **6:** 213.
27. DOUGHERTY, R.F. & A. WHITE. 1945. Functional alterations in lymphoid tissue induced by adrenal cortical secretion. Am. J. Anat. **77:** 81–116.
28. COHEN, J.J. 1972. Thymus-derived lymphocytes sequestered in the bone marrow of hydrocortisone-treated mice. J. Immunol. **108:** 841–844.
29. FAUCI, A.S. & D.C. DALE. 1974. The effect of *in vivo* hydrocortisone on subpopulations of human lymphocytes. J. Clin. Invest. **53:** 240–246.
30. FAUCI, A.S. 1976. Mechanisms of corticosteroid action on lymphocyte subpopulations. II. Differential effects of *in vivo* hydrocortisone, prednisone, and dexamethasone on *in vitro* expression of lymphocyte function. Clin. Exp. Immunol. **24:** 54–62.
31. HARRIS, T.J., T.J. WALTMAN, S.M. CARTER & A.S. MAISEL. 1995. Effect of prolonged catecholamine infusion on immunoregulatory function: implications in congestive heart failure. J. Am. Coll. Cardiol. **26:** 102–109.
32. LANDMANN, R., F.B. MULLER, C.H. PERINI, *et al.* 1984. Changes of immunoregulatory cells induced by psychological and physical stress: relationship to plasma catecholamines. Clin. Exp. Immunol. **58:** 127–135.
33. SCHEDLOWSKI, M., A. FALK, A. ROHNE, *et al.* 1993. Catecholamines induce alterations of distribution and activity of human natural killer (NK) cells. J. Clin. Immunol. **13:** 344–351.
34. BENSCHOP, R.J., M. RODRIGUEZ-FEUERHAHN & M. SCHEDLOWSKI. 1996. Catecholamine-induced leukocytosis: early observations, current research, and future directions. Brain Behav. Immun. **10:** 77–91.
35. CARLSON, S.L., S. FOX & K.M. ABELL. 1997. Catecholamine modulation of lymphocyte homing to lymphoid tissues. Brain Behav. & Immun. **11:** 307–320.

36. KAPPEL, M., N. TVEDE, H. GALBO, *et al.* 1991. Evidence that the effect of physical exercise on NK cell activity is mediated by epinephrine. J. Appl. Physiol. **70:** 2530–2534.
37. BLECHA, F., R.A. BARRY & K.W. KELLEY. 1982. Stress-induced alterations in delayed-type hypersensitivity to SRBC and contact sensitivity to DNFB in mice. Proc. Soc. Exp. Biol. Med. **169:** 239–246.
38. BILBO, S.D., F.S. DHABHAR, K. VISWANATHAN, *et al.* 2002. Short day lengths augment stress-induced leukocyte trafficking and stress-induced enhancement of skin immune function. Proc. Natl. Acad. Sci. USA **99:** 4067–4072.
39. COE, C.L., G. LUBACH & E. W.B. 1989. Immunological consequences of maternal separation in infant primates. *In* Infant Stress and Coping. M. Lewis & J. Worobey, Eds. Jossey-Bass Inc. New York, NY.
40. DHABHAR, F.S. & B.S. MCEWEN. 1999. Enhancement of the immunization/sensitization phase of cell-mediated immunity: the role of acute stress & adrenal stress hormones. Neuroimmunomodulation **6:** 213.
41. VISWANATHAN, K., S.D. BILBO & F.S. DHABHAR. 2002. Acute stress administered before primary immunization or before challenge enhances skin cell mediated immunity to keyhole limpet hemocyanin (KLH). Brain Behav. Immun. **16:** 222.
42. WOOD, P.G., M.H. KAROL, A.W. KUSNECOV & B.S. RABIN. 1993. Enhancement of antigen-specific humoral and cell-mediated immunity by electric footshock stress in rats. Brain Behav. Immun. **7:** 121–134.
43. PERSOONS, J.H.A., F. BERKENBOSCH, K. SCHORNAGEL, *et al.* 1995. Increased specific IgE production in lungs after the induction of acute stress in rats. J. Allergy Clin. Immunol. **95:** 765–770.
44. CARR, D.J., T.W. WOOLLEY & J.E. BLALOCK. 1992. Phentolamine but not propranolol blocks the immunopotentiating effect of cold stress on antigen-specific IgM production in mice orally immunized with sheep red blood cells. Brain Behav. Immun. **6:** 50–63.
45. SABISTON, B.H., J.E.M. STE ROSE & B. CINADER. 1978. Temperature stress and immunity in mice. J. Immunogenet. **5:** 197–212.
46. SOLOMON, G.F. 1969. Stress and antibody response in rats. Int. Arch. Allergy **35:** 97–104.
47. BLECHA, F. & K.W. KELLEY. 1981. Effects of cold and weaning stressors on the antibody-mediated immune response of pigs. J. Anim. Sci. **53:** 439–447.
48. COCKE, R., J.A. MOYNIHAN, N. COHEN, *et al.* 1993. Exposure to conspecific alarm chemosignals alters immune responses in BALB/c mice. Brain Behav. Immun. **7:** 36–46.
49. BERKENBOSCH, F., D.A. WOLVERS & R. DERIJK. 1991. Neuroendocrine and immunological mechanisms in stress-induced immunomodulation. J. Steroid Biochem. Mol. Biol. **40:** 639–647.
50. DANES, R.A. & B.A. ARANEO. 1989. Contrasting effects of glucocorticoids on the capacity of T cells to produce the growth factors interleukin 2 and interleukin 4. Eur. J. Immunol. **19:** 2319–2325.
51. GAJEWSKI, T.F., S.R. SCHELL, G. NAU & F.W. FITCH. 1989. Regulation of T-cell activation: differences among T-cell subsets. Immunol. Rev. **111:** 79–110.
52. MOSMANN, T.R. & R.L. COFFMAN. 1989. TH1 and TH2 cells: different patterns of lymphokine secretion lead to different functional properties. Ann. Rev. Immunol. **7:** 145–173.
53. MASON, D. 1991. Genetic variation in the stress response: susceptibility to experimental allergic encephalomyelitis and implications for human inflammatory disease. Immunol. Today **12:** 57–60.
54. GRAYSON, J., N.J. DOOLEY, I.R. KOSKI & R.M. BLAESE. 1981. Immunoglobulin production induced in vitro by glucocorticoid hormones: T cell-dependent stimulation of immunoglobulin production without B cell proliferation in cultures of human peripheral blood lymphocytes. J. Clin. Invest. **68:** 1539–1547.
55. WU, C.Y., M. SARFATI, C. HEUSSER, *et al.* 1991. Glucocorticoids increase the synthesis of immunoglobulin E by interleukin 4-stimulated human lymphocytes. J. Clin. Invest. **87:** 870–877.
56. RINNER, I., K. SCHAUENSTEIN, H. MANGGE, *et al.* 1992. Opposite effects of mild and severe stress on *in vitro* activation of rat peripheral blood lymphocytes. Brain Behav. Immun. **6:** 130–140.

57. Jain, S. & J.R. Stevenson. 1991. Enhancement by restraint stress of natural killer cell activity and splenocyte responsiveness to concanavalin A in Fischer 344 rats. Immunol. Invest. **20:** 365–376.
58. Shurin, M.R., D. Zhou, A. Kusnecov, *et al.* 1994. Effect of one or more footshocks on spleen and blood lymphocyte proliferation in rats. Brain Behav. Immun. **8:** 57–65.
59. Lyte, M., S.G. Nelson & B. Baissa. 1990. Examination of the neuroendocrine basis for the social conflict-induced enhancement of immunity in mice. Physiol. Behav. **48:** 685–691.
60. Shurin, M.R., A. Kusnecov, E. Hamill, *et al.* 1994. Stress-induced alteration of polymorphonuclear leukocyte function in rats. Brain Behav. Immun. **8:** 163–169.
61. Millar, D.B., J.R. Thomas, N.D. Pacheco & F.M. Rollwagen. 1993. Natural killer cell cytotoxicity and T-cell proliferation is enhanced by avoidance behavior. Brain Behav. Immun. **7:** 144–153.
62. Wiegers, J.G., J.M.H.M. Reul, F. Holsboer & E.R. De Kloet. 1994. Enhancement of rat splenic lymphocyte mitogenesis after short term exposure to corticosteroids in vitro. Endocrinology **135:** 2351–2357.
63. Wiegers, G.J., M.S. Labeur, I.E. Stec, *et al.* 1995. Glucocorticoids accelerate anti-T cell receptor-induced T cell growth. J. Immunol. **155:** 1893–1902.
64. Broug-Holub, E. & G. Kraal. 1996. Dose- and time-dependent activation of rat alveolar macrophages by glucocorticoids. Clin. Exp. Immunol. **104:** 332–336.
65. Renz, H., A. Henke, P. Hofmann, *et al.* 1992. Sensitization of rat alveolar macrophages to enhanced TNF-α release by in vivo treatment with dexamethasone. Cellular Immunol. **144:** 249–257.
66. LeMay, L.G., A.J. Vander & M.J. Kluger. 1990. The effects of psychological stress on plasma interleukin-6 activity in rats. Physiol. & Behav. **47:** 957–961.
67. Zhou, D., A. W. Kusnecov, M. R. Shurin, *et al.* 1993. Exposure to physical and psychological stressors elevates plasma interleukin **6:** relationship to the activation of the hypothalamic-pituitary-adrenal axis. Endocrinology **133:** 2523–2530.
68. Maes, M., D. Hendriks, G. Van, *et al.* 1997. Effects of psychological stress on serum immunoglobulin, complement and acute phase protein concentrations in normal volunteers. Psychoneuroendocrinology **22:** 397–409.
69. Abbas, A.K., A.H. Lichtman & J.S. Pober. 2000. Cellular and Molecular Immunology, 4th Ed. W.B. Saunders. Philadelphia.
70. Fleshner, M., K.T. Nguyen, C.S. Cotter, *et al.* 1998. Acute stressor exposure both suppresses acquired immunity and potentiates innate immunity. Am. J. Physiol. **275:** R870–878.
71. Rhinehart, J.J., A.L. Sagone, S.P. Balcerzak, *et al.* 1975. Effects of corticosteroid therapy on human monocyte function. N. Engl. J. Med. **292:** 236–241.
72. Moynihan, J.A. & S.Y. Stevens. 2001. Mechanisms of stress-induced modulation of immunity in animals. *In* Psychoneuroimmunology, 3rd Ed. R. Ader, D.L. Felten & N. Cohen, Eds. Academic Press. San Diego.
73. Lyte, M., S.G. Nelson & M.L. Thompson. 1990. Innate and adaptive immune responses in a social conflict paradigm. Clin. Immunol. Immunopathol. **57:** 137–147.
74. Sadeghi, R., C.M. Hawrylowicz, Y. Chernajovsky & M. Feldmann. 1992. Synergism of glucocorticoids with granulocyte macrophage colony stimulating factor (GM-CSF) but not interferon gamma or interleukin-4 on induction of HLA class II expression on human monocytes. Cytokine **4:** 287–297.
75. Kiecolt-Glaser, J.K., R. Glaser, S. Gravenstein, *et al.* 1996. Chronic stress alters the immune response to influenza virus vaccine in older adults. Proc. Natl. Acad. Sci. USA **93:** 3043–3047.
76. Sheridan, J.F. 1998. Stress-induced modulation of anti-viral immunity: normal cousins Memorial Lecture 1997. Brain Behav. Immun. **12:** 1–6.
77. Cohen, S. & R.B. Herbert. 1996. Health psychology: psychological factors and physical disease from the perspective of human psychoneuroimmunology. Annu. Rev. Psychol. **47:** 113–142.
78. Basso, A.M., M. Depiante-Depaoli, L. Cancela & V. Molina. 1993. Seven-day variable-stress regime alters cortical β-adrenoreceptor binding and immunologic responses: reversal by imipramine. Pharmacol. Biochem. Behav. **45:** 665–672.

79. EDWARDS, E.A. & L.M. DEAN. 1977. Effects of crowding of mice on humoral antibody formation and protection to lethal antigenic challenge. Psychosom. Med. **39:** 19–24.
80. BARTROP, R., L. LAZARUS, E. LUCKHURST, *et al.* 1977. Depressed lymphocyte function after bereavement. The Lancet **8016:** 834–836.
81. WISTAR, R. & W.H. HILDEMANN. 1960. Effect of stress on skin transplantation immunity in mice. Science **131:** 159–160.
82. BONNEAU, R.H., J.F. SHERIDAN, N. FENG & R. GLASER. 1991. Stress-induced effects on cell-mediated innate and adaptive memory components of the murine immune response to herpes simplex virus infection. Brain Behav. Immun. **5:** 274–295.
83. BROWN, D.H. & B.S. ZWILLING. 1994. Activation of the hypothalamic-pituitary-adrenal axis differentially affects the anti-mycobacterial activity of macrophages from BCG-resistant and susceptible mice. J. Neuroimmunol. **53:** 181–187.
84. MCEWEN, B.S. 2002. The end of stress as we know it. :239. Dana Press. Washington, DC.
85. SEPHTON, S.E., R.M. SAPOLSKY, H.C. KRAEMER & D. SPIEGEL. 1998. Absence of diurnal cortisol variation predicts early breast cancer mortality. Preprint. Neuroimmunomodulation **5:** 45.

The Role of Neural Inflammation in Asthma and Chronic Obstructive Pulmonary Disease

GUY F. JOOS, KATELIJNE O. DE SWERT, VANESSA SCHELFHOUT, AND ROMAIN A. PAUWELS

Department of Respiratory Diseases, Ghent University Hospital, De Pintelaan 185, B 9000 Ghent, Belgium

ABSTRACT: The tachykinins substance P and neurokinin A are found within airway nerves and immune cells. They have various effects on the airways that can contribute to the changes observed in asthma and chronic obstructive pulmonary disease. Both tachykinin NK_1 and NK_2 receptors have been involved in the bronchoconstriction and the proinflammatory changes induced by substance P and neurokinin A. Tachykinin NK_1 and NK_2 receptor antagonists have activity in various animal models of allergic asthma and chronic bronchitis. It is suggested that dual NK_1/NK_2 and triple $NK_1/NK_2/NK_3$ tachykinin receptor antagonists have potential in the treatment of obstructive airway diseases.

KEYWORDS: substance P; neurokinin A; tachykinins; asthma; neurogenic airway inflammation; tachykinin receptor antagonists

INTRODUCTION

Substance P and neurokinin A are members of the tachykinin peptide family, consisting of mammalian and nonmammalian tachykinins.[1] These neuropeptides are synthesized by sensory neurons and subsequently stored in the terminal parts of the axon collaterals. The tachykinins are potent vasodilators and contractors of smooth muscle. In studies on rodent airways, substance P and neurokinin A have been implicated as the neurotransmitters mediating the excitatory part of the nonadrenergic, noncholinergic (NANC) nervous system.[2] These noncholinergic excitatory nerves can be activated by mechanical and chemical stimuli, generating antidromic impulses and a local axon reflex which leads to noncholinergic bronchoconstriction and neurogenic inflammation.[2]

Substance P and neurokinin A have various effects that could contribute to the changes observed in asthma and chronic obstructive pulmonary disease (COPD). These include smooth muscle contraction, submucosal gland secretion, vasodilatation, increase in vascular permeability, stimulation of cholinergic nerves, stimulation of mast cells, stimulation of B and T lymphocytes, stimulation of macrophages,

Address for correspondence: Prof. Dr. Guy F. Joos, Department of Respiratory Diseases, Ghent University Hospital, De Pintelaan 185, B-9000 Ghent, Belgium. Voice: 32 9 240 2359; fax: 32 9 240 2341.
guy.joos@rug.ac.be

Ann. N.Y. Acad. Sci. 992: 218–230 (2003). © 2003 New York Academy of Sciences.

chemoattraction of eosinophils and neutrophils, and the vascular adhesion of neutrophils.[3,4] Substance P and neurokinin A interact with the different targets in the airways by stimulation of tachykinin NK_1, NK_2, and NK_3 receptors.[5] The physiological activity of both exogenously administered and endogenously released neuropeptides is modulated through enzymatic cleavage and inactivation by peptidases. In human airways, two major peptidases are neutral endopeptidase (NEP, also called enkephalinase, E.C.3.4.24.11), which is predominantly present in airway epithelium, and angiotensin-converting enzyme (ACE, E.C.3.14.5.1), present within the pulmonary endothelium.[6]

In the present article an update on the role of tachykinins and their receptors in asthma and chronic obstructive pulmonary disease is given.

NEURONAL AND NON-NEURONAL SOURCES OF TACHYKININS IN THE AIRWAYS

SP and NKA are contained in a distinct subpopulation of primary afferent nerves that are characterized by sensitivity to capsaicin. Substance P and neurokinin A are present in nerve profiles, found beneath and within the epithelium, around blood vessels and submucosal glands, and within the bronchial smooth muscle layer.[7–9] Using confocal laser scanning microscopy and immunohistochemistry for the protein gene product 9.5 (PGP-IR), Lamb and Sparrow demonstrated an arrangement of epithelial nerves in human bronchi which was very similar to that of porcine nerves containing sensory neuropeptides. An apical layer of varicose processes terminated in enlarged varicosities, and these fibers encircled goblet cells. These processes arose from fibers that had crossed the epithelium from a basal plexus that was supplied by nerve bundles in the lamina propria. As in other studies, substance P-immunoreactive nerves were faintly stained in human bronchi.[10]

Tachykinins have been measured in bronchoalveolar lavage (BAL), induced sputum, and plasma. Various studies have shown that tachykinins can be released into the airways after exposure to allergen, ozone, or hypertonic saline solution. Nieber *et al.* found a significantly larger amount of substance P in bronchoalveolar lavage fluid of atopic compared to nonallergic subjects. After intrasegmental provocation with allergen, a significant increase in BAL substance P levels was observed.[11] Heaney *et al.* also recovered neurokinin A from BAL fluid from normal and asthmatic patients. Neurokinin A was increased in the asthmatic patients 4 hours after inhalation challenge with house dust mite.[12] Exposure of healthy individuals to ozone increased the concentration of substance P in BAL fluid[13] and decreased the immunoreactivity for substance P, assessed on bronchial biopsies.[14] Nasal application of hypertonic saline also induced release of substance P.[15]

Although increased amounts of tachykinins have been recovered from airways, there has been debate about a possible upregulation of substance P–containing nerves in patients with asthma or COPD. In tissue obtained at autopsy, after lobectomy and at bronchoscopy, both the number and the length of substance P–immunoreactive nerve fibers was increased in airways of subjects with asthma, when compared to airways of subjects without asthma.[16] However, Howarth *et al.* could not identify any substance P–containing nerves in endobronchial biopsies from patients with mild asthma.[17] More recently, in an extensive study on 49 asthmatic patients, including 16 patients with severe asthma, Chanez and colleagues did not find evidence for an upregulation of substance P–containing nerves in asthma. Nerves were present in most of the endobronchial biopsy specimens, as demonstrated by the neural marker PGP 9.5, and were found within and below the epithelium and adjacent to smooth muscle, glands, and blood vessels. However, nerves positive for substance P and calcitonin gene-related peptide (CGRP) were rarely found in the biopsy specimens, and no increase in patients with asthma was observed.[18] On the other hand, it was observed that substance P–like immunoreactivity was decreased in tracheal tissue of asthmatic subjects studied at autopsy. This may reflect augmented release of substance P, followed by degradation.[19] Lucchini *et al.* studied lung tissue obtained at thoracotomy from patients with chronic bronchitis. The lung tissue in chronic bronchitis did not contain more nerves, and did not show a change in the amount of substance P– or CGRP-containing nerves. In contrast, the density of vasoactive intestinal peptide (VIP)-containing nerves was significantly higher in the glands of patients with chronic bronchitis compared to control subjects.[20]

In recent years, it has become clear from both animal and human studies that immune cells may form an additional source of tachykinins.[4,21] Evidence for the production of substance P by eosinophils (mouse, man), monocytes and macrophages (rat, man), lymphocytes (man), and dendritic cells (mouse) has been reported. Inflammatory stimuli such as lipopolysaccharide (LPS) can upregulate the concentration of tachykinins in these cells.[22,23] These findings can help to explain the paradox between the relatively few SP- and NKA-containing nerves observed in human airways and the recovery of SP and NKA from sputum and BAL fluid.[24,12] Thus, increased amounts of immune cells attracted to the inflamed airways might be responsible for an increased content of substance P and neurokinin A in patients with asthma or COPD. Moreover, the release of tachykinins from these inflammatory cells might further stimulate and activate these cells in an autocrine or paracrine fashion. Indeed, these inflammatory cells produce and secrete substance P and possess tachykinin NK_1 receptors on their membrane.[22]

It is also possible that substance P is produced by epithelial or endothelial cells.[4] Chu and colleagues reported staining for substance P in the epithelium on biopsy specimens. In comparison to control subjects, patients with asthma showed a significantly higher expression of substance P in the epithelium but not in the submucosa. It is of interest to note that in their study the epithelial expression of substance P was correlated with the epithelial mucus content.[25]

TACHYKININ AIRWAY RECEPTORS

Most of the biological actions of tachykinins are mediated via activation of one of the three tachykinin receptors, denoted NK_1, NK_2 and NK_3. The NK_1, NK_2 and NK_3 tachykinin receptors have the highest affinity for substance P, neurokinin A, and neurokinin B, respectively. There is, however, a much wider crosstalk between natural tachykinin peptides and their receptors than originally recognized: for instance, it is presently accepted that NKA is a high-affinity and effective endogenous ligand for NK_1 receptors at many synapses and/or neuroeffector junctions.[5] A novel member of the tachykinin receptor family was recently discovered, and termed NK_4.

The tachykinins SP and NKA interact with the targets on the airways by specific tachykinin receptors. The tachykinin NK_1 and NK_2 receptor have been characterized in human airways, both pharmacologically and by cloning. *In vitro* studies on isolated human bronchi and bronchioli have reported that tachykinin NK_2 receptors are present on smooth muscle of both large and small airways and mediate part of the bronchoconstrictor effect of tachykinins. Tachykinin NK_1 receptors are localized on smooth muscle of small airways and are responsible for a transient, low-intensity contraction.[26,27] Most of the proinflammatory effects of substance P are mediated by the tachykinin NK_1 receptor (reviewed in Advenier *et al.*[28]). The tachykinin NK_3 receptor has been recently demonstrated in guinea pig airways, where it mediates citric acid–induced cough and changes in airway responsiveness induced by substance P and citric acid. Moreover, the tachykinin NK_3 receptor mediates the neurokinin-induced facilitation of synaptic neurotransmission in parasympathetic ganglia.[29]

Smoking increases the tachykinin NK_1 receptor mRNA.[30] In asthmatics the expression of the tachykinin NK_2 receptor mRNA is increased.[31] Glucocorticoids can reduce the level of tachykinin receptor mRNA.[32] Using antibodies to the tachykinin NK_1 and NK_2 receptors, Mapp and colleagues found expression of both tachykinin receptors in bronchial glands, bronchial vessels, and bronchial smooth muscle. Receptors were occasionally found in nerves (NK_1) and in inflammatory cells (NK_2) such as T lymphocytes, macrophages, and mast cells. The distribution of both tachykinin NK_1 and NK_2 receptors was similar in the tissues examined from nonsmokers, asymptomatic smokers, symptomatic smokers with normal lung function, and symptomatic smokers with chronic airflow limitation.[33] In a study on endobronchial biopsies by Chu and colleagues, immunoreactivity for the tachykinin NK_1 receptor was found in the epithelium and submucosa. The NK_1 receptor expression was mainly seen on cell surfaces of the upper half of the epithelial layer. Goblet cells appeared to be the cells with the strongest staining. In the submucosa the tachykinin NK_1 receptor was primarily localized on the endothelial cells of the blood vessels, the surfaces of inflammatory cells, and some smooth muscle cells. In this study the expression of substance P as well as the tachykinin NK_1 receptor was significantly higher in the epithelium of asthmatic subjects.[25]

BRONCHOCONSTRICTOR EFFECT OF TACHYKININS

Tachykinins are potent contractors of airways. This has been demonstrated both *in vitro* and *in vivo*, both in animal and in human airways. The *in vitro* contractile effect of substance P and neurokinin A has been studied extensively. Substance P contracts human bronchi and bronchioli,[34,35] but is less potent than histamine or acetylcholine.[36] Neurokinin A is a more potent constrictor of human bronchi than substance P and was reported to be, on a molar base, two to three orders of magnitude more potent than histamine or acetylcholine.

It has long been thought that only tachykinin NK_2 receptors are involved in contraction of isolated human airways.[37] However, in small-diameter bronchi (~1 mm in diameter), in addition to a robust NK_2 tachykinin receptor-mediated contraction, tachykinins also cause contraction via NK_1 tachykinin receptor stimulation. The NK_1-mediated contraction of small bronchi appears to be mediated by prostanoids.[26] In an extensive study on medium-sized human isolated bronchi (2–5 mm in diameter) the specific NK_1 receptor agonist [Sar^9,$Met(O_2)^{11}$]SP was found to induce contraction in about 60% of the preparations, an effect that was not mediated by prostanoids, but from a direct activation of smooth muscle receptors and release of inositol phosphate.[27] So, it appears that in both small- and medium-sized human bronchi, part of the contraction induced by tachykinins is mediated by tachykinin NK_1 receptors.

The *in vivo* bronchoconstrictor effect of substance P and neurokinin A, administered by inhalation or intravenous infusion, has been reported by several groups. In these studies, neurokinin A was found to be a more potent bronchoconstrictor than substance P. Patients with asthma are hyperresponsive to substance P and neurokinin A (reviewed in Ref. 38). The bronchoconstrictor effect of inhaled substance P and neurokinin A in asthmatics can be prevented by pretreatment with sodium cromoglycate and nedocromil sodium.[39,40] This has led us to postulate that substance P and neurokinin A are indirect broncoconstrictors in man. This indirect bronchoconstrictor effect could arise from an effect on inflammatory cells (e.g., mast cells) and/or nerves. In experimental animals, tachykinins are able to cause acetylcholine release from postganglionic cholinergic airway nerve endings[41,42] and to activate mast cells.[43,44] The exact mechanism of tachykinin-induced bronchoconstriction in man is, however, not yet known. In some patients cholinergic mechanisms do play a role.[45] Histamine, however, does not seem to be involved as pretreatment with different H_1 receptor antagonists (astemizole and terfenadine) did not inhibit neurokinin A–induced bronchoconstriction.[45,46] We recently were able to demonstrate that leukotrienes mediate part of the bronchoconstrictor effect of neurokinin A: the cysLT1 receptor antagonist zafirlukast partially inhibited bronchoconstriction induced by inhaled neurokinin A in patients with asthma.[47]

PLASMA EXTRAVASATION

Ablation of sensory nerves by capsaicin pretreatment abolishes airways plasma extravasation induced by a variety of mediators and stimuli, including histamine, serotonin, and cigarette smoke.[48,49] Tachykinin NK_1 receptors that mediate neurogenic plasma extravasation have been visualized on postcapillary endothelial cells.[50] Once plasma extravasation occurs, leukocytes initiate a process that results in slowing down their velocity, rolling on and adhering to the venular endothelium. The involvement of tachykinin NK_1 receptors in the neurogenic plasma extravasation in the central airways of rats and guinea-pigs has been demonstrated by the use of selective tachykinin receptor agonists and antagonists. The tachykinin NK_1 receptors are also implicated in the extravasation caused by hypertonic saline, bradykinin, antigen challenge, or acetylcholine. Tachykinin NK_2 receptors mediate part of the neurogenic plasma extravasation in the secondary bronchi and intraparenchymal airways of the guinea-pig.[51–57]

Using antibodies directed against the tachykinin NK_1 receptor protein, Bowden and colleagues have demonstrated that in the rat trachea tachykinin NK_1 receptors are present on the endothelial cells of the postcapillary venules. These receptors are internalized in endosomes upon binding with substance P. They also observed an increase in the number of tachykinin NK_1 receptor immunoreactive endosomes when the vagus nerve is electrically stimulated, indicating that substance P released by activation of the sensory nerves has a direct effect on the tachykinin NK_1 receptors on postcapillary venular endothelium.[50] In addition to the direct effects of tachykinins on the venular endothelium, indirect mechanisms involving mast cell activation and serotonin (5-HT) release participate in the tachykinin-induced plasma exudation in the respiratory tract of some animal species. In rabbit airways, involvement of 5-HT receptors and arachidonic acid derivates in the tachykinin-induced increase in vascular permeability has been suggested.[54,55] Neurogenic plasma protein extravasation in rat airways involves the activation of tachykinin NK_1 receptors. In F344 but not in BDE rats, an additional indirect mechanism, involving mast cell activation, 5-HT release, and stimulation of 5-HT_2 receptors, participates in this process.[56,57]

Microvascular leakage can now be measured in human airways. A particularly interesting approach is the "dual induction" model: first substance P is inhaled and then sputum is induced by inhalation of hypertonic saline solution. In this way, Van Rensen and colleagues demonstrated that inhalation of substance P induced significant increases in the levels of alpha_2-macroglobulin, ceruloplasmin, and albumin in induced sputum.[58]

PLASTICITY OF TACHYKINERGIC AIRWAY INNERVATION AND ROLE OF NEUROTROPHINS

Allergic airway inflammation may increase the amount of substance P and neurokinin A in the airways, by increasing the number of nerves, and/or by increasing the nonneuronal sources of these tachykinins. One of the factors known to increase the expression of substance P is nerve growth factor (NGF). Nerve growth factor (NGF) belongs to the family of neurotrophins. Neurotrophins control the survival, differentiation, and maintenance of neurons in the peripheral and central nervous system. Under physiological conditions, neurotrophins are produced by nerve-associated cells like glial cells or Schwann cells and by nerve cells themselves, while during inflammation neurotrophins can also be produced by fibroblasts, mast cells, macrophages, and T and B cells [for review see Bonini *et al.*[59] and Braun *et al.*[60]]. In a study performed by Virchow and colleagues, a significant increase in the neurotrophins NGF, brain-derived neurotrophic factor, and neurotrophin-3 was observed in BAL fluid, obtained 18 hours after segmental allergen provocation in patients with asthma.[61] Mice with NGF overexpression from a lung-specific promoter were shown to have an increased number of tachykinin-containing sensory nerve fibers in the airways.[62,63] When NGF is injected in the tracheal wall of guinea-pigs, the substance P expression in airway neurons is enhanced. Moreover, a phenotypic switch in the nature of vagal sensory neurons producing this neuropeptide was observed: large, capsaicin-insensitive nodose neurons become substance P–positive.[64]

One of the factors that might upregulate NGF expression in human airways is inflammation. Indeed, incubation of isolated human airway smooth muscle cells with the pro-inflammatory cytokine interleukin-1beta increased NGF production in a dose-dependent way.[65] Another factor of importance might be respiratory infection: rat airways infected with respiratory syncytial virus (RSV) doubled the expression of NGF.[66]

TACHYKININS AND ALLERGIC AIRWAY INFLAMMATION

Tachykinins have a wide array of immunomodulatory effects that might contribute to inflammatory processes in the airways,[4,21] It is well known that SP can degranulate rat, murine, and some human mast cells, causing release of histamine, 5-HT, and TNF-α. Both receptor-dependent (NK_1) and receptor-independent mechanisms are involved.[44,67]

In several animal models tachykinins were found to be involved in antigen-induced bronchoconstriction, airway inflammation, and enhanced bronchial responsiveness. In a murine model of lung inflammation, an increased SP-content in the BAL fluid and an increased NK_1 receptor mRNA expression in BAL lymphocytes and alveolar macrophages was observed. Furthermore, the tachykinin NK_1 receptor antagonist CP96345 significantly reduced the number of granulocytes and lymphocytes in BAL after antigen-challenge in sensitized mice.[68] In conscious, unrestrained guinea-pigs, the NK_1 receptor is involved in both the development of antigen-induced airway hyperresponsiveness to histamine and the antigen-induced infiltration of eosinophils, neutrophils, and lymphocytes.[69] On the other hand, the NK_2 receptor is involved in the development of the antigen-induced late reaction.[70] The effect of allergen challenge has also been studied in the Brown Norway (BN) rat model.[71] So from animal studies, it seems that both the tachykinin NK_1 and the NK_2 receptor are involved in antigen-induced airway effects. In addition, it is possible that tachykinin NK_3 receptors are also involved in this process: aerosol administration of the tachykinin NK_3 receptor antagonist SR142801 caused a significant reduction in neutrophil and eosinophil influx in the airways of ovalbumin-sensitized and -challenged mice.[72] At present it is not known whether similar mechanisms operate in human airways: probably an answer to this question will come from studies with dual NK_1/NK_2 or triple NK_1/NK_2/NK_3 tachykinin receptor antagonists.

TACHYKININ ANTAGONISTS: A NEW THERAPY FOR ASTHMA OR COPD?

Studies on rodents have demonstrated that a number of strategies are possible to interfere with the action of sensory neuropeptides in the airways: (1) depletion of neuropeptides within nerves (e.g., by the neurotoxin capsaicin); (2) inhibition of the release of sensory neuropeptides [e.g., by β_2-adrenoceptor agonist, theophylline, cromoglycate, or phophodiesterase (PDE4) inhibitors]; and (3) inhibition of tachykinin receptors by receptor antagonists.[73]

In animal models tachykinins and their receptors have been involved in airway responses to nonspecific stimuli. Both the NK_1 and the NK_2 tachykinin receptor have been involved in airway contraction induced by cold air, hyperventilation, and cigarette smoke, in plasma extravasation induced by hypertonic saline bronchoconstriction, and in airway hyperresponsiveness induced by viruses, IL-5 and nerve growth factor.[74] The tachykinin NK_1 receptor also promotes ozone-induced lung inflammation.[63] Viral infection causes an upregulation of the tachykinin NK_1 receptor, leading to enhanced neurogenic inflammation.[75] In recent years, the tachykinin NK_3

receptor was found to be involved in citric acid–induced cough and enhanced bronchial responsiveness.[76,77]

At the present time clinical trials with at least four tachykinin antagonists have been performed and reported: FK224, a cyclic peptide tachykinin antagonist for NK_1 and NK_2 receptors; CP-99,994, a non-peptide NK_1 tachykinin receptor antagonist; FK888, a peptidic tachykinin NK_1 receptor antagonist; and SR48968 (saredutant), a non-peptide NK_2 tachykinin receptor antagonist. In our center we recently completed two additional studies, one with the bicyclic peptidic tachykinin NK_2 receptor antagonist MEN 11420 (nepadutant) and one with the dual NK_1/NK_2 tachykinin receptor antagonist DNK333A.

FK244, 4 mg given by metered dose inhaler, was shown to inhibit bradykinin-induced bronchoconstriction and cough in nine asthmatics.[78] These findings suggested that bradykinin causes bronchoconstriction by release of tachykinins from sensory nerves. However, in a similar study, using a lower dose, FK224 had no effect on bradykinin-induced bronchoconstriction.[79] Moreover, we have studied the effect of inhaled FK224 on NKA-induced bronchoconstriction in 10 mild asthmatic patients.[80] Inhaled FK224 had no effect on baseline lung function and offered no protection against NKA-induced bronchoconstriction.

Fahy *et al.* studied the effect of the non-peptide NK_1 tachykinin receptor antagonist CP-99,994 on hypertonic saline-induced bronchoconstriction in 14 patients with mild asthma.[81] Compared to placebo, it had no effect on bronchoconstriction and cough induced by hypertonic saline solution. However it remains to be proved whether this compound at the given dose is able to block the airway responses induced by inhaled SP or NKA.

The NK_1 tachykinin receptor antagonist FK888 has been studied in exercise-induced asthma.[82] Inhalation of FK888 in nine asthmatic subjects had no effect on baseline lung function. While pretreatment with FK888 did not attenuate the maximal decrease in lung function, it did reduce the time of recovery from exercise-induced bronchoconstriction.

The NK_2 tachykinin receptor antagonist SR 48968 (saredutant) (100 mg *per os*) caused a significant inhibition of NKA-induced bronchoconstriction, with a mean 3–5-fold shift of the dose–response curve for NKA to the right.[83] Administration of saredutant for 9 days (100 mg *per os*, each day) did not, however, affect baseline airway caliber or bronchial responsiveness to adenosine.[84] In a recently completed study we found that the NK_2 tachykinin receptor antagonist MEN 11420 (nepadutant) (2 and 8 mg i.v.) shifted the dose–response curve for NKA to the right, in a similar way as observed in the study with SR 48968.[85] These studies are the first to demonstrate activity of a tachykinin NK_2 receptor antagonist demonstrated in airways of man. It is, however, clear that although these agents are potent antagonists *in vitro,*[37,86] their potential to inhibit the bronchoconstrictor effect of neurokinin A in patients with asthma is rather limited. We think that this can be explained by an additional involvement of tachykinin NK_1 receptors in the bronchoconstrictor effect of neurokinin.[26,27] This idea is supported by our recent findings with a dual NK_1/NK_2 receptor antagonist. In a study on 19 patients with asthma, DNK333A, a newly developed NK_1/NK_2 receptor tachykinin receptor antagonist, was able to shift the dose-response curve to inhaled neurokinin A to a large extent (4.8 doubling doses).[87] So, by inhibiting both the tachykinin NK_1 and the NK_2 receptor, a better protection against the bronchoconstrictor effect of NKA was observed.

CONCLUSIONS AND FUTURE PERSPECTIVES

Tachykinins are produced in human airways and mimic various features of asthma and COPD. So, tachykinin receptor antagonists have potential in the treatment of asthma and COPD. However, development of tachykinin receptor antagonists for airways diseases has been rather slow and up to now somehow disappointing. This is in contrast to the extensive and overwhelming preclinical data suggesting a role for tachykinins in asthma and possibly COPD. There are several explanations for this apparent paradox:

1. The lack of efficacy can be easily explained by the low potency or defective pharmacokinetics of the compounds tested so far. Potent tachykinin receptor antagonists have only recently become available and some of them have not been considered for application in airways diseases, but for depression or emesis.[88]
2. Blocking either the NK_1 or the NK_2 receptor is probably an insufficient approach, as most of the effects of tachykinins in the airways are mediated by more than one tachykinin receptor.
3. In the application of a new tachykinin receptor antagonist to airways diseases, it is crucial that one first demonstrates that the antagonist is indeed able to block airway effects of an agonist (e.g., substance P or neurokinin A). This allows to determine the *in vivo* activity of the antagonist under consideration and to determine dose and dosing frequency for further clinical study.

So, in conclusion, the arrival of more potent, and low-molecular single and dual or even triple tachykinin recetor antagonists[89,90] should allow us to obtain a final judgment on the role of tachykinins in airway diseases such as asthma and COPD.

REFERENCES

1. Severini, C., G. Improta, G. Falconieri-Erspamer, et al. 2002. The tachykinin peptide family. Pharmacol. Rev. **54:** 285–322.
2. Barnes, P.J. 1986. Asthma as an axon reflex. Lancet **i:** 242–244.
3. Joos, G.F., P.R. Germonpre, J.C. Kips, *et al.* 1994. Sensory neuropeptides and the human lower airways: present state and future directions Eur. Respir. J. **7:** 1161–1171.
4. Maggi, C.A. 1997. The effects of tachykinins on inflammatory and immune cells. Regul. Pept. **70:** 75–90.
5. Maggi, C.A. 2000. The troubled story of tachykinins and neurokinins Trends Pharmacol. Sci. **21:** 173–175.
6. Di Maria, G.U., S. Bellofiore & P. Geppetti. 1998. Regulation of airway neurogenic inflammation by neutral endopeptidase. Eur. Respir. J. **12:** 1454–1462.
7. Lundberg, J.M., T. Hökfelt, C.-R. Martling, *et al.* 1984. Substance P-immunoreactive sensory nerves in the lower respiratory tract of various mammals including man. Cell Tissue Res. **235:** 251–261.
8. Luts, A., R. Uddman, P. Alm, *et al.* 1993. Peptide-containing nerve fibers in human airways: distribution and coexistence pattern. Int. Arch. Allergy Immunol. **101:** 52–60.
9. Sheldrick, R.L.G., K.F. Rabe, A. Fischer, *et al.* 1995. Further evidence that tachykinin-induced contraction of human isolated bronchus is mediated only by NK2 receptors. Neuropeptides **29:** 281–292.

10. LAMB, J.P. & M.P. SPARROW. 2002. Three-dimensional mapping of sensory innervation with substance p in porcine bronchial mucosa: comparison with human airways Am. J. Respir. Crit. Care Med. **166:** 1269–1281.
11. NIEBER, K., C.R. BAUMGARTEN, R. RATHSACK, *et al.* 1992. Substance P and β-endorphine-like immunoreactivity in lavage fluids of subjects with and without allergic asthma. J. Allergy Clin. Immunol. **90:** 646–652.
12. HEANEY, L.G., L.J.M. CROSS, L.P.A. MCGARVEY, *et al.* 1998. Neurokinin A is the predominant tachykinin in human bronchoalveolar lavage fluid in normal and asthmatic subjects Thorax **53:** 357–362.
13. HAZBUN, M.E., R. HAMILTON, A. HOLIAN & W.L. ESCHENBACHER. 1993. Ozone-induced increases in substance P and 8-epi-prostaglandin F2a in the airways of human subjects. Am. J. Respir. Cell Mol. Biol. **9:** 568–572.
14. KRISHNA, M.T., D.R. SPRINGALL, Q.-H. MENG, *et al.* 1997. Effects of ozone on epithelium and sensory nerves in the bronchial mucosa of healthy humans. Am. J. Respir. Crit. Care Med. **156:** 943–950.
15. BARANIUK, J.N., M. ALI, A. YUTA, *et al.* 1999. Hypertonic saline nasal provocation stimulates nociceptive nerves, substance P release, and glandular mucous exocytosis in normal humans. Am. J. Respir. Crit. Care Med. **160:** 655–662.
16. OLLERENSHAW, S.L., D. JARVIS, C.E. SULLIVAN & A.J. WOOLCOCK. 1991. Substance P immunoreactive nerves in airways from asthmatics and nonasthmatics Eur. Respir. J. **4:** 673–682.
17. HOWARTH, P.H., D.R. SPRINGALL, A.E. REDINGTON, *et al.* 1995. Neuropeptide-containing nerves in endobronchial biopsies from asthmatic and nonasthmatic subjects. Am. J. Respir. Cell Mol. Biol. **3:** 288–296.
18. CHANEZ, P., D. SPRINGALL, A.M. VIGNOLA, *et al.* 1998. Bronchial mucosal immunoreactivity of sensory neuropeptides in severe airway diseases. Am. J. Respir. Crit. Care Med. **158:** 985–990.
19. LILLY, C.M., T.R. BAI, S.A. SHORE, *et al.* 1995. Neuropeptide content of lungs from asthmatic and nonasthmatic patient.s Am. J. Respir. Crit. Care Med. **151:** 548–553.
20. LUCCHINI, R.E., F. FACCHINI, G. TURATO, *et al.* 1997. Increased VIP-positive nerve fibers in the mucous glands of subjects with chronic bronchitis. Am. J. Respir. Crit. Care Med. **156:** 1963–1968.
21. JOOS, G.F. & R.A. PAUWELS. 2000. Pro-inflammatory effects of substance P: new perspectives for the treatment of airway diseases? Trends Pharmacol. Sci. **21:** 131–133.
22. GERMONPRE, P.R., G.R. BULLOCK, B.N. LAMBRECHT, *et al.* 1999. Presence of substance P and neurokinin 1 receptors in human sputum macrophages and U-937 cells. Eur. Respir. J. **14:** 776–782.
23. LAMBRECHT, B.N., P.R. GERMONPRE, E.G. EVERAERT, *et al.* 1999. Endogenously produced substance P contributes to lymphocyte proliferation induced by dendritic cells and direct TCR ligation. Eur. J. Immunol. **29:** 3815–3825.
24. TOMAKI, M., M. ICHINOSE, M. MIURA, *et al.* 1995. Elevated substance P content in induced sputum from patients with asthma and patients with chronic bronchitis. Am. J. Respir. Crit. Care Med. **151:** 613–617.
25. CHU, H.W., M. KRAFT, J.E. KRAUSE, *et al.* 2000. Substance P and its receptor neurokinin 1 expression in asthmatic airways. J. Allergy Clin. Immunol. **106:** 713–722.
26. NALINE, E., M. MOLIMARD, D. REGOLI, *et al.* 1996. Evidence for functional tachykinin NK1 receptors on human isolated small bronchi. Am. J. Physiol. **271:** L763–767.
27. AMADESI, S., J. MOREAU, M. TOGNETTO, *et al.* 2001. NK1 receptor stimulation causes contraction and inositol phosphate increase in medium size human isolated bronchi. Am. J. Respir. Crit. Care Med. **163:** 1206–1211.
28. ADVENIER, C., V. LAGENTE & E. BOICHOT. 1997. The role of tachykinin receptor antagonists in the prevention of bronchial hyperresponsiveness, airway inflammation and cough. Eur. Respir. J. **10:** 1892–906.
29. CANNING, B.J., S.M. REYNOLDS, L.U. ANUKWU, *et al.* 2002. Endogenous neurokinins facilitate synaptic transmission in guinea pig airway parasympathetic ganglia. Am. J. Physiol. Regul. Integr. Comp. Physiol. **283:** R320–R330.
30. ADCOCK, I.M., M. PETERS, C. GELDER, *et al.* 1993. Increased tachykinin receptor gene expression in asthmatic lung and its modulation by steroids. J. Mol. Endocrinol. **11:** 1–7.

31. BAI, T.R., D. ZHOU, T. WEIR, *et al.* 1995. Substance P (NK1)- and neurokinin A (NK2)-receptor gene expression in inflammatory airway disease. Am. J. Physiol. **269:** L309–L317.
32. KATSUNUMA, T., J.C.W. MAK & P.J. BARNES. 1998. Glucocorticoids reduce tachykinin NK2 receptor expression in bovine tracheal smooth muscle. Eur. J. Pharmacol. **344:** 99–106.
33. MAPP, C.E., D. MIOTTO, F. BRACCIONI, *et al.* 2000. The distribution of neurokinin-1 and neurokinin-2 receptors in human central airways. Am. J. Respir. Crit. Care Med. **161:** 207–215.
34. FINNEY, M.J.B., J.A. KARLSSON & C.G.A. PERSSON. 1985. Effects of bronchoconstrictors and bronchodilators on a novel human small airway preparation. Br. J. Pharmacol. **85:** 29–36.
35. ADVENIER, C., E. NALINE, G. DRAPEAU & D. REGOLI. 1987. Relative potencies of neurokinins in guinea-pig trachea and human bronchus. Eur. J. Pharmacol. **139:** 133–137.
36. MARTLING, C.-R., E. THEODORSSON-NORHEIM & J.M. LUNDBERG. 1987. Occurrence and effects of multiple tachykinins; substance P, neurokinin A and neuropeptide K in human lower airways. Life Sci. **40:** 1633–1643.
37. ADVENIER, C., E. NALINE, L. TOTY, *et al.* 1992. Effects on the isolated human bronchus of SR 48968, a potent and selective nonpeptide antagonist of the neurokinin A (NK2) receptors. Am. Rev. Respir. Dis. **146:** 1177–1181.
38. JOOS, G.F., P.R. GERMONPRÉ, J.C. KIPS, *et al.* 1994. Sensory neuropeptides and the human lower airways: present state and future directions. Eur. Respir. J. **7:** 1161–1171.
39. CRIMI, N., F. PALERMO, R. OLIVERI, *et al.* 1988. Effect of nedocromil on bronchospasm induced by inhalation of substance P in asthmatic subjects. Clin. Allergy **18:** 375–382.
40. JOOS, G.F., R.A. PAUWELS & M.E. VAN DER STRAETEN. 1989. The effect of nedocromil sodium on the bronchoconstrictor effect of neurokinin A in subjects with asthma. J. Allergy Clin. Immunol. **83:** 663–668.
41. TANAKA, D.T. & M.M. GRUNSTEIN. 1984. Mechanisms of substance P-induced contraction of rabbit airway smooth muscle. J. Appl. Physiol. **57:** 1551–1557.
42. SZAREK, J.L., J.Z. ZHANG & C.A. GRUETTER. 1993. 5-HT2 receptors augment cholinergic nerve-mediated contraction of rat bronchi. Eur. J. Pharmacol. **231:** 339–346.
43. FEWTRELL, C.M.S., J.C. FOREMAN, C.C. JORDAN, *et al.* 1982. The effects of substance P on histamine and 5-hydroxytryptamine release in the rat. J. Physiol. **330:** 393–411.
44. JOOS, G.F. & R.A. PAUWELS. 1993. The in vivo effect of tachykinins on airway mast cells in the rat. Am. Rev. Respir. Dis. **148:** 922–926.
45. CRIMI, N., F. PALERMO, R. OLIVERI, *et al.* 1990. Influence of antihistamine (astemizole) and anticholinergic drugs (ipratropium bromide) on bronchoconstriction induced by substance P. Ann. Allergy **65:** 115–120.
46. CRIMI, N., R. OLIVERI, R. POLOSA, *et al.* 1993. The effect of oral terfenadine on neurokinin-A induced bronchoconstriction. J. Allergy Clin. Immunol. **91:** 1096–1098.
47. JOOS, G., V. VAN DE VELDE, V. SCHELFHOUT & R. PAUWELS. 2001. The leukotriene receptor antagonist zafirlukast inhibits neurokinin-A induced bronchoconstriction in patients with asthma. Am. J. Respir. Crit. Care Med. **163:** A418.
48. LUNDBERG, J.M. & A. SARIA. 1983. Capsaicin-induced desensitization of airway mucosa to cigarette smoke, mechanical and chemical irritants. Nature **302:** 215–253.
49. SARIA, A., J.M. LUNDBERG, G. SKOFITSCH & F. LEMBECK. 1983. Vascular protein leakage in various tissues induced by substance P, capsaicin, bradykinin, serotonin, histamine and by antigen challenge. Naunyn-Schmiedeberg's Arch. Pharmacol. **324:** 212–218.
50. BOWDEN, J.J., A.M. GARLAND, P. BALUK, *et al.* 1994. Direct observation of substance P-induced internalization of neurokinin 1 (NK1) receptors at sites of inflammation. Proc. Natl. Acad. Sci. USA **91:** 8964–8968.
51. QIAN, Y., X. EMONDS-ALT & C. ADVENIER. 1993. Effects of capsaicin, (+/-)-CP 96,345 and SR 48968 on the bradykinin-induced airways microvascular leakage in guinea-pigs. Pulm. Pharmacol. **6:** 63–67.
52. DELAY-GOYET, P., A. FRANCO-CERCEDA, S.F. GONSALVES, *et al.* 1992. CP-96,345 antagonism of NK1 receptors and smoke-induced protein extravasation in relation to its cardiovascular effects. Eur. J. Pharmacol. **222:** 213–218.

53. BERTRAND, C., P. GEPPETTI, J. BAKER, *et al.* 1993. Tachykinins, via NK1 receptor activation, play a relevant role in plasma protein extravasation evoked by allergen challenge in the airways of sensitized guinea-pigs. Regul. Pept. **46:** 214–216.
54. DELAUNOIS, A., P. GUSTIN & M. ANSAY. 1993. Role of neuropeptides in acetylcholine-induced edema in isolated and perfused rabbit lungs. J. Pharmacol. Exp. Ther. **266:** 483–491.
55. DELAUNOIS, A., P. GUSTIN & M. ANSAY. 1993. Effects of capsaicin on the endothelial permeability in isolated and perfused rabbit lungs. Fund. Clin. Pharmacol. **7:** 81–91.
56. GERMONPRÉ, P.R., G.F. JOOS, E. EVERAERT, *et al.* 1995. Characterization of neurogenic inflammation in the airways of two highly inbred rat strains. Am. J. Respir. Crit. Care Med. **152:** 1796–1804.
57. GERMONPRÉ, P.R., G.F. JOOS, K. MEKEIRELE & R.A. PAUWELS. 1997. Role of the 5-HT receptor in neurogenic inflammation in Fisher 344 rat airways. Eur. J. Pharmacol. **324:** 249–255.
58. VAN RENSEN, E.L., P.S. HIEMSTRA, K.F. RABE & P.J. STERK. 2002. Assessment of microvascular leakage via sputum induction: the role of substance P and neurokinin A in patients with asthma. Am. J. Respir. Crit. Care Med. **165:** 1275–1279.
59. BONINI, S., A. LAMBIASE, F. LEVI-SCHAFFER & L. ALOE. 1999. Nerve growth factor: an important molecule in allergic inflammation and tissue remodelling. Int. Arch. Allergy Immunol. **118:** 159–162.
60. BRAUN, A., M. LOMMATZSCH & H. RENZ. 2000. The role of neurotrophins in allergic bronchial asthma. Clin. Exp. Allergy **30:** 178–186.
61. VIRCHOW, J.C., P. JULIUS, M. LOMMATZSCH, *et al.* 1998. Neurotrophins are increased in bronchoalveolar lavage fluid after segmental allergen provocation. Am. J. Respir. Crit. Care Med. **158:** 2002–2005.
62. HOYLE, G.W., R.G. GRAHAM, J.B. FINKELSTEIN, *et al.* 1998. Hyperinnervation of the airways in transgenic mice overexpressing nerve growth factor. Am. J. Respir. Cell Mol. Biol. **18:** 149–157.
63. GRAHAM, R.M., M. FRIEDMAN & G.W. HOYLE. 2001. Sensory nerves promote ozone-induced lung inflammation in mice Am. J. Respir. Crit Care Med. **164:** 307–313.
64. HUNTER, D.D., A.C. MYERS & B.J. UNDEM. 2000. Nerve Growth factor-induced phenotypic switch in guinea pig airway sensory neurons. Am. J. Respir. Crit. Care Med. **161:** 1985–1990.
65. FREUND, V., F. PONS, V. JOLY, *et al.* 2002. Upregulation of nerve growth factor expression by human airway smooth muscle cells in inflammatory conditions. Eur. Respir. J. **20:** 458–463.
66. HU, C., K. WEDDE-BEER, A. AUAIS, *et al.* 2002. Nerve growth factor and nerve growth factor receptors in respiratory syncytial virus-infected lungs. Am. J. Physiol. Lung Cell Mol. Physiol. **283:** L494–L502.
67. JOOS, G.F., R.A. LEFEBVRE, G. BULLOCK & R.A. PAUWELS. 1997. Role of 5-hydroxytryptamine and mast cells in the tachykinin-induced contraction of rat trachea *in vitro*. Eur. J. Pharmacol. **338:** 259–268.
68. KALTREIDER, H.B., S. ICHIKAWA, P.K. BYRD, *et al.* 1997. Upregulation of neuropeptides and neuropeptide receptors in a murine model of immune inflammation in lung parenchyma. Am. J. Respir. Cell Mol. Biol. **16:** 133–144.
69. SCHUILING, M., A. ZUIDHOF, J. ZAAGSMA & H. MEURS. 1999. Involvement of tachykinin NK1 receptor in the development of allergen-induced airway hyperreactivity and airway inflammation in conscious, unrestrained guinea-pigs. Am. J. Respir. Crit. Care Med. **159:** 423–430.
70. SCHUILING, M., A. ZUIDHOF, H. MEURS & J. ZAAGSMA. 1999. Role of tachykinin NK2-receptor activation in the allergen-induced late asthmatic reaction, airway hyperreactivity and airway inflammation cell influx in conscious, unrestrained guinea-pigs. Br. J. Pharmacol. **127:** 1030–1038.
71. MAGHNI, K., R. TAHA, W. AFIF, *et al.* 2000. Dichotomy between neurokinin receptor actions in modulating allergic airway responses in an animal model of helper T cell type 2 cytokine-associated inflammation. Am. J. Respir. Crit. Care Med. **162:** 1068–1074.

72. NÉNAN, S., N. GERMAIN, V. LAGENTE, *et al.* 2001. Inhibition of inflammatory cell recruitment by the tachykinin NK_3-receptor antagonist, SR 14280, in a murine model of asthma. Eur. J. Pharmacol. **421:** 210–205.
73. LUNDBERG, J.M. 1996. Pharmacology of Cotransmission in the Autonomic Nervous System: integrative aspects on amines, neuropeptides, adenosine triphosphate, amino acids and nitric oxide. Pharmacol. Rev. **48:** 113–178.
74. JOOS, G.F., K.O. DE SWERT & R.A. PAUWELS. 2001. Airway inflammation and tachykinins: prospects for the development of tachykinin receptor antagonists. Eur. J Pharmacol. **429:** 239–250.
75. PIEDIMONTE, G. 2001. Neural mechanisms of respiratory syncytial virus-induced inflammation and prevention of respiratory syncytial virus sequelae. Am. J. Respir. Crit. Care Med. **163:** S18–S21.
76. DAOUI, S., C. COGNON, E. NALINE & X. EDMONDS-ALT. 1998. Involvement of tachykinin NK3 receptors in citric acid-induced cough and bronchial responses in guinea pigs. Am. J. Respir. Crit. Care Med. **158:** 42–48.
77. DAOUI, S., E. NALINE, V. LAGENTE, *et al.* 2000. Neurokinin B- and specific tachykinin NK(3) receptor agonists-induced airway hyperresponsiveness in the guinea-pig. Br. J. Pharmacol. **130:** 49–56.
78. ICHINOSE, M., N. NAKAJIMA, T. TAKAHASHI, *et al.* 1992. Protection against bradykinin-induced bronchoconstriction in asthmatic patients by neurokinin receptor antagonist Lancet **340:** 1248–1251.
79. SCHMIDT, D., R.A. JORRES, K.F. RABE & H. MAGNUSSEN. 1996. Reproducibility of airway response to inhaled bradykinin and effect of the neurokinin receptor antagonist FK-224 in asthmatic subjects. Eur. J. Clin. Pharmacol. **50:** 269–273.
80. JOOS, G.F., J. VAN SCHOOR, J.C. KIPS & R.A. PAUWELS. 1996. The effect of inhaled FK244, a tachykinin NK-1 and NK-2 receptor antagonist, on neurokinin A-induced bronchoconstriction in asthmatics. Am. J. Respir. Crit. Care Med. **153:** 1781–1784.
81. FAHY, J.V., H.H. WONG, P. GEPPETTI, *et al.* 1995. Effect of an NK1 receptor antagonist (CP-99,994) on hypertonic saline-induced bronchoconstriction and cough in male asthmatic subjects. Am. J. Resp. Crit. Care Med. **152:** 879–884.
82. ICHINOSE, M., M. MIURA, H. YAMAUCHI, *et al.* 1996. A neurokinin 1-receptor antagonist improves exercise-induced airway narrowing in asthmatic patients. Am. J. Respir. Crit. Care Med. **153:** 936–941.
83. VAN SCHOOR, J., G. JOOS, B. CHASSON, *et al.* 1998. The effect of the NK2 receptor antagonist SR48968 (saredutant) on neurokinin A-induced bronchoconstrction in asthmatics. Eur. Respir. J. **12:** 17–23.
84. KRAAN, J., H. VINK-KLOOSTER & D.S. POSTMA. 2001. The NK-2 receptor antagonist SR 48968C does not improve adenosine hyperresponsiveness and airway obstruction in allergic asthma. Clin. Exp. Allergy **31:** 274–278.
85. JOOS, G., V. SCHELFHOUT, V. VAN DE VELDE & R. PAUWELS. 2001. The effect of the tachykinin NK2 receptor antagonist MEN11420 (nepadutant) on neurokinin A-induced bronchoconstriction in patients with asthma. Am. J. Respir. Crit. Care Med. **163:** A628.
86. CATALIOTO, R.-M., M. CRISCUOLI, P. CUCCHI, *et al.* 1998. MEN 11420 (Nepadutant), a novel glycosylated bicyclic peptide tachykinin NK2 receptor antagonist. Br. J. Pharmacol. **123:** 81–91.
87. JOOS, G., W. VINCKEN, R.E. LOUIS, *et al.* 2001. The effect of the dual NK1/NK2 tachykinin receptor antagonist DNK333A on neurokinin A-induced bronchoconstriction in patients with asthma. Am. J. Respir. Crit. Care Med. **163:** A628.
88. DIEMUNSCH, P. & L. GRELOT. 2000. Potential of substance P antagonists as antiemetics Drugs **60:** 533–546.
89. RUMSEY, W.L., D. AHARONY, R.A. BIALECKI, *et al.* 2001. Pharmacological characterization of ZD6021: a novel, orally active antagonist of the tachykinin receptors. J. Pharmacol. Exp. Ther. **298:** 307–315.
90. ANTHES, J.C., R.W. CHAPMAN, C. RICHARD, *et al.* 2002. SCH 206272: a potent, orally active tachykinin NK(1), NK(2), and NK(3) receptor antagonist. Eur. J. Pharmacol. **450:** 191–202.

Endocrine and Immune Responses to Stress in Chronic Inflammatory Skin Disorders

ANGELIKA BUSKE-KIRSCHBAUM AND DIRK H. HELLHAMMER

Department of Psychobiology, University of Trier, Trier, Germany

ABSTRACT: Atopy is a genetically and environmentally determined condition predisposing to different forms such as atopic dermatitis (AD) or allergic asthma (AA). Both AD and AA are considered to be multifactorial diseases; however, distinct immunologic abnormalities have been described that play a crucial role. There is growing evidence that immunoglobulin-E hypersecretion and activation of the predominantly T-helper-2 (TH2)-like T cell subset trigger allergic inflammatory processes and cause the disease to become chronic. In the present paper, data suggesting reduced hypothalamic-pituitary-adrenal (HPA) axis responsiveness in patients with AD and AA are summarized, and the potential etiologic significance of a hyporeactive HPA axis is discussed. We propose that because of defective HPA axis, immunoregulation under stressful conditions is ineffective in patients with atopic conditions, leading to aberrant immune responses and subsequent exacerbation of the disease. Further research into the role of the HPA axis in atopy may elucidate the cause of stress-induced exacerbation of atopic symptoms and may be of clinical relevance.

KEYWORDS: stress; atopic dermatitis; psoriasis; hypothalamic-pituitary-adrenal (HPA) axis; sympathetic-adrenomedullary (SAM) system; psychoneuroimmunology

INTRODUCTION

Atopic dermatitis (AD) is a chronic inflammatory skin disease characterized by symptoms such as dry and eczematous skin lesions, lichenification, and an often torturing pruritus. There is general agreement that AD is a multifactorial disease triggered by multiple factors such as genetic predisposition, allergens, altered vascular reactivity, or microbial organisms.[1] However, despite expanding research efforts in this field, the pathogenesis of AD is still obscure and not fully understood. In the last two decades, a growing number of reports point to the relevance of an underlying immunoregulatory abnormality in AD.[2] In AD patients, exposure to environmental allergens leads to B cell activation and profound secretion of allergen-specific immunoglobulin-E (IgE). IgE antibodies bind to high-affinity IgE receptors on mast cells and basophils that are present in various tissues, particularly the skin. Subseqent allergen contact leads to cross-linking of receptor-bound IgE molecules, triggering the release of proinflammatory mediators (i.e., histamines).

Address for correspondence: Dr. Angelika Buske-Kirschbaum, Department of Psychobiology, University of Trier, Trier, Germany.

Ann. N.Y. Acad. Sci. 992: 231–240 (2003). © 2003 New York Academy of Sciences.

These substances are known to initiate immediate hypersensitivity reactions characterized by redness of the skin, erythema, and itching.[3] Several lines of evidence, however, have extablished that the immediate hypersensitivity reaction is only part of a larger response, called the "late phase response," leading to chronic local inflammation of the skin predominantly mediated by eosinophils. It could be demonstrated that Langerhans cells express high-affinity IgE receptors and that binding of IgE stimulates Langerhans cells to fragment and present allergen to T cells, mainly to the T-helper-2 (TH2)-like T cell subset.[4] There is broad acceptance that a predominant stimulation of TH2 cells and a subsequent release of mainly TH2-derived cytokines, such as interleukin-4 (IL-4), IL-5, IL–10, and IL-13, plays a critical role in the maintenance of AD and in its chronicity. IL-4 and IL-13 stimulate IgE synthesis and induce B cells to switch from other Ig isotypes to IgE. They further induce expression of VCAM-1, leading to the adhesion and recruitment of eosinophils to the inflammatory site. IL-5 activates eosinophils to secrete toxic proteins that are known to be mainly responsible for the tissue damage found in AD.[5,6]

Besides profound immunoregulatory abnormalities, an increasing number of reports underscore the relevance of psychological factors such as stress in AD.[7] Early clinical findings indicate that 50–70% of persons with AD experienced severe stress or trauma before the onset of the disease.[8] These reports are in line with more recent findings suggesting that increased levels of everyday stress are associated with aggravation of AD symptoms 24 hours late.[9] The relevance of psychosocial stress in triggering AD is further emphasized by the positive effect of psychological interventions including stress management or relaxation training, which were shown to lead to significant improvement in AD symptoms.[10,11] Although it is well established that the severity of AD is promoted by stress, the underlying mechanisms of stress-induced exacerbation of AD symptoms remains to be determined.

A potential hint as to *how* stress may affect chronic allergic inflammatory processes comes from psychoneuroimmunologic findings.[12] Research has demonstrated that stress affects atopy-relevant immune responses such as IgE production, degranulation of cutanous mast cells, leukocyte adhesion, secretion of TH1/TH2-derived cytokines, or eosinphil activation and migration.[13–17] In this functional neuroimmunologic network, the hypothalamus-pituitary-adrenal (HPA) axis has been most frequently discussed as one major pathway through which the central nervous system (CNS) exerts its influence on immune processes under stressful conditions.[18] The immunoregulatory relevance of the HPA axis has been further emphasized in that an appropriate HPA axis response to stress is even necessary to control the immune system and to prevent an immune process, such as an inflammatory response, from reaching a level that may be damaging to the host.[19,20] This assumption is strongly supported by animal data showing that blunted responsiveness of the HPA axis to stress is closely linked to increased susceptibility to inflammatory disease.[21,22]

Regarding these data it may be intriguing to postulate that also in chronic *allergic* inflammation, reduced HPA axis responsiveness may be a significant factor. It may be speculated that the inability of the atopic patient to exert an appropriate HPA axis response and thus to generate an adequate regulatory (immunosuppressive) signal for the immunologic target cell may increase the risk for aberrant immune functioning, especially under stressful conditions. This model could explain the often described stress-related exacerbation of allergic inflammation and subsequently of atopic symptoms.

In a series of studies our laboratory followed this line of reasoning to investigate HPA axis function under stress in chronic allergic disease. In the first study, children with AD were confronted with a standardized laboratory stressor (Trier Social Stress Test for Children, TSST-C) including free speech and mental arithmetic in front of a panel. The TSST-C was adapted from the "Trier-Social-Stress-Test" (TSST), which has been demonstrated in numerous studies to significantly stimulate the HPA axis and the sympathetic adrenomedullary (SAM) system.[23] As expected, control subjects showed a significant increase in cortisol levels in response to the stressor; however, a significantly blunted cortisol response was observed in children with AD (FIG. 1A). No difference between the two groups could be observed in heart rate responses to the stress test or in personality aspects including emotional excitability, anxiety, self-conviction, or ambition in school.[24] These findings suggest that the adrenocortical response to stress is attenuated in patients with AD, which is in line with previous reports by Ruprecht and coworkers.[25,26] They reported reduced cortisol levels to a corticotropin-releasing hormone (CRH) challenge as well as an increased number of glucocorticoid receptors in the peripheral lymphocytes of adults with AD. These findings support the idea of a hyporesponsive HPA axis and a potentially compensatory upregulation of glucocorticoid binding sites due to the long-term reduced action of endogenous cortisol in persons with AD.

Regarding these findings, the question arises of whether a hyporesponsive HPA axis is a characteristic feature of skin atopy or whether it is generally linked to chronic allergic inflammatory processes. Following this question, we recently investigated HPA axis responsiveness in children with allergic asthma (AA). AA is a chronic disorder of the airways characterized by airway inflammation and airflow obstruction. The immunopathology of AA parallels the immunopathology of AD in that IgE-mediated inflammation, TH2-cell-predominant immune responses, and eosinophilia have been described.[27] AA is often considered a chronic bronchial inflammatory condition of the "atopic triad."[28] We found that when exposed to psychosocial stress, children with AA showed significantly blunted cortisol responses compared to those of a non-atopic control group (FIG. 1B). Again, no differences could be determined in heart rate responses to the stressor or in psychological variables such as subjective stress experience or subjective well-being after the stressor.[29]

These data strongly support the idea that reduced HPA axis reactivity as found in patients with AD probably does not reflect a specific phenomenon linked to skin atopy, but rather is a general phenomenon associated with allergic inflammation regardless of the target organ.

The finding of a dysfunctional HPA axis also in asthmatic patients may be of clinical significance. Increasing data suggest exacerbation of AA symptoms after stress. Various acute stressful situations, such as watching stressful film sequences[30] or being confronted with stressful interactions,[31] are reported to worsen respiratory capacity in AA patients. In parallel to the model just described for AD patients, it may be hypothesized that the failure of AA patients to render an adequate immunoregulatory HPA axis response to stress may facilitate atopy-relevant immunologic changes, leading to exacerbation of AA and its chronicity. To further strenghten this model we investigated whether in patients with AD with hyporeactivity of the HPA axis to stress, aberrant immune responses and further worsening of atopic symptoms can be observed. Adult AD patients were exposed to the TSST. Blood and saliva samples were obtained before and after the stress test as well as 24 hours later at

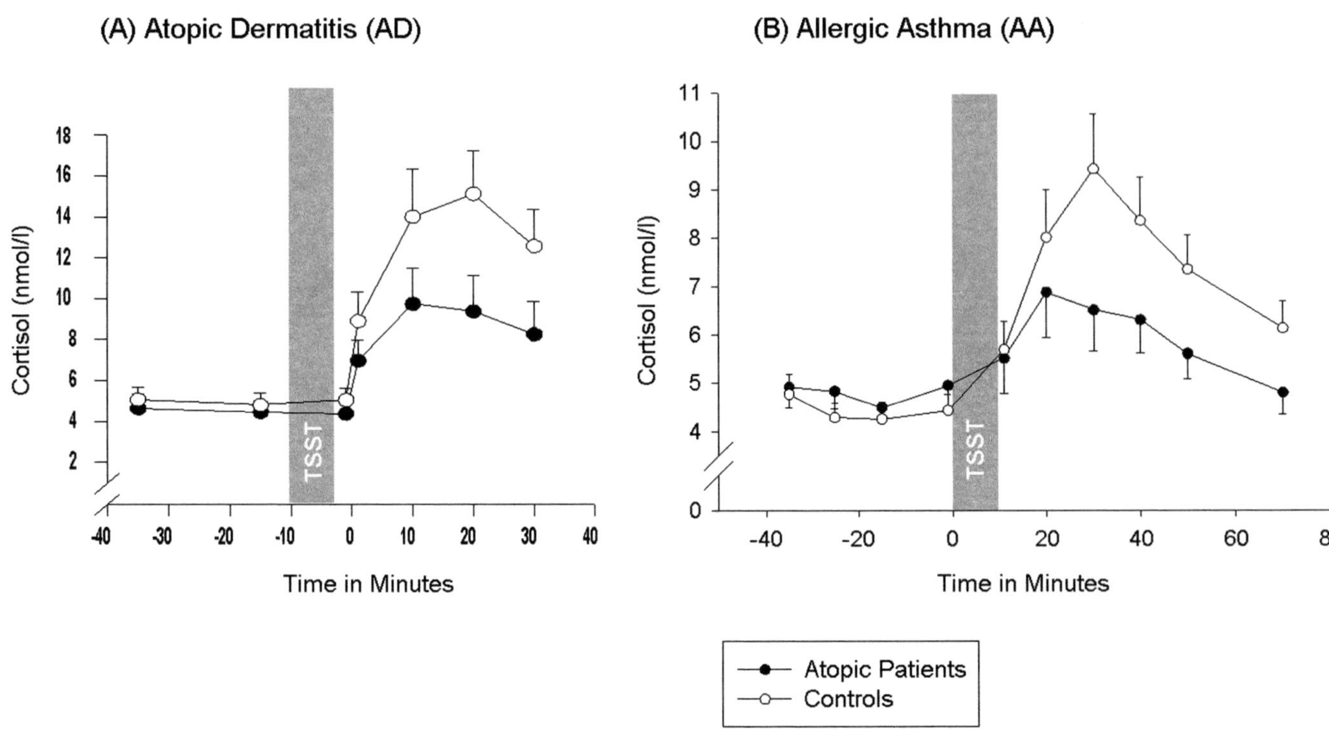

FIGURE 1. Alteration of cortisol levels in response to psychosocial stress (TSST-C) in (**A**) children with atopic dermatitis (AD) and (**B**) children with allergic asthma and non-atopic controls.

identical time points under resting conditions. Again, in this study, HPA axis responsiveness was significantly reduced in AD patients as indicated by a blunted cortisol level and, moreover, a blunted ACTH response to the stressor[32] (FIG. 2). The latter observation supports the idea that dysfunction of the HPA axis may be located at the suprapituitary side. This would be in line with animal data suggesting deficient paraventricular nucleus CRH mRNA levels in LEW/N rats, which are characterized by a hyporesponsivenss of the HPA axis and high vulnerability to inflammatory disease.[33]

Most interesting, however, is that under stress, distinct immunologic alterations, such as a significant increase in eosinophil number and IgE levels, were found in subjects with AD but not in control subjects (FIG. 3).[34] These immune changes may be of clinical relevance. Eosinophils are considered to play a crucial role in AD, and recruitment and activation of eosinophils are assumed to precede exacerbation of AD.[5,6] When activated, eosinophils can secrete cytotoxic mediators that are positively correlated with disease severity and that have been described as contributing to tissue injury.[35] IgE is widely accepted as a key molecule in AD and enables immediate hypersensitivity reactions by stimulating mast cells and basophils. It further propagates the recruitment and activation of atopy-relevant TH2-cells initiating the late phase response and chronicity of the disease.[3,4]

The finding of increased eosinophil numbers and IgE levels in response to stress in AD patients, but not in healthy control subjects, is intriguing because it could be an additional piece in the puzzle of how stress may affect the atopic condition. From these data it could be speculated that when being stressed, atopic patients show an attenuated HPA axis response, leading to reduced ACTH and cortisol release. This hyporesponsiveness of the HPA axis is accompanied by a "shift" towards an immune profile known to trigger chronic allergic inflammation. The potential pathological relevance of these immune changes is underlined by the observation that 24 hours after the stress test, significant worsening of the skin condition in our AD subjects could be determined.[34]

It is important to keep in mind, however, that our data linking attenuated HPA axis responsiveness to chronic allergic inflammation in AA and AD are of a correlational nature. It stilll remains to be determined whether attenuated reactivity of the HPA axis in patients with AD represents a (genetically determined) predisposition of the individual that may contribute to the development of atopy, or alternatively, whether attenuated HPA axis reactivity is a consequence of long-term chronic inflammation. The latter assumption would be supported by findings demonstrating activation of the HPA axis by proinflammatory cytokines with later downregulation of the system in chronic inflammatory conditions.[18,36] With this in mind we studied newborns with atopic predisposition as defined by a positive family history of atopy (at least one parent was atopic) and elevated IgE levels (IgE>kU/l) in cord blood. With this study we tested whether a hyporeactive HPA axis can be observed early in life before the onset of (potential) allergic inflammation and therefore may be of etiologic significance. In contrast to our expectations, we found that newborns with a predisposition to atopy showed *elevated* cortisol responses to venipuncture stress when compared to newborns without atopic predisposition.[37] Venipuncture has often been demonstrated to induce significant activation of the HPA axis and lead to marked release of cortisol.[38] Combining the data may be puzzling. One may wonder what the potential link might be between the previous observations of *hypo*reactivity

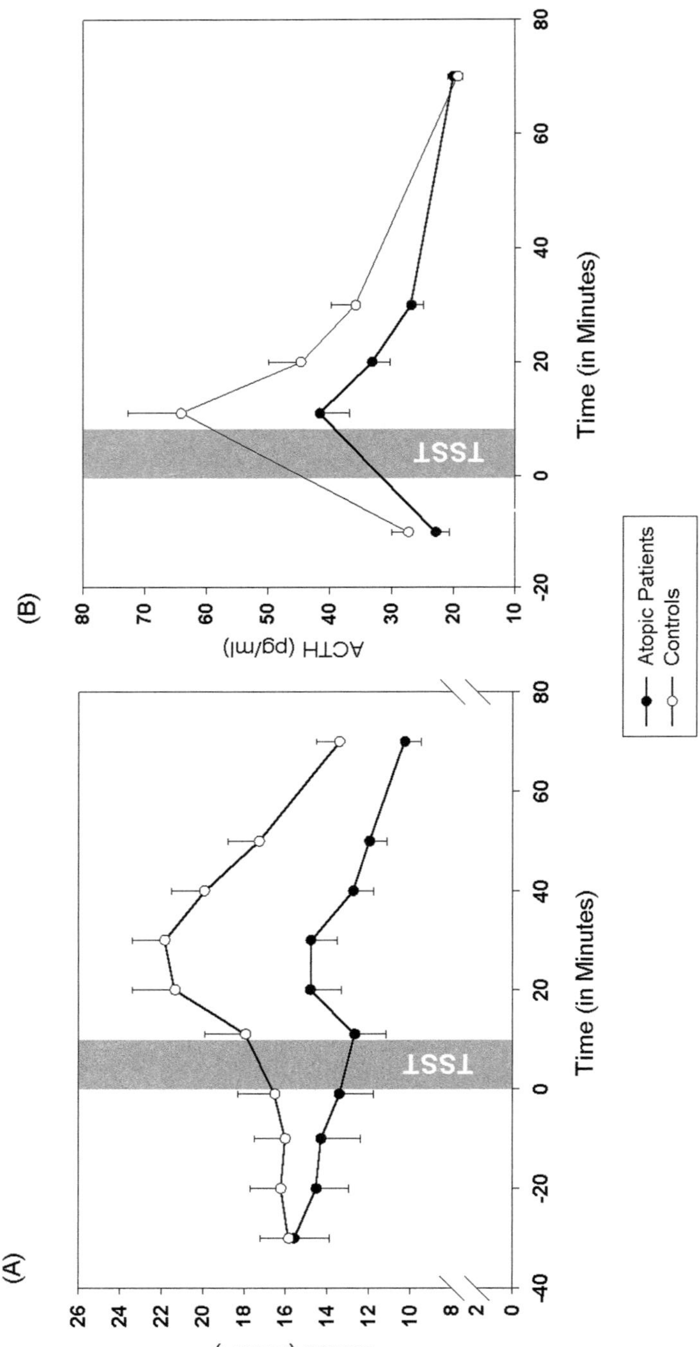

FIGURE 2. Changes of cortisol (**A**) and ACTH (**B**) levels in response to psychosocial stress (TSST) in patients with atopic dermatitis and non-atopic controls.

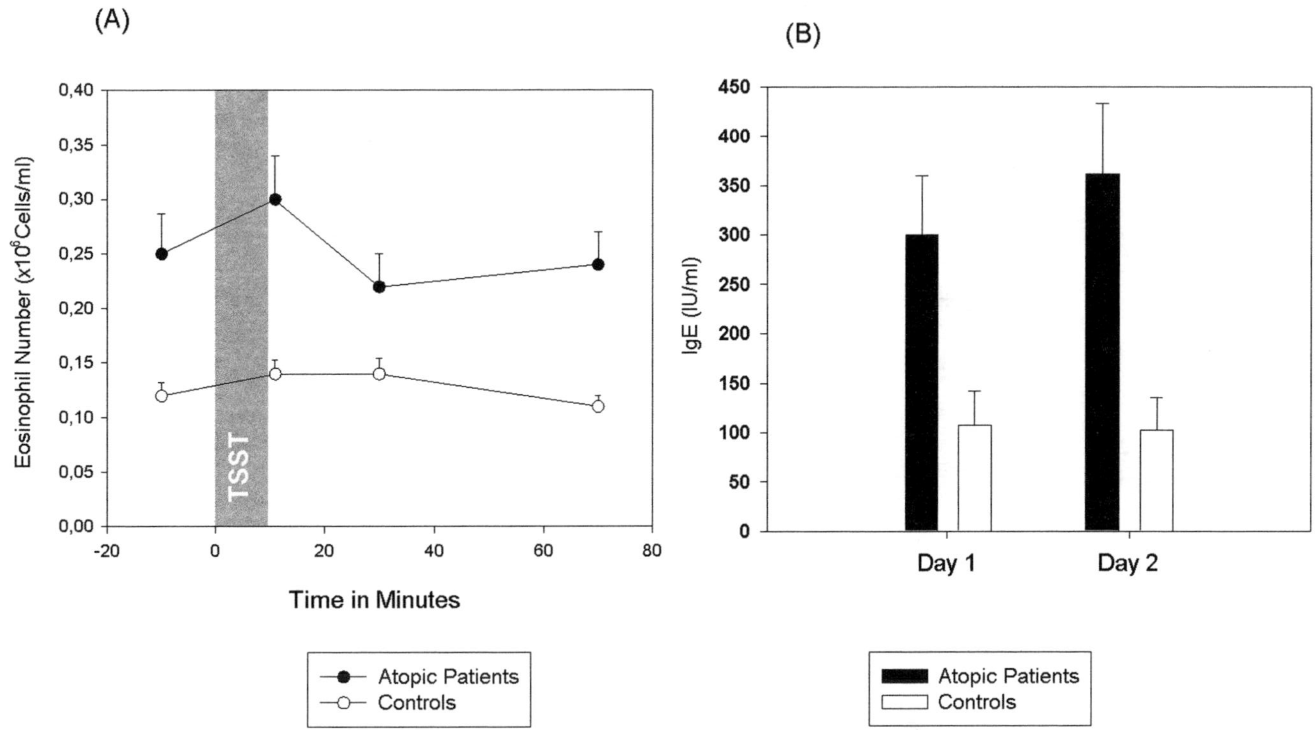

FIGURE 3. Changes in **(A)** eosinophil number and **(B)** IgE levels in response to psychosocial stress (TSST) in patients with atopic dermatitis (AD) and non-atopic controls.

of the HPA axis in persons with long-term AD and the observation of *hyper*reactivity of the system in newborns with atopic predisposition. To fit the two findings together, it could be speculated that with the onset of the disease and/or its becoming chronic, the HPA axis may switch from a hyper- to a hyporeactive state. To date, no convincing data are available to support this hypothesis. However, there are reports suggesting that the long-term release of proinflammatory cytokines (as observed after onset of allergic inflammation) can diminish HPA axis responsiveness due to increased negative feedback produced by persistently increased endogenous cortisol concentrations.[36,39] Alternatively, psychological factors such as chronic stress or altered maternal behavior (increased licking and grooming) have been emphasized to be linked to a blunted HPA axis responsiveness in animals.[40,41] Although these animal data are difficult to transfer to human beings, they provide evidence that the magnitude of the HPA axis response is associated with the experience of chronic stress or a distinct (overprotective) mother-child interaction. Both factors, however, an increased everyday stress level and an altered mother-child interaction characterized by overprotection, have been described for the atopic patient.[42]

In this article, reduced HPA axis responsiveness as indicated by low ACTH and cortisol responses after stress was described in atopic patients. We suggested that the dysfunction of the HPA axis in these patients may be located at the suprapituitary side and may be a common feature of the atopic condition independent of the target organ being affected. Regarding the immunoregulatory relevance of the HPA axis, we proposed a psychoendocrine-immunologic pathway, which may explain how stress can affect atopic symptoms. In this model we speculated that a disminished HPA axis response may result in altered immune functions and, subsequently, in increased vulnerability to develop or exacerbate allergic inflammation. Because the HPA axis is significantly involved in the adaptive stress response, aggravation of disease can mainly be expected under stress. This model was supported by our data showing that stress can result in atopy-relevant immune changes with subsequent exacerbation of atopic symptoms. It is important to note, however, that data of a hyporesponsive HPA axis in atopic patients can be correlated, and the etiologic significance of a dysfunctional HPA axis remains to be determined. Is a hyporeactive HPA axis really involved in the pathogenesis of atopy or is it one additional symptom resulting from a long-term disease process or even an epiphenomenon without clinical relevance? We found that altered HPA axis reactivity, that is, increased responsiveness of the system, is linked to an atopic disposition, suggesting that alteration of HPA axis functioning is evident before the onset of an ongoing inflammatory response. Does this mean that patients with atopic conditions show a genetically determined hypersensitivity of the HPA axis that alters in a hyporesponsive system due to psychological, immunologic, or other factors linked to chronic disease?

It is clear that additional research is necessary to further elucidate the significance of the HPA axis in chronic allergic inflammatory disease. Interdisciplinary research strategies may help to further clarify the psychoendocrine-immune pathways being involved in stress-induced exacerbation of the disease, which may lead to new disease concepts and promising therapeutic regimens.

ACKNOWLEDGMENT

This work was supported by Deutsche Forschungsgemeinschaft Grant He 1013/13-1.

REFERENCES

1. LEUNG, D.Y. 2000. Atopic dermatitis: new insights and opportunities for therapeutic interventions. J. Allergy Clin. Immunol. **105:** 860–876.
2. LEUNG, D.Y. 1999. Pathogenesis of atopic dermatitis. J. Allergy Clin. Immunol. **104:** S99–S108.
3. BOGUNIEWICZ, M. 1997. Advances in the understanding and treatment of atopic dermatitis. Curr. Opin. Pediatr. **9:** 577–581.
4. EEDY, D.J. 2001. What's new in atopic dermatitis? Br. J. Dermatol. **145:** 380–384.
5. LEUNG, D.Y. & N.A. SOTER. 2001. Cellular and immunologic mechanisms in atopic dermatitis. J. Am. Acad. Dermatol. **44:** S1–S12.
6. GREWE, M., C.A.F.M. BRUUIJNZEEL-KOOMEN, E. SCHÖPF, *et al.* 1998. A role for Th1 and Th2 cells in the immunopathogenesis of atopic dermatitis. Immunol. Today **19:** 359–361.
7. BUSKE-KIRSCHBAUM, A., A. GEIBEN & D.H. HELLHAMMER. 2001. Psychobiological aspects of atopic dermatitis: an overview. Psychother. Psychosom. **70:** 6–16.
8. BROWN, D.G. 1972. Stress as a precipitant factor of eczema. J. Psychosom. Res. **16:** 321–327.
9. KING, R.M. & G.V. WILSON. 1991. Use of a diary technique to investigate psychosomatic relations in atopic dermatitis. J. Psychosom. Res. **35:** 697–706.
10. EHLERS, A., U. STANGIER & U. GIELER. 1995. Treatment of atopic dermatitis: a comparison of psychological and dermatological approaches to relapse prevention. J. Consult. Clin. Psychol. **63:** 624–635.
11. MELIN, L., T. FREDERIKSEN, P. NOREN, *et al.* 1986. Behavioral treatment of scratching in patients with atopic dermatitis. Br. J. Dermatol. **115:** 467–474.
12. ADER, R., D.L. FELTEN & N. COHEN. 2000. Psychoneuroimmunology. Academic Press. San Diego.
13. PERSOONS, J.H., F. BERKENBOSCH, K. SCHORNAGE, *et al.* 1995. Increased specific IgE production in lungs after the induction of acute stress in rats. J. Allergy Clin. Immunol. **95:** 765–770.
14. SINGH, L.K., N. ALEXACOS, R. LETOURNEAU, *et al.* 1999. Acute immobilization stress triggers skin mast cell degranulation via corticotropin releasing hormone, neurotensin and substance P: a link to neurogenic skin disorders. Brain Behav. Immunol. **13:** 225–239.
15. SCHMID-OTT, G., B. JAEGER, C. ADAMEK, *et al.* 2001. Levels of circulating CD8 (+) T lymphocytes, natural killer cells and eosinophils increase upon acute psychosocial stress in patients with atopic dermatitis. J. Allergy Clin. Immunol. **107:** 171–177.
16. GOEBEL, M.U. & P.J. MILLS. 2000. Acute psychological stress and exercise and changes in the peripheral leukocyte adhesion expression and density. Psychosom. Med. **62:** 664–670.
17. PAIK I.H., K.Y. TOH, C. LEE, *et al.* 2000. Psychological stress may induce increased humoral and decreased cellular immunity. Behav. Med. **26:** 139–141.
18. CHROUSOS, G.P. 1995. The hypothalamus-pituitary-adrenal axis and immune mediated inflammation. N. Engl. J. Med. **332:** 1351–1362.
19. STERNBERG, E.M. 2001. Neuroendocrine regulation of autoimmune/inflammatory disease. J. Endocrinol. **169:** 429-435.
20. CHROUSOS, G.P. 2000. Stress, chronic inflammation, and emotional and physical well-being: concurrent effects and chronic sequelae. J. Allergy Clin. Immunol. **106:** S275–S291.
21. STERNBERG, E.M., J.M. HILL, G.P. CHROUSSOS, *et al.* 1989. Inflammatory mediator-induced hypothalamic-pituitary-adrenal axis activation is defective in streptococcal cell wall arthritis-susceptible Lewis rats. Proc. Natl. Acad. Sci. USA **86:** 2374–2378.
22. TONELLI, L., J.I. WEBSTER, K.L. RAPP, *et al.* 2001. Neuroendocrine responses regulating susceptibility and resistance to autoimmune/inflammatory disease in inbred rat strains. Immunol. Rev. **184:** 203–211.
23. KIRSCHBAUM, C., K.M. PIRKE & D.H. HELLHAMMER. 1993. The "Trier Social Stress Test:" a tool for investigating psychobiological stress responses in a laboratory setting. Neuropsychobiology **28:** 76–81.

24. Buske-Kirschbaum, A., S. Jobst, A. Wustmans, *et al.* 1997 Attenuated free cortisol response to psychosocial stress in children with atopic dermatitis. Psychosom. Med. **59:** 419–426.
25. Rupprecht, M., O.P. Hornstein, D. Schlüter, *et al.* 1995. Cortisol, corticotropin, and β-endorphin responses to corticotropin-releasing hormone in patients with atopic eczema. Psychoneuroendocrinology **20:** 543–551.
26. Rupprecht, M., R. Rupprecht, H.U. Koch, *et al.* 1991. Elevated glucocorticoid receptor concentrations before and after glucocorticoid treatment in atopic dermatitis. Dermatologica **183:** 100–105.
27. Maddox, L. & D.A. Schwartz. 2002. The pathophysiology of asthma. Annu. Rev. Med. **53:** 477–498.
28. Oettgen, H.C. & R.S. Geha. 1999. IgE in asthma and atopy: cellular and molecular connections. J. Clin. Invest. **104:** 829–835.
29. Buske-Kirschbaum, A., K. von Auer, S. Krieger, *et al.* 2003. Blunted cortisol responses to psychosocial stress in asthmatic children: a general feature of atopic disease? Psychosom. Med. In press.
30. Ritz, T., A. Steptoe, S. DeWilde, *et al.* 2000. Emotions and stress increase respiratory resistance in asthma. Psychosom. Med. **62:** 401–412.
31. Kolbe, J., J. Garrett, M. Vamos, *et al.* 1994. Influences on trends in asthma morbidity and mortality: the New Zealand experience. Chest **106:** S211–S215.
32. Buske-Kirschbaum, A., A. Geiben, H. Höllig, *et al.* 2002. Altered responsiveness of the hypothalamus-pituitary-adrenal axis and the sympathetic adrenomedullary system to stress in patients with atopic dermatitis. J. Clin. Endocrinol. Metab. **87:** 4245–4251.
33. Calogero, A.E., E.M. Sternberg, G. Bagdy, *et al.* 1992. Neurotransmitter-induced hypothalamus-pituitary-adrenal axis responsiveness is defective in inflammatory disease-susceptible Lewis rats: *in vivo* and *in vitro* studies suggesting globally defective hypothalamic secretion of corticotropin-releasing hormone. Neuroendocrinology **55:** 600–608.
34. Buske-Kirschbaum, A., A. Gierens, H. Höllig, *et al.* 2002. Stress-induced immunomodulation is altered in patients with atopic dermatitis. J. Neuroimmunol. **129:** 161–167.
35. Martin, L.B., H. Kita, K.M. Leiferman, *et al.* 1996. Eosinophils in allergy: role in disease, degranulation, and cytokines. Int. Arch. Allergy Immunol. **109:** 207–215.
36. Turnbull, A.V. & C.L. Rivier. 1999. Regulation of the hypothalamus-pituitary-adrenal axis by cytokines: actions and mechanisms of action. Physiol. Rev. **79:** 1–71.
37. Buske-Kirschbaum A., S. Fischbach, W. Rauh, *et al.* 2003. Increased responsiveness of the hypothalamus-pituitary-adrenal (HPA) axis to stress in newborns with atopic disposition. Submitted.
38. Mantagos, S., A. Koulouris & A. Vagenakis. 1991. A simple stress test for evaluation of hypothalamus-pituitary-adrenal axis during the first 6 months of life. J. Clin. Endocrinol. Metab. **72:** 214–216.
39. Mastorakos, G., G.P. Chrousos & J.S. Weber. 1993. Recombinant interleukin-6 activates the hypothalamic-pituitary-adrenal axis in humans. J. Clin. Endocrinol. Metab. **77:** 1690–1694.
40. Francis, D.D. & M.J. Meaney. 1999. Maternal care and the development of stress responses. Curr. Opin. Neurobiol. **9:** 128–134.
41. Murison, R. & A.M. Milde. 1999. Long-term effects of two animal stress procedures on corticosterone: models for PTSD [Abstr.]. Int. Soc. Psychoneuroendocrinol.
42. Varni, J.W. & J.L. Wallander. 1988. Pediatric chronic disabilities. *In* Handbook of Pediatric Psychology. D.K. Routh, Eds. Guilford Press. New York.

Neurotrophins in Allergic Airway Dysfunction

What the Mouse Model Is Teaching Us

MAREK LOMMATZSCH,[a] ARMIN BRAUN,[b] AND HARALD RENZ[c]

[a]*Department of Pneumology, University of Rostock, 18055 Rostock, Germany*

[b]*Fraunhofer Institute of Toxicology and Experimental Medicine, 30625 Hannover, Germany*

[c]*Department of Clinical Chemistry and Molecular Diagnostics, Philipps-University of Marburg, 35043 Marburg, Germany*

ABSTRACT: Neurotrophins such as nerve growth factor (NGF) and brain-derived neurotrophic factor (BDNF) are potent mediators of neuronal plasticity in the adult. There is increasing evidence that they regulate a variety of immune functions as well. Thus, neurotrophins are candidate molecules for neuroimmune interactions in allergic bronchial asthma, where elevated neurotrophin levels have been reported. In a mouse model of allergic airway inflammation we have identified macrophages and lymphocytes as additional cellular sources of NGF and BDNF in the inflamed lung. There was an unusual time course of BDNF in bronchoalveolar lavage fluid. BDNF levels peaked 1 week after the last allergen challenge, and did not correlate with the time course of the inflammatory response. In a series of experiments using blocking anti-NGF and anti-BDNF antibodies, we have shown that NGF specifically enhances inflammation and the allergic early-phase response. In contrast, BDNF influenced chronic airway obstruction and local neuronal hyperreactivity without affecting inflammation. Using transgenic mice overexpressing NGF in the airway epithelium, we have confirmed the data obtained from anti-NGF experiments. Allergen-challenged NGF overexpressors displayed a markedly augmented airway inflammation, early-phase response, and sensory irritation compared to wild-type mice. Studies with p75-NTR (–/–) knockout mice showed that these NGF effects are at least in part mediated by the low-affinity neurotrophin receptor. Thus, our experiments suggest that NGF and BDNF have a profound, but differential impact on allergic airway dysfunction.

KEYWORDS: allergy; asthma; neurotrophins; nerve growth factor (NGF); brain-derived neurotrophic factor (BDNF); airway; hyperresponsiveness

INTRODUCTION

Allergic bronchial asthma is characterized by two main clinical features: variable airway obstructions following allergen challenge (allergen-induced airway obstruc-

Address for correspondence: Marek Lommatzsch, M.D., Department of Pneumology, University of Rostock, Ernst-Heydemann-Str. 6, 18055 Rostock, Germany. Voice: 0049-381-494-7461; fax: 0049-381-494-7392.
marek.lommatzsch@med.uni-rostock.de

Ann. N.Y. Acad. Sci. 992: 241–249 (2003).

tion) and a long-lasting exaggerated bronchoconstrictor response to unspecific stimuli (airway hyperresponsiveness).[1] The pathogenesis of allergen-induced airway obstruction has been defined over the last two decades. After allergic sensitization, repeated allergen exposures lead to chronic allergic airway inflammation, characterized by an influx of eosinophils, mast cells, and allergen-specific T cells, a Th2-type cytokine pattern, and airway remodeling.[2] Allergen challenges are thought to induce an IgE-mediated release of mast cell mediators, which directly or indirectly lead to airway smooth muscle contraction. Following an immediate airway obstruction (early-phase response), a late airway obstruction occurs hours or days after allergen challenge (late-phase response).[1]

The mechanisms of airway hyperresponsiveness in response to unspecific stimuli are far less understood.[3] The idea that airway hyperresponsiveness may be directly linked to the current degree of allergic airway inflammation (e.g., eosinophil infiltration) has not been confirmed in recent clinical and experimental studies.[4,5] This is in keeping with the old finding that airway hyperresponsiveness can persist over several months after the last allergen challenge in human asthmatics.[6] Therefore, current hypotheses on airway hyperresponsiveness focus on structural and functional changes of resident cells in the lung.[7] These changes include epithelial cell dysfunction, hypertrophy and receptor changes of airway smooth muscle, and neuronal hyperreactivity.[8] Dependent on the reagent chosen for the measurement of airway hyperresponsiveness, different pathways can be detected. Methacholine, directly acting on airway smooth muscle cells via muscarinic receptors, predominantly reflects changes in smooth muscle function.[9] Capsaicin, specifically acting on sensory neurons, reflects changes in pulmonary afferents.[10] Finally, substances acting on a variety of pulmonary cell types (e.g., histamine, serotonin, or leukotrienes) detect several pathways of bronchial hyperresponsiveness.[11,12] In this review, we focus on the pathogenesis of neuronal dysfunction in allergic asthma, with specific regard to neurotrophins and their contribution to altered airway reactivity in a mouse model of allergic bronchial asthma.

NEUROTROPHINS IN NEUROIMMUNE INTERACTIONS

For ethical reasons, it is impossible to obtain neurons from the brainstem or ganglia of living asthmatics in order to define the neurons' specific contribution to airway dysfunction. Therefore, neuronal changes in asthma have been predominantly studied in animal models. It has been shown that both sensory and motor neurons innervating the lung display long-lasting functional changes following allergen challenge.[13] In a series of *in vivo* and *ex vivo* studies, Undem and Fischer have demonstrated profound sensory hyperreactivity in guinea-pigs following experimental allergic inflammation.[14] This hyperreactivity has been correlated to a specific upregulation of tachykinins in lung-innervating sensory neurons of the jugular and nodose ganglia.[15] Even phenotype switching in lung-innervating sensory neurons was demonstrated following allergic airway inflammation.[16] However, the specific contribution of tachykinins to the pathogenesis of sensory hyperreactivity is not clearly defined yet.[17] On the other hand, functional changes in parasympathetic efferents have been shown, including muscarinic receptor changes and altered neurotransmitter release and transmission.[13]

Although characteristics of neuronal hyperreactivity have been explored in the last years, there have been no concepts on possible links between the inflammatory network and neuronal dysfunction in asthma. Recently, neurotrophins have been identified as candidate mediators in this neuroimmune crosstalk.[18] Neurotrophins are known as essential target-derived survival and differentiation factors of the peripheral nervous system in prenatal stages.[19] Though recent studies suggest that neurons may require neurotrophins for survival even after birth,[20] neurotrophins seem to have a predominantly functional role in the adult. It has been demonstrated for a variety of neuronal subpopulations that neurotrophins are potent regulators of synaptic plasticity, neurotransmitter/neuropeptide production, and excitability.[21–23] Especially long-lasting changes in neuronal activity were attributed to neurotrophins, since a single exposure with a neurotrophin can alter neuronal function for hours or even days.[24,25]

Neurotrophins exert their effects via specific high-affinity receptors, including trkA for nerve growth factor (NGF), trkB for brain-derived neurotrophic factor (BDNF), and neurotrophin-4 (NT-4) and trkC for neurotrophin-3 (NT-3). In addition, all neurotrophins can act via the low-affinity p75-neurotrophin-receptor (p75-NTR).[26] Notably, the interaction of high- and low-affinity neurotrophin receptors on the cell surface can induce completely different intracellular signals compared to an activation of either a high- or low-affinity receptor alone.[27] Neurotrophin receptors are not only found on neurons, but also on a variety of immune cells. Neurotrophins influence mast cell degranulation, lymphocyte differentiation, and the chemotaxis of granulocytes (for review see Braun *et al.*[18] and Carr *et al.*[28]). Thus, neurotrophins represent a group of mediators capable of acting on both immune cells and neurons in inflammatory processes. In 1998, we demonstrated for the first time enhanced neurotrophin levels in bronchoalveolar lavage (BAL) fluids of human asthmatics after segmental allergen challenge.[29]

NEUROTROPHIN EXPRESSION IN A MOUSE MODEL OF ASTHMA

To analyze the cellular sources of enhanced neurotrophin production in asthma, we turned to a well-established mouse model of experimental asthma. In this model, mice are intraperitoneally sensitized to a specific allergen (ovalbumin). This sensitization results in high allergen-specific IgE-levels. Mice are then repeatedly challenged with allergen via aerosol. They develop airway inflammation, antigen-induced airway obstruction, and airway hyperresponsiveness, thus mimicking several key features of human asthma.[30] There was a constitutive expression of BDNF, but not NGF, in airway epithelium and airway smooth muscle in naive animals.[31,32] Following allergen challenge, a diffuse overexpression of NGF and BDNF in the peribronchial and perivascular infiltrate was detected in the lungs of allergen-sensitized mice.[30,32] This was paralleled by a marked increase of NGF and BDNF levels in the BAL fluids. Macrophages represented the main cellular source of enhanced neurotrophin production in murine airways.[30,32] Cell culture experiments with immune cells extracted from lung homogenates revealed that lymphocytes represent additional neurotrophin sources in mucosal infiltrates. Notably, NGF was produced by pulmonary T cells and B cells, whereas BDNF was only produced by T cells.[30,32]

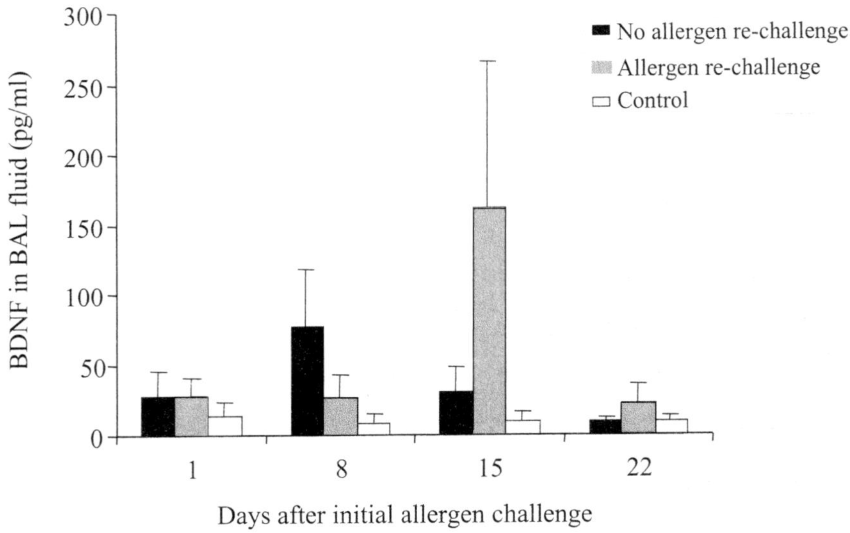

FIGURE 1. BDNF time course in BAL fluid after allergen challenge. Female Balb/c mice were intraperitoneally sensitized to ovalbumin (adsorbed at $Al(OH)_3$) on days 1, 14 and 21 and then divided into three groups. The first group was challenged with ovalbumin on days 26 and 27 and then left without any additional allergen challenge ("No allergen re-challenge"). The second group was challenged with ovalbumin on days 26 and 27 and then re-challenged on days 33 and 34 ("Allergen re-challenge"). The third group was challenged with vehicle alone (PBS) on days 26 and 27 and then left without any additional challenge ("Control"). Shown are the following time points: 1 day (day 28), 8 days (day 35), 15 days (day 42). and 22 days (day 49) after the initial allergen challenges. In every group at every time point $n>6$ animals were killed to obtain bronchoalveolar lavage fluid. Lungs were lavaged twice with 0.8 ml ice-cold PBS via the trachea. BDNF levels in centrifugated cell-free BAL fluid supernatants were measured by ELISA as described.[30] Shown are the means with each standard deviation.

Studying the time course of BDNF expression in the murine lung, we made a surprising observation. BDNF levels in BAL fluid peaked seven days after the last allergen challenge, and were still elevated after two weeks (FIG. 1). This time course of BDNF did not correlate with the time course of cell counts or Th-2 cytokines in BAL fluid (data not shown). The lack of correlation between BDNF levels and current inflammation was confirmed by allergen re-exposure experiments. Allergen re-exposure at the time point of maximum BDNF levels (1 week after the first allergen challenge) led to dramatically increased cell counts, but *decreased* BDNF levels compared to animals not re-exposed to allergen (FIG. 1). Animals re-exposed to allergen again showed a BDNF peak 1 week after the last allergen challenge. This BDNF peak was even more pronounced than the BDNF peak in the group without allergen re-challenge (FIG. 1). These observations suggest that the maximum of BDNF secretion is not occurring during progression, but during regression of airway inflammation. Thus, enhanced BDNF expression in inflammation could be part of a recently discussed "healing" mechanism, intended to protect innervating neurons from inflammatory damage.[33]

To further characterize the functional role of enhanced NGF and BDNF levels in this condition, a series of experiments using anti-NGF and anti-BDNF antibodies were carried out. In addition, we examined airway function and airway inflammation in transgenic animals overexpressing NGF specifically in the airway epithelium,[34] as well as in p75-NTR (–/–) knockout animals.[35]

NEUROTROPHINS MODULATE AIRWAY INFLAMMATION IN MICE

Allergen-challenged mice, systemically and locally treated with anti-NGF antibodies, showed decreased cell counts and Th-2 cytokine levels in BAL fluid compared to mice treated with isotype-matched control antibodies. Most profound effects of anti-NGF-treatment were observed on eosinophil counts.[36] There were no effects of anti-NGF treatment on serum IgE-levels, indicating that NGF effects were not mediated by altered IgE production. Allergen-challenged NGF overexpressors showed dramatically enhanced cell counts and Th-2 cytokine levels compared to values in wild-type animals. Again, most profound effects were observed on eosinophil counts.[36] Naive NGF overexpressors did not show airway inflammation per se. To further characterize the mechanisms of NGF action on airway inflammation, the inflammatory response of p75-NTR (–/–) knockouts was analyzed.[37] Allergen-sensitized and -challenged p75-NTR (–/–) knockouts showed decreased eosinophil counts and Th2-cytokine levels compared to wildtype animals. Both NGF overexpressors and p75-NTR (–/–) knockouts did not show altered immunoglobulin levels in the peripheral blood.[36,37]

In contrast, allergen-sensitized and -challenged mice, treated with monoclonal anti-BDNF antibodies, did not show significant changes in cell counts or cytokine levels in BAL fluid compared to animals treated with isotype-matched control antibodies (unpublished data). These experiments indicate that NGF, but not BDNF, enhances the severity of the local inflammatory response, probably involving the p75-NTR. There are at least two possible pathways of NGF action. On one hand, NGF could directly act on infiltrating immune cells, for example, influence eosinophil chemotaxis and lymphocyte activation. On the other hand, NGF may enhance local neurogenic inflammation via activation and neuropeptide upregulation in innervating neurons.

NEUROTROPHINS CONTRIBUTE TO AIRWAY DYSFUNCTION IN MICE

To analyze neurotrophin actions on murine lung function, we used *in vivo* and *in vitro* methods. *In vivo* head-out body plethysmography was used to characterize neurotrophin effects on sensory irritation, smooth muscle hyperreactivity, and airway caliber.[38,39] *In vitro* electric field stimulation of isolated tracheal segments was used to define neurotrophin effects on local neuronal reactivity in response to unspecific stimuli.[40]

Using body plethysmography, we analyzed sensory irritation, which is defined as the pause before expiration in response to capsaicin challenge ("time of break,"

TB).[38] Allergen-challenged wild-type mice show a characteristic prolongation of TB. This allergen-induced sensory irritation was markedly increased in allergen-challenged NGF overexpressors, and completely abolished in allergen-challenged p75-NTR (–/–) knockouts.[36,37] Neither anti-NGF treatment, nor NGF overexpression or p75-NTR receptor deletion had any effect on airway smooth muscle hyperreactivity as shown by measurement of the midexpiratory flow (EF_{50}) after methacholine challenge, supporting the idea that NGF specifically mediates neuronal changes in allergic airway disease.

We then analyzed neurotrophin effects on allergen-induced airflow limitation. Allergen-challenged mice show a characteristic reversible decrease in the midexpiratory flow (EF_{50}) immediately after allergen challenge (early-phase response).[40] In addition, these mice develop chronic airway obstruction 1 week after the last allergen challenge.[39] Anti-NGF treatment partly abrogated the early-phase response, but did not influence chronic airway obstruction.[36] NGF overexpressors showed an increased early-phase response.[36] Anti-BDNF treatment did not influence the allergic early-phase response, but abrogated chronic airway obstruction occurring 1week after allergen challenge (unpublished data). Thus, NGF and BDNF seem to have distinct functions in allergen-induced airway obstruction. NGF enhances the early-phase response in conjunction with an augmented local inflammatory response. By contrast, BDNF seems to have a long-lasting effect on airway tone, which is not attributable to the current degree of airway inflammation.

To define the role of neurotrophins on local neuronal hyperreactivity, a well-established model of *in vitro* electric field stimulation was used. Electrical field stimulation of isolated tracheal segments reflects local neuronal reflex activity of the airways.[41] This reflex activity is enhanced following allergen challenge, as shown by a decreased stimulation frequency needed to induce a half-maximal contraction of the

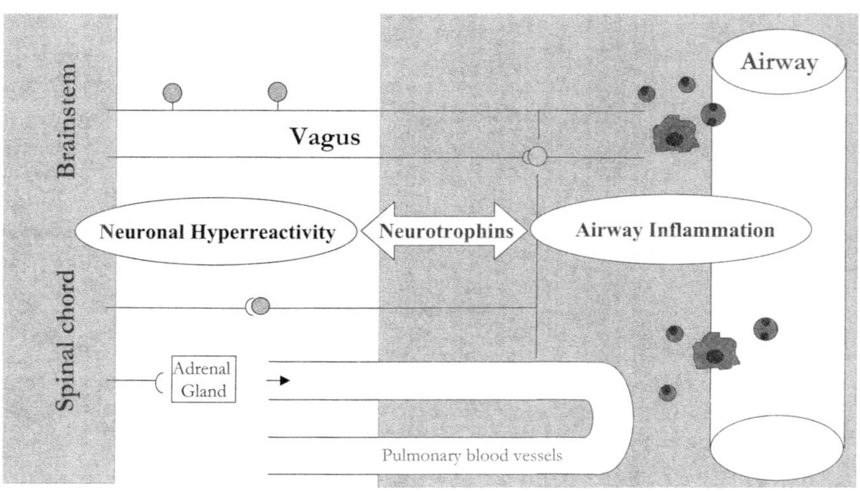

FIGURE 2. Neurotrophins represent a possible link between airway inflammation and neuronal hyperreactivity in allergic bronchial asthma.

airway (ES_{50}).[40] Anti-NGF treatment partly abrogated this hyperreactivity, whereas local NGF administration to non-allergic control animals was sufficient to induce hyperreactivity.[32,42] Anti-BDNF and BDNF treatment had a similar and even more pronounced effect on local neuronal hyperreactivity (unpublished data). Thus, both NGF and BDNF may enhance the local neuronal reflex activity in inflamed airways.

CONCLUSION

Neurotrophins such as NGF and BDNF represent a possible link between airway inflammation and airway dysfunction in allergic bronchial asthma (FIG. 2). In a mouse model of asthma, we have defined cellular sources of enhanced NGF and BDNF production in the inflamed lung. NGF enhances sensory irritability, but does not show any effect on smooth muscle hyperreactivity. These results are in keeping with reports demonstrating a specific contribution of NGF to neuronal dysfunction in guinea-pigs.[43,44] In addition, NGF has profound influences on airway inflammation itself. In contrast, BDNF seems to be a "late-phase neurotrophin," involved in the pathogenesis of long-term airway obstruction and local neuronal hyperreactivity. Thus, the data obtained from the murine asthma model suggest that NGF and BDNF have a profound, but differential impact on allergic airway dysfunction.

REFERENCES

1. BUSSE, W.W. & R.F. LEMANSKE. 2001. Asthma. N. Engl. J. Med. **344:** 350–362.
2. DJUKANOVIC, R., W.R. ROCHE, J.W. WILSON, *et al.* 1990. Mucosal inflammation in asthma. Am. Rev. Respir. Dis. **142:** 434–457.
3. HARGREAVE, F.E., J. DOLOVICH, P.M. O'BYRNE, et al. 1986. The origin of airway hyperresponsiveness. J. Allergy Clin. Immunol. **78:** 825–832.
4. LECKIE, M.J., A. TEN BRINKE, J. KHAN, *et al.* 2000. Effects of an interleukin-5 blocking monoclonal antibody on eosinophils, airway hyper-responsiveness, and the late asthmatic response. Lancet **356:** 2144–2148.
5. HOGAN, S.P., K.I. MATTHAEI, J.M.YOUNG, *et al.* 1998. A novel T cell-regulated mechanism modulating allergen-induced airways hyperreactivity in BALB/c mice independently of IL-4 and IL-5. J. Immunol. **161:** 1501–1509.
6. JUNIPER, E.F., P.A. FRITH & F.E. HARGREAVE. 1982. Long-term stability of bronchial responsiveness to histamine. Thorax **37:** 288–291.
7. LEIGH, R., R. ELLIS, J. WATTIE, *et al.* 2002. Dysfunction and remodeling of the mouse airway persist after resolution of acute allergen-induced airway inflammation. Am. J. Respir. Cell. Mol. Biol. **27:** 526–535.
8. BOCHNER, B.S., B.J. UNDEM & L.M. LICHTENSTEIN. 1994. Immunological aspects of allergic asthma. Annu. Rev. Immunol. **12:** 295–335.
9. O'CONNOR, B.J., S.D. CROWTHER, J.F. COSTELLO & J. MORLEY. 1999. Selective airway responsiveness in asthma. Trends Pharmacol. Sci. **20:** 9–11.
10. SPINA, D. 1996. Airway sensory nerves: a burning issue in asthma? Thorax **51:** 335–337.
11. ADELROTH, E., M.M. MORRIS, F.E. HARGREAVE & P.M. O'BYRNE. 1986. Airway responsiveness to leukotrienes C4 and D4 and to methacholine in patients with asthma and normal controls. N. Engl. J. Med. **315:** 480–484.
12. HARGREAVE, F.E., P. STERK, E.C. ADELROTH, *et al.* 1986. Airway responsiveness to histamine or methacholine: advances in measurement and interpretation. Respiration **50:** 72–76.
13. UNDEM, B.J., R. KAJEKAR, D.D. HUNTER & A.C. MYERS. 2000. Neural integration and allergic disease. J. Allergy Clin. Immunol. **106:** S213–220.

14. UNDEM, B.J., D.D. HUNTER, M. LIU, *et al.* 1999. Allergen-induced sensory neuroplasticity in airways. Int. Arch. Allergy Immunol. **118:** 150–153.
15. FISCHER, A., G.P. MCGREGOR, A. SARIA, *et al.* 1996. Induction of tachykinin gene and peptide expression in guinea pig nodose primary afferent neurons by allergic airway inflammation. J. Clin. Invest. **98:** 2284–2291.
16. HUNTER, D.D., A.C. MYERS & B.J. UNDEM. 2000. Nerve growth factor-induced phenotypic switch in guinea pig airway sensory neurons. Am. J. Respir. Crit. Care Med. **161:** 1985–1990.
17. JOOS, G.F., P.R. GERMONPRE & R.A. PAUWELS. 2000. Role of tachykinins in asthma. Allergy **55:** 321–337.
18. BRAUN, A., M. LOMMATZSCH & H. RENZ. 2000. The role of neurotrophins in allergic bronchial asthma. Clin. Exp. Allergy **30:** 178–186.
19. LEWIN, G.R. & Y.A. BARDE. 1996. Physiology of the neurotrophins. Annu. Rev. Neurosci. **19:** 289–317.
20. STUCKY, C., J. SHIN & G.R. LEWIN. 2002. Neurotrophin-4: a survival factor for adult sensory neurons. Curr. Biol. **12:** 1401.
21. LI, Y.X., Y. ZHANG, H.A. LESTER, *et al.* 1998. Enhancement of neurotransmitter release induced by brain-derived neurotrophic factor in cultured hippocampal neurons. J. Neurosci. **18:** 10231–10240.
22. MCALLISTER, A.K., L.C. KATZ & D.C. LO. 1999. Neurotrophins and synaptic plasticity. Annu. Rev. Neurosci. **22:** 295–318.
23. WINTER, J. 1998. Brain-derived neurotrophic factor, but not nerve growth factor, regulates capsaicin sensitivity of rat vagal ganglion neurones. Neurosci. Lett. **241:** 21–24.
24. KANG, H. & E.M. SCHUMAN. 1995. Long-lasting neurotrophin-induced enhancement of synaptic transmission in the adult hippocampus. Science **267:** 1658–1662.
25. REIBEL, S., B.VIVIEN-ROELS, B.T. LE, *et al.* 2000. Overexpression of neuropeptide Y induced by brain-derived neurotrophic factor in the rat hippocampus is long lasting. Eur. J. Neurosci. **12:** 595–605.
26. PATAPOUTIAN, A. & L.F. REICHARDT. 2001.Trk receptors: mediators of neurotrophin action. Curr. Opin. Neurobiol. **11:** 272–280.
27. CARTER, B.D. & G.R. LEWIN. 1997. Neurotrophins live or let die: does p75NTR decide? Neuron **18:** 187–190.
28. CARR, M.J., D.D. HUNTER & B.J. UNDEM. 2001. Neurotrophins and asthma. Curr. Opin. Pulm. Med. **7:** 1–7.
29. VIRCHOW, J.C., P. JULIUS, M. LOMMATZSCH, *et al.* 1998. Neurotrophins are increased in bronchoalveolar lavage fluid after segmental allergen provocation. Am. J. Respir. Crit. Care Med. **158:** 2002–2005.
30. BRAUN, A., M. LOMMATZSCH, A. MANNSFELDT, *et al.* 1999. Cellular sources of enhanced Brain-derived neurotrophic factor production in a mouse model of allergic inflammation. Am. J. Respir. Cell. Mol. Biol. **21:** 537–546.
31. LOMMATZSCH, M., A. BRAUN, A. MANNSFELDT, *et al.* 1999. Abundant production of Brain-derived neurotrophic factor by adult visceral epithelia. Implications for paracrine and target-derived neurotrophic functions. Am. J. Pathol. **155:** 1183–1193.
32. BRAUN, A., E. APPEL, R. BARUCH, *et al.* 1998. Role of nerve growth factor in a mouse model of allergic airway inflammation and asthma. Eur. J. Immunol. **28:** 3240–3251.
33. KERSCHENSTEINER, M., E. GALLMEIER, L. BEHRENS, *et al.* 1999. Activated human T cells, B cells, and monocytes produce Brain-derived neurotrophic factor in vitro and in inflammatory brain lesions: a neuroprotective role of inflammation? J. Exp. Med. **189:** 865–870.
34. HOYLE, G.W., R.M. GRAHAM, J.B. FINKELSTEIN, *et al.* 1998. Hyperinnervation of the airways in transgenic mice overexpressing nerve growth factor. Am. J. Respir. Cell Mol. Biol. **18:** 149–157.
35. LEE, K.F., E. LI, L.J. HUBER, *et al.* 1992. Targeted mutation of the gene encoding the low affinity NGF receptor p75 leads to deficits in the peripheral sensory nervous system. Cell **69:** 737–749.
36. PÄTH, G., A. BRAUN, N. MEENTS, *et al.* 2002. Augmentation of allergic early-phase reaction by nerve growth factor. Am. J. Respir. Crit. Care Med. **166:** 818–826.

37. KERZEL, S., G. PÄTH, W.A. NOCKHER, *et al.* 2003. Pan-neurotrophin receptor p75 contributes to neuronal hyperreactivity and airway inflammation in a murine model of experimental asthma. Am. J. Respir. Cell Mol. Biol. **28:** 170–178.
38. ALARIE, Y. 1998. Computer-based bioassay for evaluation of sensory irritation of airborne chemicals and its limit of detection. Arch. Toxicol. **72:** 277–282.
39. NEUHAUS-STEINMETZ, U., T. GLAAB, A. DASER, *et al.* 2000. Sequential development of airway hyperresponsiveness and acute airway obstruction in a mouse model of allergic inflammation. Int. Arch. Allergy Immunol. **121:** 57–67.
40. HERZ, U., A. BRAUN, R. RÜCKERT & H. RENZ. 1998. Various immunological phenotypes are associated with increased airway responsiveness. Clin. Exp. Allergy **28:** 625–634.
41. ANDERSSON, R.G. & N. GRUNDSTROM. 1983. The excitatory non-cholinergic, non-adrenergic nervous system of the guinea-pig airways. Eur. J. Respir. Dis. Suppl. **131:** 141–157.
42. BRAUN, A., D. QUARCOO, O. SCHULTE-HERBRÜGGEN, *et al.* 2001. Nerve growth factor induces airway hyperresponsiveness in mice. Int. Arch. Allergy Immunol. **124:** 205–207.
43. DE VRIES, A., M.C. DESSING, F. ENGELS, *et al.* 1999. Nerve growth factor induces a neurokinin-1 receptor- mediated airway hyperresponsiveness in guinea pigs. Am. J. Respir. Crit. Care Med. **159:** 1541–1544.
44. FRIBERG, S.G., C. OLGART HÖGLUND & L.E. GUSTAFSSON. 2001. Nerve growth factor increases airway responses and decreases levels of exhaled nitric oxide during histamine challenge in an in vivo guinea- pig model. Acta Physiol. Scand. **173:** 239–245.

Index of Contributors